中医临床

The plant shown on the cover is Clematis chinensis Osbeck., whose dried root and rhizome is known as wēi líng xiān (威灵仙, Radix et Rhizoma Clematidis), or Chinese clematis root. As a Chinese medicinal, it acts to dispel wind-damp, unblock the channels and collaterals, and relieve pain. Wēi líng xiān is widely used in the clinical treatment of both gout and rheumatoid arthritis.

Project Editor: Liu Shui & Zeng Chun
Copy Editor: Liang Qi
Book Designer: Li Xi
Cover Designer: Li Xi
Typesetter: Wei Hong-bo

The Clinical Practice of Chinese Medicine

Gout & Rheumatoid Arthritis

中医临床

The Clinical Practice of Chinese Medicine

Gout & Rheumatoid Arthritis

by **Deng Zhao-zhi**

Professor & Chief Physician of Chinese Internal Medicine, the Second Teaching Hospital of Guangzhou University of CM, Guangzhou, China

with co-authors

He Yi-ting, Ph.D. TCM
Chief Physician & Professor of Chinese Internal Medicine

Chen Wei, M.S. TCM
Chief Physician & Professor of Chinese Internal Medicine

Zhu Li-qun, M.S.
Chief Physician

Translated by

Wang-lei, Ph.D. TCM

Li Yi-meng, Ph.D. TCM

Edited by

Mei Li, M.S.TOM

PMPH 人民卫生出版社
PEOPLE'S MEDICAL PUBLISHING HOUSE
BEIJING • LONDON • NEW YORK

人民卫生出版社
PMPH PEOPLE'S MEDICAL PUBLISHING HOUSE

Website: http://www.pmph.com

Book Title: The Clinical Practice of Chinese Medicine:
Gout & Rheumatoid Arthritis
中医临床实用系列：痛风与类风湿性关节炎

Contact address: Bldg 3, 3 Qu, Fangqunyuan, Fangzhuang, Beijing 100078, P.R. China, phone/fax: 8610 6769 1034, E-mail: pmph@pmph.com

For text and trade sales, as well as review copy enquiries, please contact PMPH at pmphsales@gmail.com

Disclaimer

This book is for educational and reference purposes only. In view of the possibility of human error or changes in medical science, neither the author, editor, publisher, nor any other party who has been involved in the preparation or publication of this work guarantees that the information contained herein is in every respect accurate or complete. The medicinal therapy and treatment techniques presented in this book are provided for the purpose of reference only. If readers wish to attempt any of the techniques or utilize any of the medicinal therapies contained in this book, the publisher assumes no responsibility for any such actions.

It is the responsibility of the readers to understand and adhere to local laws and regulations concerning the practice of these techniques and methods. The authors, editors, and publishers disclaim all responsibility for any liability, loss, injury, or damage incurred as a consequence, directly or indirectly, of the use and application of any of the contents of this book.

First published: 2008
ISBN: 978-7-117-09485-6/R · 9486

Cataloguing in Publication Data:
A catalog record for this book is available from the CIP-Database China.

Printed in The People's Republic of China

ISBN 978-7-117-09485-6
9 787117 094856 >

About the Author

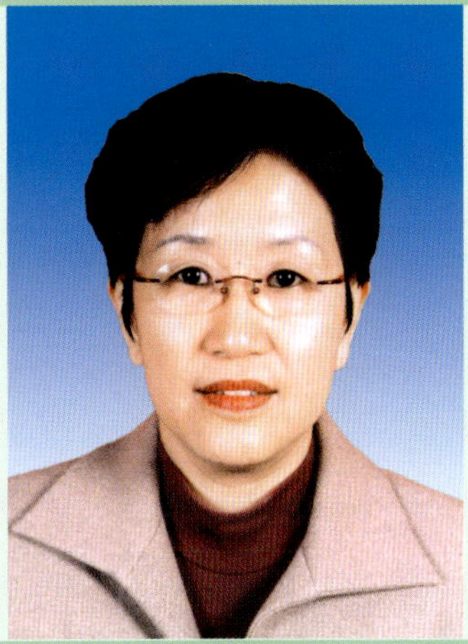

邓兆智　教授

Professor **Deng Zhao-zhi** is a medical doctor, professor, and Master's level supervisor at the Second Teaching Hospital of Guangzhou University of Chinese Medicine (also known as the Guangdong Provincial Hospital of TCM). As an expert in rheumatology, Professor Deng specializes in the diagnosis and treatment of diseases such as systemic lupus erythematosus, ankylosing spondylitis, gout, osteoarthritis, Sjogren's syndrome, erythema nodosum, scleroderma, dermatomyositis, multiple myositis, adult Still's disease, and psoriatic arthritis. Since the establishment of the field of rheumatology in 1986, an integration of Chinese and Western medical approaches has been adopted for its diagnosis and treatment. Professor Deng has studied and absorbed the experiences and essential teachings of famous veteran doctors of Chinese medicine in this field, and has incorporated the knowledge gathered from classical texts into her studies. She has a distinct perspective towards the clinical classification and differentiation of the signs and symptoms of rheumatic disease. In the past few years, the department of rheumatology has become one of the most outstanding departments in the Guangdong Provincial Hospital of TCM. The department handles the most specialized diseases, and most patients come from all over the world. The number of patient visits to this department exceeds 10,000 per year, which is the highest number of patient visits per year in the entire country. Professor Deng is a standing committee member of the rheumatism branch of the Chinese Medicine Institute and serves as the director of the rheumatology board at the Guangdong Provincial Medical Association. She is the chief editor of many monographs, and has published numerous research papers. She has conducted several scientific research projects for the State Administration of Chinese Medicine and Guangdong Natural Science Foundation. She won the Second Level Award of Technological Advancement from Guangzhou University of Chinese Medicine.

Foreword

Chinese medicine is a broad and profound art of healing. It is a well-established and comprehensive system of medicine with an ancient origin and a long rich history. Throughout the ages, it has made a significant contribution to the prosperity of the Chinese civilization. The system of pattern differentiation and treatment fully reflects the Chinese medical view of health and disease as a holistic concept, the emphasis on the body's ability to regulate itself and adapt to the environment, and the need for individualized treatment. The integration of diseases and syndromes is the consummation of treatment based on pattern differentiation; it fully displays the superior characteristic of this discipline, and has an extensive influence on the development of the art of Chinese medicine.

The intention of this series of books is to introduce accurate Chinese medical diagnosis and treatment of various diseases to overseas readers.

The Chinese edition of *The Clinical Practice of Chinese Medicine* was edited by the Second Teaching Hospital of Guangzhou University of CM (also known as Guangdong Provincial Hospital of TCM), and published by People's Medical Publishing House. When the series was published in 2000, it was widely accepted in clinical practice due to its originality, distinguishing features, richness in content, completeness, accuracy, and outstanding emphases. This series has become a trademark of standard in the eyes of Chinese and integrative medical practitioners. During the second printing of this series of books, Professor Deng Tie-tao praised, "For a series to be printed a multiple number of times, shows that it is highly regarded and has received excellent reviews." In order to keep up with the constant development of medical science, this series was revised and re-published in 2004 by People's Medical Publishing House. Due to its popularity, it has been reprinted numerous times since.

The English edition of this series of books includes 20 volumes:

- *COPD & Asthma*
- *Coronary Artery Disease & Hyperlipidemia*
- *Stroke & Parkinson's Disease*
- *Chronic Gastritis & Irritable Bowel Syndrome*
- *Diabetes & Obesity*
- *Gout & Rheumatoid Arthritis*
- *Menstrual Disorders I: Dysfunctional Uterine Bleeding & Amenorrhea*
- *Menstrual Disorders II: Premenstrual Syndrome, Dysmenorrhea & Perimenopause*
- *Endometriosis & Uterine Fibroids*
- *Pelvic Inflammatory Disease & Miscarriage*
- *Postpartum Hypogalactia & Breast Hyperplasia*
- *Male & Female Infertility*
- *Urticaria*
- *Eczema & Atopic Dermatitis*
- *Lupus Erythematosus*
- *Scleroderma & Dermatomyositis*
- *Acne & Alopecia*
- *Psoriasis & Cutaneous Pruritus*
- *Herpes Zoster & Fungal Skin Infections*
- *Chloasma & Vitiligo*

Clinical application varies by individual and by location; when this is combined with the rapid development of medical science, the treatment methods and medicinal dosages may also vary accordingly. When using these books as a reference guide, overseas readers should confirm the formulas and dosages of medicinals according to the individual health condition of the patient, as well as take into account the origin of the Chinese medicinals.

The quotes in these books were taken from various medical literature during the compilation process. We have deleted some of the contents of the original texts for the purpose of uniformity and ease in readability. We ask for the reader's forgiveness and express our respect and gratitude toward the original authors.

Due to the complicated nature of the diagnoses and treatments covered in these books, and the wide range of topics they touch upon, it is inevitable that one may encounter errors while reading through them. We respectfully welcome constructive criticism and corrections from our readers.

The clinical practice of medicine changes with the constant development of medical science. The books in this series will be revised regularly to continuously adapt to the development of traditional Chinese medicine.

Editorial Board for the English edition of
The Clinical Practice of Chinese Medicine series

Editorial Board

for the English edition of

The Clinical Practice of Chinese Medicine Series

Academic Consultants

Wu Xian-zhong

Specialist of Integrative Medicine, Academician of Chinese Academy of Engineering, Professor, Tianjin Medical University, Chairman of Tianjin Institute of Acute Abdomen Research on Integrative Medicine

Chen Ke-ji

Specialist of Cardiovascular & Aging Diseases, Academician of Chinese Academy of Science, Professor of Medicine, Xiyuan Hospital, and Institute of Aging Medicine, China Academy of Chinese Medical Science, Consultant on Traditional Medicine, WHO

Wang Yong-yan

Specialist of Chinese Internal Medicine, Academician of Chinese Academy of Engineering, Professor and former President of Beijing University of CM, and Honorary President of China Academy of Chinese Medical Science

General Coordinator

Lü Yu-bo

Professor & Vice President, Guangzhou University of CM,
President, the Second Teaching Hospital of Guangzhou University of CM

Editors-in-Chief

Luo Yun-jian

Guangdong Province Entitled Famous Chinese Medicine Physician,Professor of Chinese Internal Medicine, & former Vice President of the Second Teaching Hospital of Guangzhou University of CM

Liu Mao-cai

Guangdong Province Entitled Famous Chinese Medicine Physician,Professor of Chinese Internal Medicine, & former Vice President of the Second Teaching Hospital of Guangzhou University of CM, Former Chairman of Institute for Aging Cerebral Diseases, Guangzhou University of CM

Associate Editors-in-Chief

Xuan Guo-wei

Guangdong Province Entitled Famous Chinese Medicine Physician, Director & Professor, Department of Chinese External Medicine, Guangzhou University of CM, Former Vice President of the Second Teaching Hospital of Guangzhou University of CM

Huang Chun-lin

Professor of Chinese Internal Medicine, & former Associate-Director of the Second Institute for Clinical Research, Guangzhou University of CM

Chen Da-can

Professor of Chinese External Medicine, Vice President of the Second Teaching Hospital of Guangzhou University of CM

Chen Zhi-qiang

Professor of Chinese External Medicine, Director of the Department of Surgery, Vice President of the Second Teaching Hospital of Guangzhou University of CM

Feng Wei-bin

Professor of Chinese Internal Medicine, the Second Teaching Hospital of Guangzhou University of CM

Yang Zhi-min

Professor of Chinese Internal Medicine, Vice President of the Second Teaching Hospital of Guangzhou University of CM

Lu Chuan-jian

Professor of Chinese External Medicine, Vice President of the Second Teaching Hospital of Guangzhou University of CM

Zou Xu

Professor of Chinese Internal Medicine, Vice President of the Second Teaching Hospital of Guangzhou University of CM

MEMBERS (Listed alphabetically by name)

Deng Zhao-zhi

Professor of Chinese Internal Medicine, Guangzhou University of CM

Fan Guan-jie

Professor of Chinese Internal Medicine, Director of Department of Education, the Second Teaching Hospital of Guangzhou University of CM

Fan Rui-qiang

Professor of Chinese External Medicine, Director of Department of Dermatology, the Second Teaching Hospital of Guangzhou University of CM

Huang Jian-ling

Professor of Chinese Medicine Gynecology, Director of the First Department of Gynecology, the Second Teaching Hospital of Guangzhou University of CM

Huang Pei-xin

Professor of Chinese Internal Medicine, the Second Teaching Hospital of Guangzhou University of CM, Head of the Research Project of Cerebral Disease Treatment on Chinese Internal Medicine, Sponsored by SATCM China

Huang Sui-ping

Professor of Chinese Internal Medicine, Director of Department of Digestion, the Second Teaching Hospital of Guangzhou University of CM

Li Li-yun

Guangdong Province Entitled Famous Chinese Medicine Physician, Professor of Chinese Medicine Gynecology, the Second Teaching Hospital of Guangzhou University of CM

Liang Xue-fang

Professor of Chinese Medicine Gynecology, Director of the Third Department of Gynecology, the Second Teaching Hospital of Guangzhou University of CM

Lin Lin

Professor of Chinese Internal Medicine, Director of Department of Respiratory, the Second Teaching Hospital of Guangzhou University of CM

Lin Yi

Professor of Mastopathy in Chinese Medicine, the Second Teaching Hospital of Guangzhou University of CM, Head of the National Key Subject –Mastopathy in Chinese Medicine

Liu Wei-sheng

Master of the National Master and Apprentice Education Program, Professor of Chinese Internal Medicine, the Second Teaching Hospital of Guangzhou University of CM

Si-tu Yi

Professor of Chinese Medicine Gynecology, the Second Teaching Hospital of Guangzhou University of CM, Head of the National Key Subject – Chinese Medicine Gynecology

Wang Xiao-yun

Professor of Chinese Medicine Gynecology, Director of Department of Gynecology, Head of Teaching Division of Gynecology, the Second Teaching Hospital of Guangzhou University of CM

SPONSORED BY

The Second Teaching Hospital of Guangzhou University of CM,
also known as **Guangdong Provincial Hospital of TCM**

Preface

Rheumatology is an important topic in Chinese medicine, and is covered extensively in medical literature throughout the last several millennia, especially in the last decade. There are also records of accumulated experience in the treatment of such disorders. The combination of Chinese and Western medical treatment has been proven to be effective for the management of obstinate illnesses such as rheumatoid arthritis and ankylosing spondylitis.

The compilers of this book are veteran clinicians of Chinese medicine who have rich clinical experience in the field of rheumatology. During the composition of this book, we consulted with the members of the Editorial Committee and specialists, and collected and extracted from their experience. We also referred to literature and data of both domestic and international sources, and integrated the analyses and approaches of foreign and domestic research.

Rheumatoid arthritis is a chronic systemic disease and a non-infectious inflammatory disorder whose cause is uncertain. The disease has a long course and often leads to joint and surrounding tissue damage, varied clinical manifestations, cartilage and bone destruction, joint deformity, and functional impairment. The disease can also lead to damage of the internal organs. So far, the therapeutic effects of the treatment of RA are unsatisfactory. Most treatments only relieve the symptoms or slow down the progression of the disease, but they do not result in a complete cure. Furthermore, most of the drugs used to treat RA produce adverse effects.

Gout is a chronic disorder of purine metabolism, whose clinical features include hyperuricemia, recurrent acute gouty arthritis, fibrous nephritis, the formation of gouty tophi, functional impairment and deformity of the joints, and in most cases, uric acid imbalance. With the continuous rise of living standards, the incidence of this disease is also increasing. However, due to the lack of treatment that targets the cause of the disease, there is no radical cure for this disease. So far, Western medical treatment can only control acute episodes, provide long-term management of hyperuricemia, and reduce relapses.

The general symptoms in both conditions are associated with what is referred to in Chinese medicine as *bi* syndrome. Combined treatments utilizing Chinese medicinals, acupuncture, massage, and physical therapy show excellent results in reducing both pain and uric acid levels, while also improving joint function and lowering rates of recurrence.

This book consists of the following chapters: Overview, Chinese Medical Etiology and Pathomechanism, Chinese Medical Treatment, Prognosis, Preventive Healthcare, Clinical Experience of Renowned Physicians, Perspectives of Integrative Medicine, Selected Quotes from Classical Texts, and Modern Research. The "Overview" chapter introduces the biomedical perspective of the disease. "Chinese Medical Etiology and Pathomechanism" and "Chinese Medical Treatment" discuss the etiology, diagnosis (pattern identification), and treatment of the disease. The "Clinical Experience of Renowned Physicians" chapter consists of information extracted from medical records and insights of famous veteran doctors of Chinese medicine. "Perspectives of Integrative Medicine" introduces the predominant treatment of Chinese Medicine and the use of Western medical intervention when necessary. "Selected Quotes from Classical Texts" and "Modern Research" provide the readers with informative references.

The targeted audience of this book is primarily readers from abroad, which include teachers and students of Chinese medicine and acupuncture colleges, medical practitioners who are directly or indirectly involved in the practice of Chinese medicine, medical doctors who are interested in Chinese medicine, and lay persons. We hope that this book will help readers understand the advancement of Chinese medical treatment of rheumatoid arthritis, and promote the integration of Chinese and Western medicine. It should be noted that the use of this book cannot replace the treatment advice or suggestions of a professional healthcare practitioner. If you or anyone you know have signs and symptoms similar to those described in this book, please consult a practitioner of Chinese medicine.

During the compilation of this book, we referred to domestic and foreign papers, medical books, periodicals, and journals, which provided us with a wealth of guidance and assistance. We express our appreciation and gratitude to the authors of the original works.

Due to the nature of clinical medicine, we apologize for any outdated or incorrect information that may appear in these books. We hope that readers will not hesitate to offer their comments and suggestions on how to improve the content of this material.

Deng Zhao-zhi
January, 2008

Contents

Gout

Rheumatoid Arthritis

Gout

by **Deng Zhao-zhi**,
Professor & Chief Physician
of Chinese Internal Medicine,
the Second Teaching Hospital
of Guangzhou University of CM,
Guangzhou, China

Chen Wei,
Professor & Chief Physician
of Chinese Internal Medicine,
the Second Teaching Hospital
of Guangzhou University of CM,
Guangzhou, China

He Yi-ting,
Professor & Chief Physician
of Chinese Internal Medicine,
the Second Teaching Hospital
of Guangzhou University of CM,
Guangzhou, China

Zhu Li-qun,
Chief Physician,
the Second Teaching Hospital
of Guangzhou University of CM,
Guangzhou, China

OVERVIEW

Gout is a heterogeneous disease in which there is tissue damage resulting from long-term impairment of purine metabolism and high levels of uric acid in the blood (hyperuricemia). The clinical features of gout are hyperuricemia, recurrent attacks of acute arthritis, and needle-like uric acid crystals in the leukocytes of synovial fluid. In addition, there may be formation of hard deposits called tophi, which can lead to joint dysfunction and deformity in severe cases. Uric acid crystals in the kidney, or calculi, can give rise to gouty nephropathy. The symptoms listed above may appear separately or concurrently. Depending on the different causes of hyperuricemia, gout can be categorized as primary or secondary.

Until recently, primary gout was once thought to be closely related to a high-purine diet; now, excessive dietary purine is considered a factor of primary gout only in patients who have already been predisposed to this disease. Primary gout is linked to congenital impairment of purine metabolism. The onset of secondary gout is often attributed to high serum uric acid levels due to increased serum uric acid production or decreased excretion of uric acid through the urine as a result of renal, hematological, or cardiovascular disease.

Hyperuricemia is one of the most important biochemical bases of gout. Five to twelve percent of patients with this symptom will ultimately develop gout and invariably present with hyperuricemia during some stages throughout the course of the disease. Hyperuricemia can be confirmed by using the uricase enzyme test to accurately detect the levels of blood uric acid (BUA) in the body.

Diagnostic Criteria

- Buildup of uric acid crystals in synovial fluid.

➢ Tophi containing uric acid crystals, as confirmed by chemical testing or polarizing microscope.

➢ The diagnosis of gout requires at least 6 of the following 12 signs and symptoms:

1) Recurrent attacks of acute arthritis;

2) Inflammation reaching its peak within one day;

3) Attack of single joint arthritis;

4) Redness of the joint;

5) Pain or swelling of the first metatarsophalangeal joint;

6) Unilateral attack of arthritis of the first metatarsophalangeal joint;

7) Unilateral attack of arthritis of the tarsal bones;

8) Possible tophi;

9) Hyperuricemia (elevated uric acid in the blood);

10) Internal, asymmetrical swelling of the joint (confirmed by X-ray);

11) Cyst under the cortical plate without erosion (confirmed by X-ray);

12) Negative biological culture of the synovial fluid during attacks of arthritis.

(1) Typical Gout

Typical gout is divided into four stages: asymptomatic hyperuricemia, acute gouty arthritis, interval (or intercritical) gout, and chronic tophaceous gout.

➢ During the acute stage, the attack occurs suddenly and during the night; there is redness, swelling, and pain of the involved joint and adjacent soft tissues. This stage can last several hours, one to two days, or even months.

➢ During the intercritical stage, there is complete remission of symptoms. Usually, the first metatarsophalangeal, metatarsal, malleolus, finger, wrist, knee and elbow joints are the first to be affected when the disease flares up.

➢ In early stages of outbreaks, 85%-90% of cases present with single-joint arthritis, while only 3% exhibit multiple-joint arthritis. There may also be hydrarthrosis (water effusion into a joint cavity).

➢ Involvement of the shoulder, hip, sacroiliac, and other intervertebral joints is uncommon.

➢ A final diagnosis is confirmed by the finding of uric acid crystals in the synovial fluid extracted from the bursa mucosa.

➢ The presence of tophi is one of the characteristic pathological changes of gout, which typically form on the auricular helix, and are also frequently seen on the fingers, wrists, knees, elbows, and first metatarsophalangeal joints.

➢ Excessive uric acid levels in the blood (hyperuricemia), and increased or decreased uric acid levels in the urine.

➢ X-ray findings: In the early stage of acute arthritis, there is swelling of the soft tissue. Recurrent attacks eventually lead to destruction of the joint cartilage, irregular joint surfaces, narrowing of the inter-joint spaces, and bone damage.

(2) Gouty Nephropathy

➢ Lumbar pain and edema, high blood pressure, acidic urine (as determined by urine pH test), and gross hematuria.

➢ Low degree albuminuria, not exceeding (++).

➢ Secondary infection with symptoms such as frequent, urgent and painful urination, bacteriuria, and fever.

➢ Early stage renal dysfunction: 100% of cases present with concentrated urine due to a decrease in the kidney's ability to dilute the urine, which is an early sign of hyperuricemic nephropathy.

➢ Late stage azotemia and uremia.

(3) Uric Acid Kidney Stones

➢ Renal colic: Intermittent pain in the lumbar and epigastric regions.

The pain is located in the kidney region of the affected side, and radiates to the inguinal groove, testicle, or labium majus of the same side.

- Gross hematuria (or hematuria that is visible under microscope) that is preceded by physical activity such as exercise, cycling, physical labor, or nephric colic.
- Infection accompanied by fever and urinary bladder excitation.
- Signs of obstruction, including urinary tract pain, dysuria, interrupted urination, and in severe cases, sudden anuresis.

(4) Acute Uric Acid Nephropathy

- Extensive obstruction of the renal tubules by a large amount of uric acid crystals.
- In the initial stage, there is increased 24-hour uric acid excretion, accompanied by hematuria, leukocyturia, and multiform crystals in the urine. The initial stage will gradually progress to oliguria and anuria as the patient's condition worsens, while 24-hour uric acid excretion is either decreased or normal.

Differential Diagnosis

The acute stage of gout, which is characterized by red swollen joints, should be distinguished from other similar diseases such as rheumatoid arthritis, psoriatic arthritis, osteoarthritis, and suppurative arthritis.

(1) Rheumatoid Arthritis

Rheumatoid arthritis is more prevalent among middle-aged and young women, in which multiple joints are usually involved. There is symmetric involvement of the proximal small joints of the extremities, including the wrist, knee, and ankle joints, accompanied by elevated immunoglobulin levels and increased rheumatoid factors without evident hyperuricemia. X-ray shows erosion of articular surfaces, narrowing of inter-joint spaces, and osteoporosis. These symptoms are significantly different from the damage caused by gout.

(2) Erysipelas and Phlegmonous Cellulitis

During the acute episode of gout, there is marked redness and swelling of the soft tissues surrounding the joint, which can easily be misdiagnosed as erysipelas or phlegmonous cellulitis. However, the latter is accompanied by aversion to cold, fever, elevation of white blood cells without joint pain, and hyperuricemia.

(3) Traumatic Arthritis and Suppurative Arthritis

Trauma and fatigue can likely induce an episode of gout, which is often misdiagnosed as traumatic arthritis. However, the duration of traumatic arthritis is closely related to the duration of the trauma, and is not accompanied by hyperuricemia. When there is destruction of the tubercle in chronic gouty arthritis, or redness and swelling of the joint(s) during acute episodes, gout is sometimes misdiagnosed as suppurative arthritis or tuberculous arthritis. In either of these cases, there are no sodium uric acid crystals in the synovial fluid or bodily excretions, though a large amount of white blood cells are present. A culture of the synovial fluid will reveal pathogenic bacteria.

(4) Psoriatic Arthritis

Asymmetric involvement of the distal joints of the toes or fingers and bone absorption is common in psoriatic arthritis. Hyperuricemia exists in approximately 20% of all cases, making it hard to distinguish from gout. However, the former involves distal toe or finger joints and the hip joint, with widened inter-joint spaces. X-ray reveals a hat-like appearance of the distal toe or finger joints.

(5) Bone Tumor

In gout, the deposition of sodium uric acid in the bones causes multiple erosion-like destruction of the bone (and thus fractures), as well as swelling and deformity of the tubercle. It can easily be misdiagnosed as bone tumor and the affected fingers, toes, or limbs would consequently be amputated. However, in bone tumor, the course of disease is persistent, and there are neither episodes of redness, swelling and acute pain nor evident hyperuricemia. A biopsy can easily differentiate between these two conditions.

(6) Pseudogout Arthritis

The acute stage of pseudogout arthritis resembles gout. Primary pseudogout is uncommon, and usually affects the knee joint of elderly patients. Blood uric acid levels are not elevated. X-ray shows calcification of the cartilage or deposits of calcium pyrophosphate dihydrate (CPPD) crystals in the synovial fluid.

(7) Other Types of Arthritis

The acute stage of gouty arthritis should be differentiated from systemic lupus erythematosus (SLE), Wright's syndrome, and hypertrophic arthritis. Blood uric acid levels are usually normal in these types of arthritis. A combination of clinical data, laboratory tests, and X-ray results is helpful in determining the correct diagnosis.

Treatment

The aim of clinical treatment is to prevent or ease acute episodes of gout; to prevent the recurrence of arthritis; to lessen the deposits of uric acid in the body; to prevent the formation of uric acid calculi; and to reduce the required doses of anti-urate medication and ease their side effects.

➢ General Treatment

Prevent obesity or overweightness. Avoid or limit the consumption of purine-rich foods such as animal organs, seafood, meat, or soups and sauces that contain these ingredients. The patient should eat more alkaline foods such as vegetables, fruits, potatoes, watermelon, and Chinese waxgourd. Avoid taking medications that hinder or reduce uric acid excretion, such as aspirin, diuretics, phenylbutazone, nicotinic acid, and vitamins B_1 and B_{12}. Avoid alcohol, hot pepper, curry, and black pepper.

➢ **Optional Measures**

During acute episodes, patients are advised to lay down and rest with the affected limb elevated, and avoid putting weight on the affected joints. Immediate administration of colchicine will produce remarkable effects. The patient should take 0.5 mg per hour or 1 mg every 2 hours until the symptoms are relieved or adverse effects surface; or, take up to a maximum of 6 mg, discontinuing if there is no alleviation of symptoms. Another alternative is to take 0.5 mg, 3 times a day, for 3 to 4 days and either reduce the dose or stop taking the medicine as soon as the symptoms are relieved. For those with gastrointestinal symptoms as a side effect of oral administration, an intravenous administration of 2 mg of colchicine with 10 ml of normal saline is suggested (for over 5 minutes). If necessary, 1 mg of colchicine can be administered again after 6 hours, with the total dosage not exceeding 4mg. Non-steroidal anti-inflammatory drugs (NSAIDs) such as piroxicam, indometacin, naproxen, ibuprofen, phenylbutazone, oxyphenbutazone, or ketoprofen can also be given. If all of the above measures produce no noticeable effects, glucocorticoids are suggested; prescribe 10 mg of prednisone (given orally) 3-4 times a day, or, give intravenous injections of 10-20 mg of dexamethasone for 3 to 5 days, reducing the dosage or terminating the medication after the symptoms have been relieved. If a single joint is involved, 5-20 mg of triamcinolone acetonide is injected into the joint to relieve pain.

➢ **Treatment in the Interval and Chronic Stages**

During the interval and chronic stages, allopurinol is administered to inhibit uric acid synthesis while probenecid, sulfinpyrazone, and benzbromarone are prescribed to promote uric acid excretion. Drugs that promote the elimination of uric acid should not be prescribed together with drugs that inhibit the uric acid excretion, such as salicylic acid, thiadiazine diuretics, furosemide, and ethacrynic acid. For patients with hyperuricemia, drugs that lower uric acid should be prescribed to stabilize blood uric acid levels.

- **Acute Renal Failure**

In cases of acute renal failure due to uric acid nephropathy, 40-100 mg of furosemide (a diuretic) is administered while simultaneously replenishing body fluids and correcting metabolic acidosis. Afterwards, a daily dose of allopurinol is given at 8mg (per kg of body weight), which is reduced to 100-300 mg per day after 3-4 days. Hemodialysis should be performed if necessary.

CHINESE MEDICAL ETIOLOGY AND PATHOMECHANISM

From the Chinese medical perspective, the main causes of gout include congenital constitutional insufficiency and dysfunction of the spleen and kidney, and are related to factors such as heredity, constitution, diet, external contraction, environment, and fatigue. Liver and kidney deficiency and failure of the spleen to transform and transport are the root of this disease, while wind, cold, dampness, heat, phlegm turbidity, and obstruction of the channels by static blood are the branch. The pathomechanism of this disease is a combination of root deficiency and branch excess. In the initial stages of gout, pathological changes involve the limbs, joints and channels, which later give way to erosion of the sinews and bones and damage to the *zang-fu* organs.

Gout is mainly attributed to the disorders of the kidney, liver and spleen. The kidney is the root of congenital constitution, and is responsible for storing original yin, containing original yang, and controlling qi transformation and water metabolism; the liver stores blood and governs the sinews, and is the basis of resistance to fatigue. Liver and kidney depletion leads to deficiency of essence and blood and causes the sinews, bones, and channels to be deprived of nourishment. The kidney controls urine and stool; its dysfunction leads to the internal accumulation of damp-turbidity. Failure of the spleen to transform and transport causes the internal generation of phlegm turbidity.

Exposure to wind, cold, damp, or heat evil; taxation fatigue; internal damage by the seven emotions; excessive consumption of alcohol; damage due to an irregular diet; and traumatic joint injuries can all cause phlegm turbidity to pour into the joints, flesh and bones. This, in turn, will obstruct the flow of qi and blood, giving rise to redness, swelling, heat, and pain of the joints and flesh; numbness; heaviness; and inhibited bending and stretching, all of which constitute the signs and symptoms of gout.

According to the difference in pathogenic factors, predominant evil, or constitutional factors, gout can be divided into categories of *bi* (痹) syndrome caused by the following: wind-damp, cold-damp, or damp-heat. Long-term invasion of wind, cold, and dampness can transform into heat, which can give rise to wind-damp-heat *bi* or damp-heat *bi*. Over a long period of time, stasis obstruction in the blood vessels causes congealing of body fluids as well as phlegm turbidity and blood stasis obstruction of the channels and collaterals, resulting in joint swelling, deformity, stiffness, petechia and nodules (surrounding the affected joints), and damage to the *zang-fu* organs. When combined with other *zang-fu* syndromes, the condition can be both complex and severe.

CHINESE MEDICAL TREATMENT

The main principle in the Chinese medical treatment of gout is treatment based on pattern differentiation. Symptoms may vary with the different stages of the disease, thus treatment should be planned accordingly. The acute arthritis stage usually manifests as wind-damp-heat *bi* or damp-heat *bi*; hence, treatment calls for clearing heat, eliminating dampness, unblocking the collaterals, and relieving pain. The chronic arthritis stage often manifests as wind-cold-damp *bi*, wind-damp *bi*, cold-damp *bi*, phlegm-stasis obstruction, or liver and kidney insufficiency. The combination of internal and external treatment on the basis of pattern identification, namely acupuncture and medicinals, can result in the improvement of symptoms and lead to a clinical cure.

Pattern Differentiation and Treatment

The treatment principle of gout is treating the branch during the onset and treating the root during remission. Depending on the different clinical manifestations, it is necessary to dispel wind and eliminate dampness; clear heat or dissipate cold; flush out phlegm; transform stasis; regulate and tonify the liver and kidney; unblock the collaterals; and relieve pain.

(1) Wind-damp-heat *Bi*

【Syndrome Characteristics】

Sudden onset; marked redness, swelling and pain of the joint; attacks occur more frequently at night; involvement of one or more joints; accompanied by fever, aversion to wind, thirst, vexation, chest fullness, headache, sweating, scanty dark urine, constipation, a yellowish or greasy tongue coating, and a wiry, slippery, and rapid pulse.

【Treatment Principle】

Clear heat, unblock the collaterals, dispel wind, and eliminate dampness.

【Commonly Used Medicinals】

To clear heat and drain fire, use *shēng shí gāo* (raw Gypsum Fibrosum), *huáng bǎi* (Cortex Phellodendri Chinensis), *lián qiào* (Fructus Forsythiae), and *lóng dǎn cǎo* (Radix et Rhizoma Gentianae); to dispel wind and eliminate dampness, use *fáng jǐ* (Radix Stephaniae Tetrandrae), *shēng yì yǐ rén* (raw Semen Coicis), *dú huó* (Radix Angelicae Pubescentis), *cāng zhú* (Rhizoma Atractylodis), *tǔ fú líng* (Rhizoma Smilacis Glabrae), *hǔ zhàng* (Rhizoma Polygoni Cuspidati), and *qín jiāo* (Radix Gentianae Macrophyllae); to unblock the collaterals and relieve pain, use *rěn dōng téng* (Caulis Lonicerae Japonicae), *chuān niú xī* (Radix Cyathulae), *dāng guī* (Radix Angelicae Sinensis), *chuān mù guā* (Fructus Chaenomelis), *wǔ jiā pí* (Cortex Acanthopanacis), and *dì lóng* (Pheretima).

【Representative Formula】

Modified *Bái Hǔ Guì Zhī Tāng* (白虎桂枝汤)

【Ingredients】

生石膏	shēng shí gāo	30-60g	Gypsum Fibrosum (raw)
知母	zhī mǔ	12g	Rhizoma Anemarrhenae
桂枝	guì zhī	10g	Ramulus Cinnamomi
粳米	jīng mǐ	12g	Oryza sativa L.
甘草	gān cǎo	6g	Radix et Rhizoma Glycyrrhizae

Boil the above ingredients in 500ml water until reduced to a 100ml decoction. Take warm, 1 batch a day, divided into two doses.

【Formula Analysis】

The nature of *shēng shí gāo* (raw Gypsum Fibrosum) is very cold, and hence it is excellent for clearing heat; the nature of *zhī mǔ* (Rhizoma Anemarrhenae) is cold and moistening, allowing it to assist *shí gāo* (Gypsum Fibrosum) in clearing heat; *jīng mǐ* (Oryza sativa L.) and *gān cǎo* (Radix et Rhizoma Glycyrrhizae) can harmonize the middle *jiao*, benefit the stomach, and prevent damage to the middle *jiao* from the cold nature of *shēng shí gāo* (raw Gypsum Fibrosum) and *zhī mǔ* (Rhizoma

Anemarrhenae). The combination of the four medicinals can clear heat, eliminate vexation, nourish the stomach, and engender fluids; *guì zhī* (Ramulus Cinnamomi) can course wind and unblock the collaterals. *Bái Hŭ Guì Zhī Tāng* (白虎桂枝汤), as a whole, can clear heat, unblock the collaterals, dispel wind, eliminate dampness, and relieve pain.

【Modifications】

➢ For scanty dark urine, *tŭ fú líng* (Rhizoma Smilacis Glabrae) 15g, *bì xiè* (Rhizoma Dioscoreae Hypoglaucae) 15g, *zé lán* (Herba Lycopi) 12g, *máo dōng qīng* (Ilex Pubescens) 15g, *yì yĭ rén* (Semen Coicis) 20g, *zé xiè* (Rhizoma Alismatis) 10g, and *chē qián zĭ* (Semen Plantaginis) 12g can be added to drain turbidity, transform stasis, and promote urination to facilitate the excretion of uric acid.

➢ For excessive heat, *huáng băi* (Cortex Phellodendri Chinensis) 10g, *liăng miàn zhēn* (Radix Zanthoxyli) 15g, and *rĕn dōng téng* (Caulis Lonicerae Japonicae) 15g can be added to clear heat and unblock the collaterals.

➢ For severe pain and swelling, add *tŭ fú líng* (Rhizoma Smilacis Glabrae) 15g, *yì yĭ rén* (Semen Coicis) 20g, *qín jiāo* (Radix Gentianae Macrophyllae) 15g, *hăi tóng pí* (Cortex Erythrinae) 15g, *rŭ xiāng* (Olibanum) 6g, *mò yào* (Myrrha) 6g, *quán xiē* (Scorpio) 5g, and *wú gōng* (Scolopendra) 3g to eliminate dampness, quicken the collaterals, unblock *bi*, and relieve pain.

➢ For impairment of the body fluids by intense heat, add *shēng dì* (Radix Rehmanniae Recens) 15g, *xuán shēn* (Radix Scrophulariae) 12g, and *mài dōng* (Radix Ophiopogonis) 15g, or use modified *Xī Jiăo Săn* (犀角散) to nourish yin, clear heat, and increase body fluids.

➢ For severe pain of the lower extremities, add medicinals such as *niú xī* (Radix Achyranthis Bidentatae) 15g, *dú huó* (Radix Angelicae Pubescentis) 15g, and *mù guā* (Fructus Chaenomelis) 12g to unblock the joints.

➢ For severe pain of the upper extremities, add *qiāng huó* (Rhizoma et Radix Notopterygii) 15g, *jiāng huáng* (Rhizoma Curcumae Longae) 12g, and *wēi líng xiān* (Radix et Rhizoma Clematidis) 12g to course and unblock the channels and collaterals of the upper extremities.

➢ If the condition is mainly attributed to damp-heat *bi*, use a modified combination of *Sì Miào Wán* (四妙丸) plus *Lóng Dǎn Xiè Gān Tāng* (龙胆泻肝汤). It can clear heat, eliminate dampness, unblock the collaterals, and relieve pain.

(2) Wind-cold-damp *Bi*

【Syndrome Characteristics】

Swelling and pain of the joint(s) with inhibited bending and stretching; subcutaneous nodules or tophi; a thin white or greasy white tongue coating; and a wiry and tight, or soggy and moderate pulse. If wind evil is predominant, there will be wandering pain, aversion to wind, and fever. If cold is predominant, there will be severe joint pain of fixed location. If dampness is predominant, there will be joint heaviness and pain of fixed location, and numbness of the skin.

【Treatment Principle】

Dispel wind, dissipate cold, eliminate dampness, and unblock the collaterals.

【Commonly Used Medicinals】

Qiāng huó (Rhizoma et Radix Notopterygii), *dú huó* (Radix Angelicae Pubescentis), *fáng fēng* (Radix Saposhnikoviae), *má huáng* (Herba Ephedrae), *xì xīn* (Radix et Rhizoma Asari), *zhì chuān wū* (Radix Aconiti Praeparata), and *zhì fù zǐ* (Radix Aconiti Lateralis Praeparata) can be used to dispel wind and dissipate cold. *Yì yǐ rén* (Semen Coicis), *cāng zhú* (Rhizoma Atractylodis), *fú líng* (Poria), and *fáng jǐ* (Radix Stephaniae Tetrandrae) can fortify the spleen and remove dampness. *Guì zhī* (Ramulus Cinnamomi), *sāng zhī* (Ramulus Mori), *dāng guī* (Radix Angelicae Sinensis), *chuān mù guā* (Fructus Chaenomelis), *jiāng huáng* (Rhizoma Curcumae Longae), *wēi líng xiān* (Radix et Rhizoma Clematidis), and *dì lóng* (Pheretima) can unblock the collaterals and relieve pain.

【Representative Formula】

Yì Yǐ Rén Tāng (薏苡仁汤)

【Ingredients】

羌活	qiāng huó	15g	Rhizoma et Radix Notopterygii
独活	dú huó	15g	Radix Angelicae Pubescentis
防风	fáng fēng	12g	Radix Saposhnikoviae
苍术	cāng zhú	12g	Rhizoma Atractylodis
当归	dāng guī	9g	Radix Angelicae Sinensis
川芎	chuān xiōng	10g	Rhizoma Chuanxiong
桂枝	guì zhī	9g	Ramulus Cinnamomi
麻黄	má huáng	6g	Herba Ephedrae
薏苡仁	yì yǐ rén	20g	Semen Coicis
制川乌	zhì chuān wū	9g	Radix Aconiti Praeparata
生姜	shēng jiāng	6g	Rhizoma Zingiberis Recens
甘草	gān cǎo	6g	Radix et Rhizoma Glycyrrhizae

Boil the above ingredients in 500ml water until reduced to a 100ml decoction. Take warm, 1 batch a day.

【Formula Analysis】

Qiāng huó (Rhizoma et Radix Notopterygii), *dú huó* (Radix Angelicae Pubescentis), and *fáng fēng* (Radix Saposhnikoviae) can dispel wind, overcome dampness, and quicken the collaterals. *Chuān wū* (Radix Aconiti), *má huáng* (Herba Ephedrae), and *guì zhī* (Ramulus Cinnamomi) can warm the channels, dissipate cold, and unblock the collaterals. *Yì yǐ rén* (Semen Coicis) and *cāng zhú* (Rhizoma Atractylodis) are used to fortify the spleen to leach out dampness. *Dāng guī* (Radix Angelicae Sinensis) and *chuān xiōng* (Rhizoma Chuanxiong) are used to nourish and invigorate blood. *Shēng jiāng* (Rhizoma Zingiberis Recens) and *gān cǎo* (Radix et Rhizoma Glycyrrhizae) are prescribed to fortify the spleen and harmonize the middle *jiao*. The formula, as a whole, dispels wind, dissipates cold, removes dampness, and unblocks the collaterals.

【Modifications】

➢ For prevalence of wind, *hǎi fēng téng* (Caulis Piperis Kadsurae) 20g and *qín jiāo* (Radix Gentianae Macrophyllae) 15g can be added to dispel wind and unblock the collaterals.

➢ For prevalence of cold, medicinals such as *fù zǐ* (Radix Aconiti Lateralis Praeparata) 6g, *gān jiāng* (Rhizoma Zingiberis) 6g, and *xì xīn* (Radix et Rhizoma Asari) 3g can be added, or modified *Wū Tóu Tāng* (乌头汤) can be prescribed to warm the channels and dissipate cold.

➢ For prevalence of dampness, *fáng jǐ* (Radix Stephaniae Tetrandrae) 10g, *bì xiè* (Rhizoma Dioscoreae Hypoglaucae) 15g, *mù guā* (Fructus Chaenomelis) 12g, and *tiān xiān téng* (Herba Aristolochiae) 10g can be added to strengthen the formula's ability to remove dampness and unblock the collaterals.

➢ For subcutaneous nodules or tophi, add medicinals that dispel phlegm, dissolve stones, and unblock the collaterals, such as *tiān nán xīng* (Rhizoma Arisaematis) 10g and *páo shān jiǎ* (blast-fried Squama Manis) 10g.

(3) Phlegm-stasis Obstruction

【Syndrome Characteristics】

Chronic, recurrent attacks of joint pain that is sometimes severe and sometimes mild. The pain may be stabbing and at a fixed location. There is swelling and, in severe cases, stiffness and deformity of the joints, inhibited bending and stretching, subcutaneous nodules, darkening of the skin (or the skin color remains unchanged), or the formation of fistulas. The pulse is wiry, or deep and rough. The tongue may be pale and enlarged, or dusky purple with a thin white or white greasy coating.

【Treatment Principle】

Invigorate blood and transform stasis; flush out phlegm and unblock the collaterals.

【Commonly Used Medicinals】

Táo rén (Semen Persicae), *hóng huā* (Flos Carthami), *dāng guī* (Radix Angelicae Sinensis), *chuān xiōng* (Rhizoma Chuanxiong), *rŭ xiāng* (Olibanum), and *mò yào* (Myrrha) are used to invigorate blood and transform stasis. *Fú líng* (Poria), *chén pí* (Pericarpium Citri Reticulatae), *bàn xià* (Rhizoma Pinelliae), and *zhú rú* (Caulis Bambusae in Taenia) are used to flush out phlegm and leach out dampness. *Guì zhī* (Ramulus Cinnamomi), *sāng zhī* (Ramulus Mori), *dāng guī* (Radix Angelicae Sinensis), *chuān xiōng* (Rhizoma Chuanxiong), *yán hú suŏ* (Rhizoma Corydalis), *wēi líng xiān* (Radix et Rhizoma Clematidis), and *wú gōng* (Scolopendra) unblock the channels and relieve pain.

【Representative Formula】

Táo Hóng Yĭn (桃红饮) plus *Èr Chén Tāng* (二陈汤)

【Ingredients】

桃仁	táo rén	15g	Semen Persicae
红花	hóng huā	10g	Flos Carthami
当归	dāng guī	12g	Radix Angelicae Sinensis
川芎	chuān xiōng	15g	Rhizoma Chuanxiong
茯苓	fú líng	15g	Poria
陈皮	chén pí	6g	Pericarpium Citri Reticulatae
法半夏	fă bàn xià	12g	Rhizoma Pinelliae Praeparatum
威灵仙	wēi líng xiān	15g	Radix et Rhizoma Clematidis
甘草	gān căo	6g	Radix et Rhizoma Glycyrrhizae

Boil the above ingredients in 500ml water until reduced to a 100ml decoction. Take warm, 1 batch a day.

【Formula Analysis】

Táo rén (Semen Persicae) and *hóng huā* (Flos Carthami) expel stasis and move blood. *Chuān xiōng* (Rhizoma Chuanxiong) enters the blood aspect and is used to regulate the qi within the blood. *Dāng guī* (Radix Angelicae

Sinensis) is used to tonify and invigorate blood. *Fă bàn xià* (Rhizoma Pinelliae Praeparatum) which is acrid, warm and dry in nature, is used to dry dampness and transform phlegm. *Chén pí* (Pericarpium Citri Reticulatae) regulates qi, dries dampness, normalizes qi, and disperses phlegm. *Fú líng* (Poria) fortifies the spleen, leaches out dampness, and transforms phlegm. *Wēi líng xiān* (Radix et Rhizoma Clematidis), which is acrid, dispersing, warm, and unblocking in nature, is fierce and moving and enters the 12 channels. *Gān căo* (Radix et Rhizoma Glycyrrhizae) harmonizes the middle *jiao*. The combination of the two formulas can invigorate blood, transform stasis, flush out phlegm, and unblock the collaterals.

【Modifications】

➢ For subcutaneous nodules, *tiān nán xīng* (Rhizoma Arisaematis) 10g and *bái jiè zĭ* (Semen Sinapis) 10g can be added to transform phlegm and dissipate nodules.

➢ For severe joint pain, add *máo dōng qīng* (Ilex Pubescens) 15g, *rŭ xiāng* (Olibanum) 6g, *mò yào* (Myrrha) 6g, *jī xuè téng* (Caulis Spatholobi) 15g, *yán hú suŏ* (Rhizoma Corydalis) 12g, *dì lóng* (Pheretima) 10g, or use modified *Xuè Fŭ Zhú Yū Tāng* (血府逐瘀汤) to move qi, invigorate blood, dispel stasis, and relieve pain.

➢ For severe swelling of the joint, add *fáng jĭ* (Radix Stephaniae Tetrandrae) 10g, *tŭ fú líng* (Rhizoma Smilacis Glabrae) 15g, *huá shí* (Talcum) 15g, and *chē qián zĭ* (Semen Plantaginis) 12g to promote water flow, transform dampness, and disperse swelling.

➢ For chronic and unremitting joint pain with possible stiffness and deformity, add *quán xiē* (Scorpio) 5g, *wú gōng* (Scolopendra) 3g, *wū shāo shé* (Zaocys) 10g, and *páo shān jiă* (blast-fried Squama Manis) 10g to track down wind and remove evil, unblock *bi*, and relieve pain.

➢ For open and ruptured phlegm nodules, *huáng qí* (Radix Astragali) 20g can be added to tonify qi, draw out toxins, and engender flesh.

(4) Liver and Kidney Insufficiency

【Syndrome Characteristics】

Recurrent attacks of joint pain that lasts for days without recovery. The pain is sometimes severe and sometimes mild, and there may be joint deformity. Accompanying symptoms include soreness of the lumbus and knees, dizziness, tinnitus, weakness and fatigue, and a deep, thready, wiry and forceless pulse.

【Treatment Principle】

Boost the liver and kidney, tonify qi and blood, dispel wind and dampness, and relieve obstruction and pain.

【Commonly Used Medicinals】

Sāng jì shēng (Herba Taxilli), *niú xī* (Radix Achyranthis Bidentatae), *qín jiāo* (Radix Gentianae Macrophyllae), and *bái sháo* (Radix Paeoniae Alba) boost the liver and kidney. *Dāng guī* (Radix Angelicae Sinensis), *chuān xiōng* (Rhizoma Chuanxiong), *dǎng shēn* (Radix Codonopsis), *huáng qí* (Radix Astragali), and *shú dì* (Radix Rehmanniae Praeparata) tonify qi and blood. *Dú huó* (Radix Angelicae Pubescentis), *fáng fēng* (Radix Saposhnikoviae), *fáng jǐ* (Radix Stephaniae Tetrandrae), *fú líng* (Poria), and *wǔ jiā pí* (Cortex Acanthopanacis) dispel wind and dampness. *Yán hú suǒ* (Rhizoma Corydalis), *jiāng huáng* (Rhizoma Curcumae Longae), *wū shāo shé* (Zaocys), and *luò shí téng* (Caulis Trachelospermi) remove obstruction and relieve pain.

【Representative Formula】

Dú Huó Jì Shēng Tāng (独活寄生汤)

【Ingredients】

独活	dú huó	15g	Radix Angelicae Pubescentis
桑寄生	sāng jì shēng	20g	Herba Taxilli
杜仲	dù zhòng	15g	Cortex Eucommiae
牛膝	niú xī	12g	Radix Achyranthis Bidentatae
细辛	xì xīn	3g	Radix et Rhizoma Asari

秦艽	qín jiāo	12g	Radix Gentianae Macrophyllae
茯苓	fú líng	15g	Poria
肉桂	ròu guì	5g	Cortex Cinnamomi
防风	fáng fēng	12g	Radix Saposhnikoviae
川芎	chuān xiōng	15g	Rhizoma Chuanxiong
党参	dǎng shēn	20g	Radix Codonopsis
当归	dāng guī	12g	Radix Angelicae Sinensis
白芍	bái sháo	15g	Radix Paeoniae Alba
熟地黄	shú dì huáng	15g	Radix Rehmanniae Praeparata
甘草	gān cǎo	6g	Radix et Rhizoma Glycyrrhizae

Boil the above ingredients in 500ml water until reduced to a 100ml decoction. Take warm, 1 batch a day.

【Formula Analysis】

Dú huó (Radix Angelicae Pubescentis), *xì xīn* (Radix et Rhizoma Asari), *fáng fēng* (Radix Saposhnikoviae), and *qín jiāo* (Radix Gentianae Macrophyllae) dispel wind, eliminate dampness, disperse cold, and relieve pain. *Sāng jì shēng* (Herba Taxilli), *dù zhòng* (Cortex Eucommiae), and *niú xī* (Radix Achyranthis Bidentatae) tonify and boost the liver and kidney while dispelling wind and dampness. *Dāng guī* (Radix Angelicae Sinensis), *chuān xiōng* (Rhizoma Chuanxiong), *shú dì huáng* (Radix Rehmanniae Praeparata), and *bái sháo* (Radix Paeoniae Alba) are used to nourish and invigorate blood. *Dǎng shēn* (Radix Codonopsis) and *fú líng* (Poria) tonify qi and fortify the spleen. *Ròu guì* (Cortex Cinnamomi) warms and unblocks the blood vessels. *Gān cǎo* (Radix et Rhizoma Glycyrrhizae) harmonizes all the medicinals. The formula, as a whole, boosts the liver and kidney, tonifies qi and blood, dispels wind and dampness, removes obstruction, and relieves pain.

【Modifications】

➢ For severe pain, add *zhì chuān wū* (Radix Aconiti Praeparata) 9g, *wū shāo shé* (Zaocys) 10g, *dì lóng* (Pheretima) 10g, *máo dōng qīng* (Ilex

Pubescens) 15g, and *hóng huā* (Flos Carthami) 10g to track down wind, unblock the collaterals, invigorate blood, and relieve pain.

- For prevalence of cold evil with severe joint pain, *fù zǐ* (Radix Aconiti Lateralis Praeparata) 6g and *gān jiāng* (Rhizoma Zingiberis) 6g can be added to warm the channels, disperse cold, and unblock the collaterals.
- For soreness and weakness of the lumbus and knees, add *xù duàn* (Radix Dipsaci) 10g and *lù jiǎo shuāng* (Cornu Cervi Degelatinatum) 10g to tonify the liver and kidney, strengthen the sinews and bones, remove obstruction, and relieve pain.
- For joint heaviness and numbness of the skin, *fáng jǐ* (Radix Stephaniae Tetrandrae) 10g, *yì yǐ rén* (Semen Coicis) 20g, *cāng zhú* (Rhizoma Atractylodis) 12g, *jī xuè téng* (Caulis Spatholobi) 15g, and *luò shí téng* (Caulis Trachelospermi) 15g can be added to dispel dampness, quicken the collaterals, and unblock obstruction.
- For pronounced yin deficiency, modified *Zuǒ Guī Yǐn* (左归饮) is prescribed to tonify yin and blood.
- For marked yang deficiency, modified *Yòu Guī Yǐn* (右归饮) or modified *Shèn Qì Wán* (肾气丸) is prescribed to tonify yang qi.

Additional Treatment Modalities

1. Chinese Patent Medicine

(1) *Xī Xiān Wán* (豨莶丸)

One pill, three times a day. For obstruction due to damp-heat.

(2) *Xī Tóng Wán* (豨桐丸)

Ten pills, twice a day. For obstruction due to damp-heat.

(3) *Hán Shī Bì Chōng Jì* (寒湿痹冲剂)

One package, three times a day. For wind-cold-damp *bi*.

(4) *Shū Jīn Huó Xuè Piàn* (舒筋活血片)

Five pills, three times a day. For phlegm-stasis obstruction.

(5) Extracts of *Léi Gōng Téng* (Radix Tripterygii Wilfordii): *Dīng Jiǎ Piàn* (丁甲片)

20mg per pill, 2-3 pills each time, three times a day. 14 days equal a course of treatment. For acute and chronic gouty arthritis.

2. Acupuncture and Moxibustion

(1) Acupuncture and Moxibustion

【Treatment Principle】

Unblock the collaterals and relieve pain.

【Main Points】

Select the acupoints that correspond to the affected joints:

- Metatarsophalangeal joints: LV 3 (*tài chōng*), SP 3 (*tài bái*), and SP 6 (*sān yīn jiāo*).
- Toe joints: SP 3 (*tài bái*), SP 2 (*dà dū*), LV 3 (*tài chōng*), and SP 6 (*sān yīn jiāo*).
- Ankle joint: LV 4 (*zhōng fēng*), BL 60 (*kūn lún*), ST 41 (*jiě xī*), GB 40 (*qiū xū*), BL 40 (*wěi zhōng*), and GB 39 (*jué gǔ*).
- Knee joint: *xī yǎn* (EX-LE 5), GB 34 (*yáng líng quán*), and LV 8 (*qū quán*) to relieve pain.
- Wrist joint: SJ 4 (*yáng chí*), SJ 5 (*wài guān*), LI 4 (*hé gǔ*), and LV 3 (*tài chōng*).
- Elbow joint: LI 4 (*hé gǔ*), LI 10 (*shǒu sān lǐ*), LI 11 (*qū chí*), and LU 5 (*chǐ zé*).
- Shoulder joint: LI 15 (*jiān yú*), SI 9 (*jiān zhēn*), GB 21 (*jiān jǐng*), and points that are tender upon palpation.

【Point Modification】

- In the case of damp-heat brewing and binding, select GB 40 (*qiū xū*), SP 2 (*dà dū*), and SP 3 (*tài bái*) to clear heat and drain dampness.

- For blood stasis obstructing the collaterals, select SP 10 (*xuè hǎi*) and BL 17 (*gé shù*) to invigorate blood and unblock the collaterals.
- For phlegm turbidity obstruction, select ST 40 (*fēng lóng*) and BL 20 (*pí shù*) to dispel phlegm and transform turbidity.
- For liver and kidney deficiency, select KI 3 (*tài xī*) and SP 6 (*sān yīn jiāo*) to tonify the liver and kidney.

【Manipulation】

Wind-cold-damp *bi* should be treated with acupuncture and moxibustion. Wind-damp-heat *bi* can be treated with acupuncture but not moxibustion. Long-term *bi* syndrome with deficiency of right qi is better treated with moxibustion. Use drainage during the acute phase; use even drainage and supplementation during remission. Retain the needles for 15 minutes per session, one treatment session a day. Ten days equals a course of treatment.

(2) Acupuncture

【Treatment Principle】

Unblock the collaterals and relieve pain.

【Point Selection and Combination】

Select acupoints that correspond to the involved joints:

1) Metatarsophalangeal joints

ashi points	ā shì xuè	阿是穴
EX-LE 10	bā fēng	八风
ST 44	nèi tíng	内庭
LV 3	tài chōng	太冲

2) Ankle joint

ashi points	ā shì xuè	阿是穴
BL 60	kūn lún	昆仑
GB 40	qiū xū	丘墟

ST 41	jiě xī	解溪
KI 3	tài xī	太溪

3) Wrist joint

ashi points	ā shì xuè	阿是穴
SJ 4	yáng chí	阳池
LI 5	yáng xī	阳溪
LI 4	hé gǔ	合谷

4) Interphalangeal and metacarpophalangeal joints

ashi points	ā shì xuè	阿是穴
EX-UE 10	sì fèng	四缝
EX-UE 9	bā xié	八邪
LI 3	sān jiān	三间

5) Knee joint

EX-LE5	xī yǎn	膝眼
EX-LE4	nèi xī yǎn	内膝眼
GB 34	yáng líng quán	阳陵泉
ST 34	liáng qiū	梁丘
BL 40	wěi zhōng	委中
GB 33	xī yáng guān	膝阳关
ST 36	zú sān lǐ	足三里

【Point Modification】

- For prevalence of wind heat damp, DU 14 (*dà zhuī*), DU 12 (*shēn zhù*), and LI 11 (*qū chí*) can be added.
- For phlegm-stasis obstruction, BL 17 (*gé shù*), SP 10 (*xuè hǎi*), BL 20 (*pí shù*), PC 6 (*nèi guān*), and BL 28 (*páng guāng shù*) can be added.

【Manipulation】

Strong needle stimulation is required on DU 14 (*dà zhuī*), DU 12 (*shēn zhù*), LI 11 (*qū chí*) and back-*shu points*. Do not retain needles. Stimulate acupoints around the involved joints with triple needling (齐刺, *qí cì*, one of the twelve needling methods), central-square needling (扬刺,

yáng cì, one of the twelve needling methods), joint needling (关刺, *guān cì*, one of the five needling methods), and transport needling (输刺, *shū cì*, one of the five, nine, and twelve needling methods) to course the qi stagnation and blood stasis of the joint. Shake the needle after inserting, or use a thick needle to cause local bleeding. Treat once a day; 15 days equal a course of treatment. For severe joint swelling pain or fusiform joint, use a three-edged needle to cause local bleeding in conjunction with cupping to draw out static blood. Administer this every 2 or 3 days; 5 treatment sessions equal a course of treatment.

(3) Auricular Acupuncture

【Point Selection】

Shen men, endocrine, liver, kidney, sympathetic, and acupoints of corresponding extremities and joints.

【Manipulation】

Prick 3 to 5 acupoints each time with 0.5-inch needles and retain the needles for 30 minutes per session, one session every 2 days. Ten sessions equal a course of treatment.

3. Tui Na

Select the acupoints of the corresponding joints according to the condition of the arthritis and the location of pain. Manipulation techniques include pushing, grasping, pressing, twist, foulage and rotating. Use gentle stimulation at first, and gradually increase pressure. Administer treatment once or twice a day for 15 to 30 minutes.

【Point Selection and Combination】

DU 14	dà zhuī	大椎
GB 20	fēng chí	风池
BL 23	shèn shù	肾俞
LI 10	shǒu sān lǐ	手三里

SI 9	jiān zhēn	肩贞
LI 4	hé gŭ	合谷

【Point Modification】

➢ For pain of the lower extremities, press on acupoints such as *zú zhĭ píng* (足趾平), GB 42 (*dì wŭ huì*) and the small joints of the feet and ankle. Apply more pressure on the soles and the dorsal aspect of the spaces in between the metatarsal bones. Rotation, plucking and shaking can be applied to the toes and ankle joints to relieve pain.

➢ For pain of the upper extremities, knead on points such as LI 4 (*hé gŭ*), LI 5 (*yáng xī*), SJ 4 (*yáng chí*), tender areas of the hands, lumbus, and legs, EX-UE8 (*wài láo gōng*), and joints of the hand and wrist to unblock the collaterals and relieve pain.

【Manipulation】

Press, knead, and grasp on the three yin channels of the hand and the three yin channels of the foot for 20 minutes, once a day. Seven sessions equal a course of treatment. Suitable for all types of gout.

4. External Application

(1) *Fú Huáng Gāo* (芙黄膏): Contains equal dosages of *fú róng yè* (Folium Hibisci Mutabilis), *shēng dà huáng* (raw Radix et Rhizoma Rhei), and *chì xiăo dòu* (Semen Phaseoli), ground into a fine powder and mixed with Vaseline in the proportion of 4:6 to make a plaster. Apply to affected areas of the body, once a day. For gout due to damp-heat obstruction.

(2) *Cè băi yè* (Cacumen Platycladi) 30g, *dà huáng* (Radix et Rhizoma Rhei) 30g, *huáng băi* (Cortex Phellodendri Chinensis) 15g, *bò hé* (Herba Menthae) 15g, and *zé lán* (Herba Lycopi) 15g ground into powder and mixed with an appropriate amount of honey and water to make a paste for external use. For gout due to damp-heat accumulating and binding.

(3) *Huí Yáng Yù Lóng Gāo* (回阳玉龙膏): *Căo wū* (Radix Aconiti Kusnezoffii)

90g, *wèi jiāng* (roasted Rhizoma Zingiberis Recens) 90g, *chì sháo* (Radix Paeoniae Rubra) 30g, *bái zhǐ* (Radix Angelicae Dahuricae) 30g, *tiān nán xīng* (Rhizoma Arisaematis) 30g, and *ròu guì* (Cortex Cinnamomi) 15g are ground into a fine powder and added with four times the amount of Vaseline to make a paste. Apply to affected areas of the body. For gout due to blood stasis.

(4) Decoct *zhì chuān wū* (Radix Aconiti Praeparata) 30g, *zhì cǎo wū* (Radix Aconiti Kusnezoffii Praeparata) 30g, *mù guā* (Fructus Chaenomelis) 30g, and *hóng huā* (Flos Carthami) 30g in 2500ml of water. Use the decoction to wash the affected areas. For gout due to blood stasis obstructing the collaterals.

(5) Decoct *liǔ shù huā* (willow flower) 30g, *yín huā* (Flos Lonicerae Japonicae) 30g, *pú gōng yīng* (Herba Taraxaci) 30g, *tǔ fú líng* (Rhizoma Smilacis Glabrae) 30g, *zǐ huā dì dīng* (Herba Violae) 30g, and *shēng dà huáng* (Radix et Rhizoma Rhei) 30g in an appropriate amount of water for 30 minutes. Use the decoction to wash the affected areas of the body. For gout due to damp-heat obstruction.

5. Simple Prescriptions and Empirical Formulas

(1) Wrap *chē qián zǐ* (Semen Plantaginis) 30g and soak it in 500ml of water for 30 minutes before decocting. To be taken frequently as a substitute for tea or other beverages, one decoction per day. Suitable for all types of gout.

(2) Combine *hǔ zhàng* (Rhizoma Polygoni Cuspidati), *zhāng nǎo* (Camphor) and Vaseline with in the proportion of 100:16:280. First, crush *hǔ zhàng* (Rhizoma Polygoni Cuspidati) into a powder and filter with an 80-mesh sifter. Dissolve camphor in an appropriate amount of alcohol (50%) and then pour it into the *hǔ zhàng* powder. Heat up Vaseline until it is liquefied and pour in the powdered *hǔ zhàng*. Tightly seal the mixture in a container and let it cool down to make a paste for external use. Cut out pieces of gauze according to the size of the involved joint. Spread 2-3mm

of paste on the gauze and apply it to the affected area. Cover with bandage. Replace it twice a day until full recovery. Suitable for gout due to damp-heat and stasis obstruction.

(3) Soak 250g of *gōu téng gēn* (Radix Uncariae) in an appropriate amount of strong white spirits (distilled liquor) for one day and divide into three portions to be taken over three days. This simple remedy can regulate qi, invigorate blood, and relieve pain. For gout due to qi stagnation and blood stasis.

(4) After boiling 1 *dàn* (担 ; a unit of weight equal to 50kg) of water, pour it into a bucket and add 250g of *zhāng mù xiè* (wood shavings of Lignum Cinnamomi Camphorae). Soak the affected foot in the bucket. Keep the steam away from the face to prevent damage to the eyes. For severe cold pain of the hands and feet.

(5) Decoct *hóng huā* (Flos Carthami) 15g, *bái zhǐ* (Radix Angelicae Dahuricae) 15g, *fáng fēng* (Radix Saposhnikoviae) 15g, and *wēi líng xiān* (Radix et Rhizoma Clematidis) 10g in alcohol to invigorate blood and dispel wind. Suitable for gouty arthritis and pain of the limbs.

PROGNOSIS

The duration of gout is long. If the kidney is not involved, the patient's life-span will not be affected. With appropriate measures for prevention and treatment, patients can lead a normal life. If not treated properly, painful acute relapses can occur, and can lead to joint deformity, kidney stones, and kidney damage. The prognosis is especially poor for patients who develop renal dysfunction.

1. Transformation from Heat to Cold and from Acute to Chronic

In the initial stage, right qi is not yet debilitated, and yang qi is still vigorous. Acute stages are most likely triggered by wind-damp-heat *bi* or damp-heat *bi*. Recurrent attacks, obstinate disease, or yang qi deficiency can lead to wind-damp-cold *bi* or cold-damp *bi*, causing the disease to progress from acute to chronic.

2. Progression from the Exterior to Interior, and from Excess to Deficiency

The early stage is caused by wind, cold, dampness, and/or heat invading the channels resulting in *bi* syndrome. Recurrent attacks eventually lead to static obstruction in the blood vessels, congealing of the body fluids, and accumulation of phlegm turbidity. The disease then enters the sinews and bones, and transforms into phlegm-stasis obstruction. Over time, qi and blood is depleted and right qi is weakened, manifesting as qi and blood insufficiency and liver and kidney deficiency. The patient's poor health condition can then trigger other disorders of the *zang-fu* organs. The disease progresses from the exterior to the interior, and from excess to deficiency.

PREVENTIVE HEALTHCARE

Since the onset of gout is closely related to diet and constitution, emphasis should be placed on preventing pathogenic factors from triggering future attacks. To prevent the onset of gout, the patient should adhere to the recommended dietary guidelines and observe the following suggestions:

Lifestyle Modification

- Keep the body warm and stay away from the cold.
- Footwear should be loose and comfortable, and should not impair the blood circulation of the feet.
- Rest well and avoid strenuous physical activities.
- Avoid joint injuries.
- Pay attention to changes of the mental state. Avoid psychospiritual stimuli and emotional stress.

➢ Avoid drugs that inhibit the excretion of uric acid, e.g., thiazide diuretics, furosemide, salicylic acid, and yeast.

➢ During acute episodes, bed rest is required. Have the patient raise the affected limb to relieve pain. When the condition has improved, the patient should partake in physical and functional exercise for the limbs.

➢ Check blood uric acid levels regularly to make sure that they are below 0.38mmol/L.

➢ Check for a family history of gout; those with asymptomatic hyperuricemia should be monitored regularly. If blood uric acid levels are above 0.42mmol/L, drugs that promote the excretion of uric acid (or inhibit its production) should be prescribed to keep blood uric acid levels normal and thereby prevent the onset of gout.

Dietary Recommendation

➢ Control the diet to prevent obesity, which helps to control hyperuricemia. However, the rapid breakdown of fat tissue leads to the elevation of blood ketone bodies and lactic acid, which inhibits the excretion of blood uric acid and thus results in the acute onset of gout. Therefore, dietary control should be well planned.

➢ Limit the intake of high-purine foods such as internal organs of animals (e.g., brain, liver, kidney, and heart), thick soups (e.g., gravy, chicken, fish), sardines, pomfret, mud eel, cat fish, fish roe, unrefined wheat, brown rice, whole wheat, beans, and fermented products. Foods with low purine content such as peas, and spinach can be eaten after cooking and discarding the soup.

➢ Strict abstinence from alcoholic beverages (especially beer), cigarettes, strong tea, and coffee is advised.

➢ Drink more cow's milk and goat's milk. Eat more eggs. Limit the intake of protein (approximately 0.8-1.0g of protein per kilogram of weight per day is recommended).

➢ Increase the intake of alkaline foods such as fresh vegetables, fruits, mineral water, steamed buns, and corn congee.

➢ Drink plenty of water (more than 3000 ml a day). This helps keep urinary production above 2000 ml per 24 hours, and thus promotes the excretion of uric acid.

➢ Refrain from eating pungent, fried, baked, smoked, fragrant, or dry foods; avoid foods of high fat content and foods that produce heat and dampness.

In addition to the dietary guidelines mentioned above, the following recipes are recommended:

1) Stir-fried Bamboo Shoots

Cut 250g of bamboo shoots into thin pieces. Stir-fry them with 30ml of vegetable oil and season with some salt. Can be eaten on a daily basis during the remission stage of gout.

2) *Jiā Wèi Luó Bō Tāng* (加味萝卜汤)

Wash the radish 250g and *bǎi zǐ rén* (Semen Platycladi) 30g. Cut the radish into thin pieces, and stir-fry them with 50ml of vegetable oil. Add *bǎi zǐ rén* (Semen Platycladi) and 500ml of water, then boil until done. Add salt to taste. May be eaten daily during the acute stage of gout.

3) *Fáng Fēng Yì Mǐ Zhōu* (防风薏米粥)

Decoct *fáng fēng* (Radix Saposhnikoviae) 10g and *yì yǐ rén* (Semen Coicis) 10g with water and take once a day for a week.

This formula clears heat and removes obstruction. It is indicated for gout due to damp-heat *bi*.

4) *Táo Rén Zhōu* (桃仁粥)

桃仁	táo rén	15g	Semen Persicae
粳米	jīng mǐ	160g	Oryza sativa L. (polished round-grained non-glutinous rice)

Crush *táo rén* (Semen Persicae) 15g into a pulp. Add water, blend, and filter out the dregs to make juice. Add *jīng mǐ* (polished round-grained non-glutinous rice) 160g to this juice and cook to make porridge.

This formula invigorates blood, dispels stasis, unblocks the collaterals, and relieves pain. It is indicated for gout due to static blood and phlegm turbidity obstruction.

5) *Shǔ Yù Xiè Bái Zhōu* (薯蓣薤白粥)

山药	shān yào	100g	Rhizoma Dioscoreae
薤白	xiè bái	10g	Bulbus Allii Macrostemi
粳米	jīng mǐ	50g	Oryza sativa L. (polished round-grained non-glutinous rice)
清半夏	qīng bàn xià	30g	Rhizoma Pinelliae Concisum
黄芪	huáng qí	30g	Radix Astragali
糖	táng	as desired	sugar

Wash 50g of polished round-grained rice and add 100g of thinly sliced *shān yào* (Rhizoma Dioscoreae) 100g. Wash and add *bàn xià* (Rhizoma Pinelliae) 30g, *xiè bái* (Bulbus Allii Macrostemi) 10g, and *huáng qí* (Radix Astragali) 30g. Add sugar to taste. There is no rule regarding the serving time and amount of this recipe.

This formula boosts qi, unblocks yang, transforms phlegm, and removes obstruction. It is indicated for gout due to poor transportation (as a result of spleen deficiency) and internal generation of phlegm turbidity causing qi deficiency and phlegm obstruction.

6) *Bái Jiè Lián Zǐ Shān Yào Gāo* (白芥莲子山药糕)

白芥子粉	bái jiè zǐ fěn	5g	Semen Sinapis (powdered)
莲子粉	lián zǐ fěn	100g	Semen Nelumbinis (powdered)
鲜淮山药	xiān huái shān yào	200g	Rhizoma Dioscoreae (fresh)
陈皮	chén pí	5g	Pericarpium Citri Reticulatae
红枣肉	hóng zǎo ròu	200g	Fructus Jujubae

Peel the *huái shān yào* (Rhizoma Dioscoreae) and cut it into thin slices. Crush *hóng zǎo ròu* (Fructus Jujubae) and mix it with *lián zǐ* (Semen Nelumbinis) powder, *xiān bái jiè zǐ* (fresh Semen Sinapis) powder and thinly sliced *chén pí* (Pericarpium Citri Reticulatae). Add some water and stir to make a cake. To be taken as breakfast, 50-100g each time.

This formula boosts qi, transforms phlegm and unblocks obstruction. It is indicated for gout due to phlegm turbidity obstruction and/or spleen and stomach qi deficiency.

Regulation of Emotional and Mental Health

Gout patients should avoid mental stress and excessive fatigue. Mental stress, insomnia, excessive fatigue, and emotional stimuli may trigger attacks of gout or exacerbate the joint pain. Patients are advised to exercise regularly to maintain physical and mental fitness.

CLINICAL EXPERIENCE OF RENOWNED PHYSICIANS

Empirical Formulas

1. Zhang Rui-yi Uses *Tòng Fēng Fāng* (痛风方) to Treat Damp-heat Phlegm Obstruction

【Ingredients】

苍术	cāng zhú	15g	Rhizoma Atractylodis
黄柏	huáng bǎi	15g	Cortex Phellodendri Chinensis
蚕沙	cán shā	12g	Faeces Bombycis
木瓜	mù guā	10g	Fructus Chaenomelis
牛膝	niú xī	6g	Radix Achyranthis Bidentatae
丹参	dān shēn	15g	Radix et Rhizoma Salviae Miltiorrhizae
白芍	bái sháo	12g	Radix Paeoniae Alba
桑枝	sāng zhī	12g	Ramulus Mori

五灵脂	wǔ líng zhī	9g	Faeces Trogopterori
延胡索	yán hú suǒ	15g	Rhizoma Corydalis
路路通	lù lù tōng	15g	Fructus Liquidambaris
槟榔	bīng láng	10g	Semen Arecae
茯苓	fú líng	15g	Poria
升麻	shēng má	3g	Rhizoma Cimicifugae
甘草	gān cǎo	3g	Radix et Rhizoma Glycyrrhizae

【Treatment Principle】

Clear heat, drain dampness, move qi, and sweep phlegm.

【Formula Analysis】

Cāng zhú (Rhizoma Atractylodis), *huáng bǎi* (Cortex Phellodendri Chinensis), and *cán shā* (Faeces Bombycis) dispel wind and eliminate dampness. *Lù lù tōng* (Fructus Liquidambaris), *wǔ líng zhī* (Faeces Trogopterori), *sāng zhī* (Ramulus Mori), and *dān shēn* (Radix et Rhizoma Salviae Miltiorrhizae) dispel stasis and unblock the collaterals. *Bīng láng* (Semen Arecae) clears heat and dries dampness. *Fú líng* (Poria) and *zé xiè* (Rhizoma Alismatis) can promote water flow to remove dampness by allowing the turbid evil to be expelled through the urine. As for the dosages of *niú xī* (Radix Achyranthis Bidentatae) and *shēng má* (Rhizoma Cimicifugae), the dosage of the former is twice that of the latter. *Niú xī* is descending in nature while *shēng má* is ascending. The combination of the two regulates and harmonizes the qi dynamic.

【Modifications】

- For prevalence of heat, add *jīn yín huā* (Flos Lonicerae Japonicae), *pú gōng yīng* (Herba Taraxaci), and *dān pí* (Cortex Moutan) to clear heat.
- For severe swelling, add *zé xiè* (Rhizoma Alismatis), *fáng jǐ* (Radix Stephaniae Tetrandrae), and *qú mài* (Herba Dianthi) to relieve swelling.
- To tonify the liver and kidney in the later stages, add *guī jiǎ* (Caraoax et Plastrum Testudinis), *gǒu qǐ zǐ* (Fructus Lycii), *yín yáng huò* (Herba Epimedii), and *suǒ yáng* (Herba Cynomorii).

➢ To sweep phlegm and dissipate nodules, add *dǎn nán xīng* (Arisaema cum Bile), *fǎ bàn xià* (Rhizoma Pinelliae Praeparatum), and *zhè bèi* (Bulbus Fritillariae Thunbergii).

➢ For constitutional deficiency, add *huáng qí* (Radix Astragali) and *rén shēn* (Radix Ginseng).

[Cheng Jue-tang. *Selection of Secret and Empirical Formulas of Renowned Physicians* (名老中医秘方验方精选). Beijing: The People's Military Medical Press (人民军医出版社). 1995: 153]

2. Zhu Liang-chun Treats All Types of Gout with *Xiè Zhuó Huà Yū Tāng* (泄浊化瘀汤)

【Ingredients】

土茯苓	tǔ fú líng	45g	Rhizoma Smilacis Glabrae
萆薢	bì xiè	15g	Rhizoma Dioscoreae Hypoglaucae
威灵仙	wēi líng xiān	30g	Radix et Rhizoma Clematidis
桃仁	táo rén	10g	Semen Persicae
红花	hóng huā	10g	Flos Carthami
泽兰	zé lán	10g	Herba Lycopi
生薏苡仁	shēng yì yǐ rén	30g	Semen Coicis (raw)
全当归	quán dāng guī	10g	Radix Angelicae Sinensis (whole)
车前子	chē qián zǐ	10g	Semen Plantaginis
泽泻	zé xiè	10g	Rhizoma Alismatis

【Indications】

Downbears turbidity, discharges toxins, invigorates blood, and transforms stasis. For acute and chronic gouty arthritis and gouty nephropathy.

【Formula Analysis】

Gout is caused by turbidity, toxins, stasis and stagnation. *Tǔ fú líng* (Rhizoma Smilacis Glabrae) discharges turbidity, resolves toxins, fortifies the stomach, dries dampness, and frees the joints. *Bì xiè* (Rhizoma

Dioscoreae Hypoglaucae) separates the pure from the turbid. These two herbs are the main ingredients; they can lower blood uric acid and relieve joint pain. *Wēi líng xiān* (Radix et Rhizoma Clematidis) unblocks the collaterals, relieves pain, and dissolves uric acid. *Zé lán* (Herba Lycopi), *táo rén* (Semen Persicae), *hóng huā* (Flos Carthami), and *dāng guī* (Radix Angelicae Sinensis) are used to invigorate blood, transform stasis, and promote generation of new blood. *Shēng yì yǐ rén* (raw Semen Coicis), *zé xiè* (Rhizoma Alismatis), and *chē qián zǐ* (Semen Plantaginis) discharge turbidity and promote urination to excrete uric acid. The combination of all the medicinals discharges and transforms turbid toxins and removes stasis and binds.

【Modifications】

- If red, swollen, hot and painful joints are the main symptoms in the acute stage, add medicinals that clear heat and unblock the collaterals, i.e., *rěn dōng téng* (Caulis Lonicerae Japonicae), *jī xuè téng* (Caulis Spatholobi), and *bàn zhī lián* (Herba Scutellariae Barbatae).
- During the interval stage, widespread joint swelling, pain, stiffness and deformity, subcutaneous nodules, and exudation are usually signs of deficiency-excess complex, e.g., turbid evil complicated by dampness, stasis, or phlegm. Thus, insects and ants, whose nature is to search and pick out things, are used to transform phlegm and disperse stasis.
- The treatment of gout-induced kidney stones should employ medicinals that free strangury and expel stones. For gouty nephropathy, treatment should focus on fortifying the spleen and boosting the kidney.

[Jiang Xi, Zhu Wan-hua. Understanding the Treatment of Gout by Discharging Turbidity and Transforming Stasis (泄浊化瘀治疗痛风的经验体会). *Jiangsu Journal of Chinese Medicine* (江苏中医). 1990, (3): 7]

3. Ye Wei-hong Treats Wind-damp-heat *Bi* with *Xiāo Tòng Yǐn* (消痛饮)

【Ingredients】

当归	dāng guī	12g	Radix Angelicae Sinensis
牛膝	niú xī	15g	Radix Achyranthis Bidentatae
防风	fáng fēng	12g	Radix Saposhnikoviae
防己	fáng jǐ	15g	Radix Stephaniae Tetrandrae
泽泻	zé xiè	18g	Rhizoma Alismatis
钩藤	gōu téng	15g	Ramulus Uncariae Cum Uncis
忍冬藤	rěn dōng téng	25g	Caulis Lonicerae Japonicae
赤芍	chì sháo	18g	Radix Paeoniae Rubra
木瓜	mù guā	15g	Fructus Chaenomelis
桑枝	sāng zhī	30g	Ramulus Mori
甘草	gān cǎo	5g	Radix et Rhizoma Glycyrrhizae

【Indications】

Clears heat, disperses swelling, unblocks the collaterals, and relieves pain. For gouty arthritis of the acute stage with joint swelling and pain.

【Formula Analysis】

Gout is mainly caused by heat accumulating in the *zang-fu* and in the channels and recurrent contraction of wind, cold and dampness. *Dāng guī* (Radix Angelicae Sinensis), *chì sháo* (Radix Paeoniae Rubra), and *niú xī* (Radix Achyranthis Bidentatae) cool and invigorate the blood and relieve pain. *Gōu téng* (Ramulus Uncariae Cum Uncis), *rěn dōng téng* (Caulis Lonicerae Japonicae), and *sāng zhī* (Ramulus Mori) clear heat, resolve toxins, and unblock the collaterals. *Fáng fēng* (Radix Saposhnikoviae), *fáng jǐ* (Radix Stephaniae Tetrandrae), *zé xiè* (Rhizoma Alismatis), and *mù guā* (Fructus Chaenomelis) can dispel wind, drain dampness, and disperse swelling; use them together with medicinals that dispel wind, leach out dampness, and relieve pain to wash and fumigate the affected area. This combination of internal and external treatment has the effect of clearing heat, dispersing swelling, unblocking collaterals, and relieving pain.

【Modifications】

➢ For red, swollen and painful joints, add *huáng bǎi* (Cortex Phellodendri Chinensis) and *dì lóng* (Pheretima).

➢ For constipation, add *dà huáng* (Radix et Rhizoma Rhei); if the stool is soft, decoct it together with the other herbs; if the stool is dry, add it to the decoction towards the end of cooking.

➢ For severe pain, add *tián sān qī* (Radix et Rhizoma Notoginseng), *rǔ xiāng* (Olibanum), and *mò yào* (Myrrha).

➢ In addition, wash and fumigate the affected joint with a decoction of the following medicinals:

马钱子	mǎ qián zǐ	10g	Semen Strychni
红花	hóng huā	15g	Flos Carthami
生半夏	shēng bàn xià	20g	Rhizoma Pinelliae
王不留行	wáng bù liú xíng	40g	Semen Vaccariae
大黄	dà huáng	30g	Radix et Rhizoma Rhei
海桐皮	hǎi tóng pí	30g	Cortex Erythrinae
葱须	cōng xū	3 roots	Allii Fistulosi Radix
艾叶	ài yè	20g	Folium Artemisiae Argyi

One batch, twice a day.

[Ye Wei-hong. Using *Xiāo Tòng Yǐn* (消痛饮) to Treat 18 Cases of Gouty Arthritis (消痛饮治疗痛风性关节炎 18 例报告). *Journal of Chinese Medicine* (中医杂志). 1990, (4): 40]

4. An Yi-xian Treats Gout with Both Internal and External Methods

【Ingredients】 (for oral intake)

苦参	kǔ shēn	20g	Radix Sophorae Flavescentis
生大黄	shēng dà huáng	15g	Radix et Rhizoma Rhei (raw)
山栀	shān zhī	15g	Fructus Gardeniae
乌梅	wū méi	20g	Fructus Mume
知母	zhī mǔ	15g	Rhizoma Anemarrhenae

丹参	dān shēn	15g	Radix et Rhizoma Salviae Miltiorrhizae
赤芍	chì sháo	15g	Radix Paeoniae Rubra
白芍	bái sháo	15g	Radix Paeoniae Alba
姜黄	jiāng huáng	15g	Rhizoma Curcumae Longae
白芷	bái zhǐ	15g	Radix Angelicae Dahuricae
猪苓	zhū líng	15g	Polyporus
泽泻	zé xiè	15g	Rhizoma Alismatis
木通	mù tōng	10g	Caulis Akebiae
水蛭	shuǐ zhì	10-15g	Hirudo
薏苡仁	yì yǐ rén	20g	Semen Coicis

Divide *shēng dà huáng* (raw Radix et Rhizoma Rhei) into three equal portions and place each portion in a separate bowl. Cook all the other medicinals together and pour the finished decoction into the three bowls containing *shēng dà huáng*. Each bowl should contain approximately 150-200ml of liquid decoction. Take one bowl of decoction every time, 3 times a day. If there are less than three bowel movements a day after taking the medicine, continue with this recipe. Otherwise, discard the *shēng dà huáng* (raw Radix et Rhizoma Rhei) after the third day. The recommended length of administration is one week.

【Ingredients】 (for external use)

苦参	kǔ shēn	30g	Radix Sophorae Flavescentis
当归	dāng guī	15g	Radix Angelicae Sinensis
海桐皮	hǎi tóng pí	20g	Cortex Erythrinae
乳香	rǔ xiāng	15g	Olibanum
没药	mò yào	15g	Myrrha
山栀	shān zhī	15-20g	Fructus Gardeniae
乌梅	wū méi	20g	Fructus Mume
紫花地丁	zǐ huā dì dīng	15g	Herba Violae
青矾	qīng fán	6g	Melanteritum
白矾	bái fán	6g	Alumen
生南星	shēng nán xīng	10g	Rhizoma Arisaematis (raw)
川乌	chuān wū	10g	Radix Aconiti

草乌	cǎo wū	10g	Radix Aconiti Kusnezoffii
黄芩	huáng qín	15g	Radix Scutellariae
土茯苓	tǔ fú líng	20g	Rhizoma Smilacis Glabrae

Decoct with water and use the liquid as a cold compress or to wash the affected joint for 30 minutes each time, three times a day, in conjunction with internal medicinals for one week.

【Indications】

Drains fire and resolves toxins; drains dampness and unblocks the collaterals. This combination of internal and external medicinals treats gout due to wind-damp-heat obstruction.

【Formula Analysis】

Internal medicinals: *Kǔ shēn* (Radix Sophorae Flavescentis) and *dà huáng* (Radix et Rhizoma Rhei) clear heat and dry dampness, drain fire and resolve toxins, promote urination and bowel movement, and expel the internally accumulated damp-heat. *Shān zhī* (Fructus Gardeniae) and *zhī mǔ* (Rhizoma Anemarrhenae) are used to drain fire, resolve toxins, invigorate blood, and dry dampness. *Dān shēn* (Radix et Rhizoma Salviae Miltiorrhizae), *niú xī* (Radix Achyranthis Bidentatae), *chì sháo* (Radix Paeoniae Rubra), *bái sháo* (Radix Paeoniae Alba), and *dà shuǐ zhì* (Hirudo) invigorate blood, dispel stasis, and relieve pain. The selection of these medicinals is based on the concept that "to treat wind, first treat the blood; when the blood moves, the wind will naturally be extinguished (治风先治血，血行风自灭)." *Zhū líng* (Polyporus), *mù tōng* (Caulis Akebiae), *zé xiè* (Rhizoma Alismatis), and *yì yǐ rén* (Semen Coicis) promote water flow and leach out dampness. *Jiāng huáng* (Rhizoma Curcumae Longae) and *bái zhǐ* (Radix Angelicae Dahuricae) dry dampness, unblock the collaterals, and relieve pain. *Wū méi* (Fructus Mume), the paradoxical assistant with its sour flavor, can astringe the intestines to prevent excessive draining precipitation.

External medicinals: *Kǔ shēn* (Radix Sophorae Flavescentis), *shān zhī* (Fructus Gardeniae), *huáng qín* (Radix Scutellariae), *zǐ huā dì dīng* (Herba Violae), and *shēng nán xīng* (raw Rhizoma Arisaematis) clear heat, resolve toxins, and dry dampness. *Dāng guī* (Radix Angelicae Sinensis), *rǔ xiāng* (Olibanum), *mò yào* (Myrrha), *chuān wū* (Radix Aconiti), and *cǎo wū* (Radix Aconiti Kusnezoffii) move qi, invigorate blood, and settle pain. *Hǎi tóng pí* (Cortex Erythrinae) and *tǔ fú líng* (Rhizoma Smilacis Glabrae) unblock the collaterals and eliminate obstruction. *Qīng fán* (Melanteritum) and *bái fán* (Alumen) dry dampness and resolve toxins. *Wū méi* (Fructus Mume), the assistant medicinal, is used to relax tension. When applied as a cold compress, it is used to suppress heat.

The combined use of the internal and external formulas can eliminate external obstruction and dispel internal evils, treating both the branch and the root simultaneously.

【Modifications】

- Adding *qiāng huó* (Rhizoma et Radix Notopterygii) 15g to the internal formula can guide the effect of the medicinals to the upper extremities.
- Adding *niú xī* (Radix Achyranthis Bidentatae) 10-20g can guide the effect of the medicinals to the lower extremities.
- For marked redness and heat, add *huáng lián* (Rhizoma Coptidis) 6-12g.
- For severe pain, add *yán hú suǒ* (Rhizoma Corydalis) 12g.
- For copious phlegm, add *lái fú zǐ* (Semen Raphani) 15g.
- For constitutional deficiency, add *shēng dì* (Radix Rehmanniae Recens) 15g and *shā shēn* (Radix Glehniae) 15g.

[Yao Zhen-song, Zhou Xi-ping. Professor An Yi-xian's Treatment of Gouty Arthritis with Chinese Medicinals (安义贤教授中药治疗痛风性关节炎拾萃). *Journal of Guiyang University of Traditional Chinese Medicine* (贵阳中医学院学报). 1998, 20 (1): 9]

5. Liu Zai-peng Treats Acute Episodes of Gout with *Tòng Fēng Dìng Tòng Tāng* (痛风定痛汤)

【Ingredients】

金钱草	jīn qián cǎo	30g	Herba Lysimachiae
泽泻	zé xiè	10g	Rhizoma Alismatis
车前子	chē qián zǐ	10g	Semen Plantaginis
海藻	hǎi zǎo	15g	Sargassum
生石膏	shēng shí gāo	30g	Gypsum Fibrosum
知母	zhī mǔ	10g	Rhizoma Anemarrhenae
黄柏	huáng bǎi	10g	Cortex Phellodendri Chinensis
赤芍	chì sháo	10g	Radix Paeoniae Rubra
生地	shēng dì	15g	Radix Rehmanniae Recens
防己	fáng jǐ	10g	Radix Stephaniae Tetrandrae
地龙	dì lóng	10g	Pheretima

【Indications】

Clears heat, drains dampness, invigorates blood, and settles pain. Suitable for acute episodes of gouty arthritis.

【Formula Analysis】

Jīn qián cǎo (Herba Lysimachiae), the chief medicinal, clears heat, drains dampness, and dissolves stones. *Chē qián zǐ* (Semen Plantaginis), *zé xiè* (Rhizoma Alismatis), and *fáng jǐ* (Radix Stephaniae Tetrandrae) clear heat and promote urination to facilitate the excretion of uric acid. *Huáng bǎi* (Cortex Phellodendri Chinensis), *zhī mǔ* (Rhizoma Anemarrhenae), *chì sháo* (Radix Paeoniae Rubra), *shēng dì* (Radix Rehmanniae Recens), *shēng shí gāo* (Gypsum Fibrosum), and *dì lóng* (Pheretima) clear heat, resolve toxins, disperse swelling, and relieve pain.

【Modifications】

- For pronounced pain, add *shuǐ niú jiǎo* (Cornu Bubali) 30g to treat heat *bi*.
- For mild local redness and swelling with severe pain, add *chuān*

wū (Radix Aconiti) 3g, *cǎo wū* (Radix Aconiti Kusnezoffii) 3g, and *guì zhī* (Ramulus Cinnamomi) 10g.

➢ For pronounced subcutaneous nodules, or gouty tophi of the joints of the hand and feet or of the ear, add *shān cí gū* (Pseudobulbus Cremastrae seu Pleiones) 15g and *hǎi zǎo* (Sargassum) 15g to soften hardness and dissolve stones.

➢ For spleen deficiency leading to damp predominance manifesting as diffuse swelling of the joints, add *cāng zhú* (Rhizoma Atractylodis) 10g, *bái zhú* (Rhizoma Atractylodis Macrocephalae) 15g, and *fú líng* (Poria) 15g to fortify the spleen, assist transportation, transform dampness, and eliminate obstruction.

[Wan Tai-bao. Professor Liu Zai-peng's Experience in Treating Gout with *Tòng Fēng Dìng Tòng Tāng* (刘再朋教授"痛风定痛汤"治疗痛风经验). *Journal of Nanjing University of Traditional Chinese Medicine* (南京中医学院学报). 1994, 10(6): 18]

Selected Case Studies

1. Yin Hui-he's Case Study: Damp-heat Pouring Downward

Patient: Zheng, male, 45 years old; born in Sichuan province; had worked in Tibet since 1950.

【Initial Visit】

January 11st, 1974: Since the first episode in 1959, the condition lasted 15 years. The condition first manifested as red, swollen, and painful joints of the right foot that gradually spread to the right ankle and the left knee with recurrent attacks. The patient experienced severe pain during the attacks, as well as redness and swelling of the skin and sweating of the whole body. The condition is relatively better during the daytime and worse at night, particularly in the joints of the feet. The pain increased by itself without any touch. Sound also aggravated the pain. Local injections of morphine had no effect on the pain.

In 1966, laboratory tests conducted at Tibet Autonomous Region Hospital showed the blood uric acid level to be 6.21mg%. The diagnosis was gout without bone abnormalities. Colchicine alleviated the condition, but produced the side effects of marked dizziness and nausea. The symptoms gradually worsened and the duration of the attacks became increasingly longer each time as the time interval between attacks decreased. The patient had 5 attacks in 1973. In November, 1973, he had come to Beijing in search of better treatment and had another acute episode in December. Laboratory tests showed a blood uric acid level of 7.35mg% and a blood sedimentation rate (ESR) of 40mm/h. X-ray revealed encroachment of the first metatarsal bone of the right foot with hyperplasia, and narrowness of the metatarsal joint cavity. The diagnosis of gout had thus been confirmed.

Since the patient could not withstand colchicine and cortisone and administration of aminobenzene sulfonamide produced no change, he was treated with Chinese medicinal therapy. The patient's facial expression was one of pain and suffering. He was supported by others on his arrival to the outpatient department. He complained of pain in both legs and redness, swelling and pain of the right toe, right ankle, and left knee. He had yellowish-red urine, a thick dark-yellow and moist tongue coating, and a thready and rapid pulse.

【Pattern Differentiation】

Damp-heat pouring downward.

【Treatment Principle】

Clear heat and dry dampness.

【Prescription】

Modified *Sān Miào Tāng* (三妙汤)

【Ingredients】

苍术	cāng zhú	15g	Rhizoma Atractylodis
黄柏	huáng bǎi	12g	Cortex Phellodendri Chinensis
薏苡仁	yì yǐ rén	30g	Semen Coicis
牛膝	niú xī	12g	Radix Achyranthis Bidentatae
木瓜	mù guā	12g	Fructus Chaenomelis
青黛	qīng dài	6g	Indigo Naturalis
滑石	huá shí	15g	Talcum
知母	zhī mǔ	15g	Rhizoma Anemarrhenae
鸡血藤	jī xuè téng	30g	Caulis Spatholobi
当归	dāng guī	15g	Radix Angelicae Sinensis
赤芍	chì sháo	15g	Radix Paeoniae Rubra
萆薢	bì xiè	12g	Rhizoma Dioscoreae Hypoglaucae

The ingredients were decocted with 500ml of water until reduced to 200ml. Six batches were prescribed and taken warm, 1 batch a day.

【Second Visit】

January 18th: The pain in the legs was lessened, and the dark-yellow tongue coating began to recede. He could walk on his own without support but still had some difficulty. He was given the same formula with a few modifications: *Dāng guī* (Radix Angelicae Sinensis) was increased to 30g, and *cán shā* (Faeces Bombycis) 30g was added. A total of 6 batches were prescribed at the dosage of one batch a day.

【Third Visit】

January 28th: The symptoms of gout had basically disappeared, and the dark-yellow tongue coating had vanished. He could walk by himself without any support. *Mù tōng* (Caulis Akebiae) 9g and *sī guā luò* (Retinervus Luffae Fructus) 9g was added to the previous formula. 6 batches were prescribed at the dosage of one batch a day. The patient's condition was stabilized, and he was advised to continue taking the formula.

On March 1st, lab test revealed an ESR of 4 mm/h, which is within the normal range. On May 7th, the blood uric acid level was 6.9mg%, which was lower than before. Since the patient's condition had been stabilized, the medicinals in the above formulas were made into pills for more convenient administration.

Lab test on September 16th showed the blood uric acid level to be 4.55 mg% (normal). The patient no longer had any difficulty walking. He was advised to continue taking the pills to consolidate the therapy effect.

X-ray on November 12th revealed that the pathological change of the first metatarsal bone of the right foot had improved significantly. There was noticeable hyperplasia around the original lesion. The disease was cured.

【Comments】

Gout has been recorded in early Chinese medical texts. General reference has been made to diseases such as rheumatoid arthritis and pyogenic arthritis. The disease is more prevalent among minority ethnic groups and is considered a type of bone-deteriorating illness. The incidence of gout is rare in coastal and inland regions.

The treatment principle and prescription of medicinals are based on Chinese medical pattern identification. The marked redness, swelling, heat and pain indicate that the disease belongs to the categories of yang and heat syndromes. However, the pain of yang and heat syndromes generally affects the upper part of the body; only damp-heat has the characteristic of pouring downward. Thus, this disease is considered to be in the category of damp-heat. In addition, the thick greasy moist dark-yellow tongue coating is also attributed to dampness, which confirms the involvement damp-heat. The etiology and pathology is evident, and treatment calls for the use of *Sān Miào Wán* (三妙丸) as the ruling formula to dry dampness and clear heat. Severe pain induced by damp-heat requires medicinals that soothe the sinews and unblock the collaterals to alleviate the pain associated with the branch syndrome. By treating the branch and root simultaneously, one can achieve satisfactory results.

[Editorial department of *New Chinese Medicine. Case Studies and Discussions of Famous Physicians of Chinese Medicine* (老中医医案医话选). Guangzhou College of Chinese Medicine, Internal Publications. 1977]

2. Jiang Shi-ying's Case Study: Joint-running Disease (历节病, *Lì Jié Bìng*)

Patient: Lin, male, 15 years old.

【Initial Visit】

April 26th, 1979: The patient has had pain of the big toe since February, which was aggravated after long periods of walking, accompanied by redness and swelling of the second digit of the foot. His condition was treated as frostbite and sprain without any improvement. A follow-up examination on February 19th, 1979 revealed a blood uric acid level of 12mg%, an ESR rate of 10 mm/h, and an ASO value of under 250 units. On April 1st, the blood uric acid level was 12mg%; after the consultation, the patient agreed to be treated for gout, and was transferred to our hospital on April 26th. There was fusiform swelling of the second digit of the right foot with local reddening of the skin and tenderness. There was a protruding bony growth on the lateral aspect of the left thumb without redness and pain. The patient had a red tongue tip with thin yellow coating, and a thready and slightly wiry pulse. There were no other abnormalities.

Initial diagnosis:

Chinese medicine: joint-running disease (历节, *lì jié*)

Biomedicine: gout

The patient was treated with indomethacin.

【Second Visit】

April 30th: The second digit of the left foot was still red and swollen after administration of indometacin. The pain was the same as before, and the patient had difficulty walking. The thumb was slightly swollen and painful. The tongue was red with yellow coating. The pulse was thready, wiry, and rapid. The treatment method was switched to Chinese medicinal therapy.

【Pattern Differentiation】

Damp-heat stasis obstruction of the channels and the joints.

【Treatment Principle】

Clear heat and drain dampness; invigorate blood and move stasis; unblock the channels and quicken the collaterals.

【Ingredients】

生石膏	shēng shí gāo	20g	Gypsum Fibrosum (raw)
毛冬青	máo dōng qīng	20g	Ilex Pubescens
钩藤	gōu téng	25g	Ramulus Uncariae Cum Uncis
玄参	xuán shēn	15g	Radix Scrophulariae
防己	fáng jǐ	15g	Radix Stephaniae Tetrandrae
苍术	cāng zhú	12g	Rhizoma Atractylodis
黄柏	huáng bǎi	12g	Cortex Phellodendri Chinensis
牛膝	niú xī	12g	Radix Achyranthis Bidentatae
连翘	lián qiào	10g	Fructus Forsythiae
赤芍	chì sháo	10g	Radix Paeoniae Rubra
丹皮	dān pí	6g	Cortex Moutan

Seven batches were prescribed. Decocted with 500ml of water until reduced to 200ml. To be taken warm, 1 batch a day. The medicinals can be redecocted.

【Third Visit】

May 7th: The pain of the toes and fingers had virtually disappeared, but the local skin was still dark red. The swelling of the toes had clearly vanished. He had a good appetite and copious urination, accompanied by a red tongue with scanty coating and a thready rapid pulse. Seven batches of the following formula were prescribed and taken warm with two spoons of honey.

桑枝	sāng zhī	30g	Ramulus Mori
毛冬青	máo dōng qīng	15g	Ilex Pubescens
生石膏	shēng shí gāo	15g	Gypsum Fibrosum (raw)
黄柏	huáng bǎi	12g	Cortex Phellodendri Chinensis
玄参	xuán shēn	12g	Radix Scrophulariae
丹皮	dān pí	12g	Cortex Moutan
威灵仙	wēi líng xiān	12g	Radix et Rhizoma Clematidis
防己	fáng jǐ	12g	Radix Stephaniae Tetrandrae
吊子风	diào zǐ fēng	12g	Uncaria rhynchophylla (Miq.)Jacks.
苍术	cāng zhú	10g	Rhizoma Atractylodis
赤芍	chì sháo	10g	Radix Paeoniae Rubra
七叶莲	qī yè lián	10g	Radix Schefflerae Arboricolae

【Fourth Visit】

May 14th: The symptoms showed significant improvement, the joint swelling and pain had disappeared, and the second digit of the foot was no longer dark red. The patient was in good spirits and had a healthy appetite. The tip of the tongue was still red. The pulse was thready and slightly rapid. Blood uric acid level was 5.7mg%.

Seven batches of the following formula were prescribed:

毛冬青	máo dōng qīng	30g	Ilex Pubescens
生石膏	shēng shí gāo	25g	Gypsum Fibrosum (raw)
金银花	jīn yín huā	15g	Flos Lonicerae Japonicae
黄柏	huáng bǎi	15g	Cortex Phellodendri Chinensis
赤芍	chì sháo	12g	Radix Paeoniae Rubra
地龙	dì lóng	12g	Pheretima
防己	fáng jǐ	12g	Radix Stephaniae Tetrandrae
野菊花	yě jú huā	12g	Flos Chrysanthemi Indici
苍术	cāng zhú	12g	Rhizoma Atractylodis
知母	zhī mǔ	12g	Rhizoma Anemarrhenae
怀牛膝	huái niú xī	10g	Radix Achyranthis Bidentatae

X-ray revealed that the second toe of the right foot was of normal shape and without apparent bone erosion or hyperplasia. The joint surfaces were smooth. No remarkable pathological changes of the second toe of the right foot. PSP excretion test showed no abnormalities.

【Fifth Visit】

May 21st: No more symptoms. The patient was physically healthy and in good spirits. He had a good appetite and his bowel movement and urination were both normal. He had a red, moist tongue and a slightly thready and rapid pulse. Ten batches of the following formula were prescribed to consolidate the treatment effect.

毛冬青	máo dōng qīng	20g	Ilex Pubescens
生石膏	shēng shí gāo	20g	Gypsum Fibrosum (raw)
苍术	cāng zhú	20g	Rhizoma Atractylodis
黄柏	huáng bǎi	20g	Cortex Phellodendri Chinensis
知母	zhī mǔ	20g	Rhizoma Anemarrhenae
白芍	bái sháo	20g	Radix Paeoniae Alba
玄参	xuán shēn	15g	Radix Scrophulariae
薏苡仁	yì yǐ rén	15g	Semen Coicis
怀牛膝	huái niú xī	10g	Radix Achyranthis Bidentatae
桂枝	guì zhī	6g	Ramulus Cinnamomi

A follow-up exam on June 10th showed a blood uric acid level of 5.75 mg% and a normal hemogram. Antistreptolycin O (ASO) and ESR were also normal. The total urine uric acid over 24 hours was 1 035mg. The disease was completely cured and the patient had no recurrent attacks for 3 years.

【Comments】

Gout falls within the scope of *bi* syndromes in Chinese medicine. According to its symptoms, it is similar to joint-running disease (历节, *lì jié*) as defined by *Essentials from the Golden Cabinet* (金匮要略, *Jīn Guì Yào Lüè*), or what is called "white tiger joint-running wind (白虎历节风, *bái hǔ lì jié fēng*)" by later generations. The common cause of this disease is wind-cold-damp evil invading the channels and pouring into the joints. Over a long period of time, the pathogen can then transform into heat and damage yin, impairing the blood and qi and producing blood stasis. Long-term accumulation of dampness leads to static blood obstructing the interior, which in turn will further prolong the disease and prevent the therapeutic effect of treatment from solidifying. In this case, the pattern is determined to be damp-heat stasis obstruction of the channels and joints, and the patient should be treated according to the clinical manifestations; one should follow the common treatment principle for *bi* syndromes, which is to unblock the channels and quicken the collaterals in conjunction with clearing heat, draining dampness, invigorating blood, and moving stasis. Once the chief pattern has been determined, prescribe the appropriate formula with the necessary modifications. After about 30 batches of medicinals, the disease can be eradicated completely.

In order to treat this disease, in addition to using *Bái Hǔ Jiā Guì Zhī Tāng* (白虎加桂枝汤) to treat joint-running disease and *Sì Miào Sǎn* (四妙散) to clear heat, drain dampness, and unblock the collaterals, it is also beneficial to add *máo dōng qīng* (Ilex Pubescens) since it strongly invigorates blood and unblocks the collaterals.

[Jiang Shi-ying. *Lì Jié* (Gout); 历节 (痛风). *New Chinese Medicine* (新中医). 1984,(4): 24]

3. Zhao Fen's Case Study: Yin Depletion and Dampness Pouring Downward

Patient: Gao, male, 53 years old; university administrator.

【Initial Visit】

November 7th, 1980.

Ten years ago, the patient sprained the sole of his foot, from which he never fully healed. The patient was exposed to cold and dampness from frequent labor in the paddy field. One day, the weather was especially cold, and the ground was especially wet; the cold-damp invaded the sinews and bones and spread to the joints of the toes, metatarsus, and ankle, and eventually gave way to local redness, swelling and pain, and fever. He was unable to walk the next day, and was treated in the local hospital without any improvement. Similar attacks occurred every year ever since, most of which were brought on by overtiredness and weather changes, particularly the transition from spring to summer. The condition was exacerbated by cloudy and damp weather. The pain involved mostly the small joints of the lower extremities and would sometimes spread to the lumbus and legs. The pain was most severe around midnight. Throughout the last ten years, he had sought treatment in many places, but the condition remained sometimes mild and sometimes severe, without a complete cure. His medical history revealed that he had suffered from arteriosclerosis, coronary artery disease, dizziness, tinnitus, chest distress, palpitation, lumbar soreness, poor memory, and lassitude and weakness upon slight physical exertion. In October, 1980 the patient had a positive lactic acid test and a blood uric acid level of 10.8mg%. A follow-up exam at a hospital showed a 24-hr urine of 3 050ml and a 24-hr uric acid level of 945.5mg. X-ray showed bone destruction of the first metatarsal joints of the left foot. The diagnosis was determined to be primary gout.

During the visit, the patient had a chronic sickly complexion, an unbalanced gait, and required physical assistance in order to walk. He had a bitter taste in the mouth, a dry throat, thirst but no desire to drink, reddish tea-colored urine, dry and hard stool, and pronounced tenderness of the joints of the left ankle and toes with local redness and swelling. His tongue was dark red with thick yellow coating that was peeled in the center. His pulse was wiry, thready, and rapid.

【Pattern Differentiation】

Liver and kidney yin depletion; damp-heat pouring downward.

【Treatment Principle】

Enrich and tonify the liver and kidney, and clear and drain damp-heat. In addition, add medicinals that invigorate blood.

【Ingredients】

续断	xù duàn	12g	Radix Dipsaci
北沙参	běi shā shēn	12g	Radix Glehniae
制首乌	zhì shǒu wū	12g	Radix Polygoni Multiflori Praeparata cum Succo Glycines Sotae
桑枝	sāng zhī	12g	Ramulus Mori
忍冬藤	rěn dōng téng	12g	Caulis Lonicerae Japonicae
土茯苓	tǔ fú líng	12g	Rhizoma Smilacis Glabrae
赤芍	chì sháo	9g	Radix Paeoniae Rubra
怀牛膝	huái niú xī	9g	Radix Achyranthis Bidentatae
薏苡仁	yì yǐ rén	20g	Semen Coicis
川芎	chuān xiōng	3g	Rhizoma Chuanxiong
牡丹皮	mǔ dān pí	12g	Cortex Moutan
当归	dāng guī	6g	Radix Angelicae Sinensis
甘草	gān cǎo	5g	Radix et Rhizoma Glycyrrhizae

Six batches were prescribed and decocted with 500ml of water until reduced to 200ml of liquid. Taken warm, 1 batch a day.

【Second Visit】

Nov. 16th: The pain in the toe and ankle joints was alleviated, and the redness and swelling had improved. His bitter taste in the mouth, dry throat and thirst had improved, and his urine was clearer. He could walk and move more freely. *Fáng fēng* (Radix Saposhnikoviae) 5g was added to the previous formula and 6 batches were prescribed.

【Third Visit】

Nov. 24th: The condition continued to improve, but the palpitation and insomnia remained. The tongue was dark red with thin greasy coating that was peeled in the center. The pulse was wiry, thready, and slightly rapid. The original prescription was modified as follows: *dān pí* (Cortex Moutan) was removed and *mŭ lì* (Concha Ostreae) 21g was added (decocted first). 6 batches were prescribed.

【Fourth Visit】

Dec. 9th: The condition was fairly stable. 6 batches of the same formula were prescribed.

【Fifth Visit】

Dec. 21st: There was still mild pain in the affected areas. His appetite had decreased. Pulse and tongue manifestations were similar to those of the last visit. The following prescription was similar to the original formula with some modifications. 6 batches were prescribed.

当归	dāng guī	7g	Radix Angelicae Sinensis
忍冬藤	rěn dōng téng	12g	Caulis Lonicerae Japonicae
制首乌	zhì shǒu wū	12g	Radix Polygoni Multiflori Praeparata cum Succo Glycines Sotae
续断	xù duàn	12g	Radix Dipsaci
桑枝	sāng zhī	12g	Ramulus Mori
土茯苓	tŭ fú líng	12g	Rhizoma Smilacis Glabrae
薏苡仁	yì yĭ rén	18g	Semen Coicis
赤芍	chì sháo	6g	Radix Paeoniae Rubra
丹参	dān shēn	9g	Radix et Rhizoma Salviae Miltiorrhizae
威灵仙	wēi líng xiān	9g	Radix et Rhizoma Clematidis
牛膝	niú xī	9g	Radix Achyranthis Bidentatae
川芎	chuān xiōng	3g	Rhizoma Chuanxiong
甘草	gān căo	5g	Radix et Rhizoma Glycyrrhizae
麦芽	mài yá	30g	Fructus Hordei Germinatus
谷芽	gŭ yá	30g	Fructus Setariae Germinatus

【Sixth Visit】

Dec. 29th: The pain had vanished. The patient was able to walk without difficulty and his appetite had returned to normal. All of his symptoms had improved significantly. Blood uric acid level was 4.9mg%. X-ray showed bony changes of the metatarsal and toe joints; there was significant improvement of the toe joints. The patient was considered to be fully recovered and thus he returned to work. The original formula was simplified for long-term use to consolidate the treatment effect. A follow-up visit one year later revealed that the patient had maintained full recovery.

【Comments】

Because of the involvement of the joints and the severe pain, gout is called "white tiger joint-running disease"(白虎历节 ; *bái hŭ lì jié*). The primary treatment principle is to disperse cold-damp and open the interstices. The symptoms of this particular case bear a resemblance to a case described in Zhu Dan-xi's *Further Treatises on the Properties of Things* (格致余论 , *Gé Zhì Yú Lùn*), except that this condition lasted more than ten years, and the chronic illness had entered the blood, transformed into heat, and damaged the yin. Hence, the treatment principle of coursing wind and dispersing cold was no longer effective.

Yellow Emperor's Inner Classic (黄帝内经 , *Huáng Dì Nèi Jīng*) states: "When injured by dampness, the lower part of the body is affected first (伤于湿者， 下先受之)." Those who live in southern China are constantly exposed to an overabundance of dampness, and in this particular case the patient's condition was caused by frequent wading. The pain started in the ankle and metatarsus, indicating that the cold and dampness first affected the lower extremities. The patient had a dry mouth but no desire to drink, tea-colored urine, and local redness and swelling of the affected joints. The pain would appear during the transition from spring to summer, when the cold weather gives way to warmth. In the damp weather, the dampness evil will invariably combine with heat.

The patient suffered from this disease for ten years; he complained of dizziness, tinnitus, palpitation, lumbago, poor memory, and fatigue, which are signs and symptoms of liver and kidney yin deficiency. There is an old saying that reads: "Chronic disease often involves deficiency, and long-term pain will eventually involve the blood (久病多虚、痛久入血)." In accordance with the treatment principle "to treat wind, first treat the blood; when the blood moves, the wind will naturally be extinguished (治风先治血，血行风自灭)," *dāng guī* (Radix Angelicae Sinensis), *chì sháo* (Radix Paeoniae Rubra), and *chuān xiōng* (Rhizoma Chuanxiong) nourish and invigorate the blood. *Sāng zhī* (Ramulus Mori), *rěn dōng téng* (Caulis Lonicerae Japonicae), *dān pí* (Cortex Moutan), *yì yǐ rén* (Semen Coicis), *shā shēn* (Radix Glehniae), and *wēi líng xiān* (Radix et Rhizoma Clematidis) course wind, overcome dampness, and clear heat without damaging the body fluids. *Shú dì* (Radix Rehmanniae Praeparata), *shǒu wū* (Radix Polygoni Multiflori), and *xù duàn* (Radix Dipsaci) tonify the kidney and strengthen the lower part of the body, guiding the effect of the formula downward. *Dān shēn* (Radix et Rhizoma Salviae Miltiorrhizae), *niú xī* (Radix Achyranthis Bidentatae), *chuān xiōng* (Rhizoma Chuanxiong), and *dāng guī* (Radix Angelicae Sinensis) were combined together to enhance their ability to transform stasis. *Tǔ fú líng* (Rhizoma Smilacis Glabrae) dispels dampness, resolves toxins, and promotes the excretion of uric acid, introducing a new approach for the treatment of this disease.

In conclusion, when treating the patient with Chinese medicine, the prerequisite is to determine if the disease is acute or chronic, and deficiency or excess. For long-term disease with constitutional deficiency, one should first tonify and then treat the disease slowly. If one does not know the root and branch of the disease and still insist on using harsh formulas to course wind and invigorate blood, it would be extremely difficult to arrive at a cure.

[Edited by Lin Shu-nian and Jiang Yuan-zheng. Damp-heat *Bi*

Syndrome (Gout); 湿热痹症 (痛风). *New Chinese Medicine* (新中医). 1985, (4). 10]

4. Huang Zhen-ming's Case Study: Obstruction of Damp-heat and Blood Stasis

Patient: Ruan, female, 52 years old.

【Initial Visit】

April 18th, 1986.

The patient had been suffering from diabetes mellitus for 5 years and hypertension for 3 years. She was receiving long-term Chinese medical and biomedical treatment. Her blood sugar was maintained at around 6.7-7.3mmol/L, and her blood pressure was approximately 24/12.5 kPa. Her condition was fairly stable. In January, 1985, she suddenly experienced pain and swelling in the left big toe, and the condition was diagnosed as "rheumatoid arthritis" at a hospital. After being treated with western pharmaceutical drugs for 2 months, the condition worsened, and she developed swelling and pain of the left ankle and left wrist as well as the formation of nodules on the painful spots of the left big toe and external malleolus. The condition was sometimes mild and sometimes severe. When it was severe, there was limited range of motion in the above-mentioned joints. Lab tests showed a blood uric acid level of 1.07mmol/L, and a diagnosis of gout (acute arthritis stage) was determined. With hormone therapy, the condition improved; there was no more joint pain and she returned to her daily activities as normal. However, she had chest oppression and nausea, her blood pressure was 24/14pKa, and her urine glucose test was positive, so the drugs were discontinued. Not long afterwards, the joint pain resumed, and the patient requested to leave the hospital and visit the outpatient clinic for treatment. She visited many hospitals and received both Chinese and Western medical treatment without any effect. The nodules ached and formed ulcerative perforations that secreted a white fluid. She required physical assistance in order to walk.

On her first visit, the condition was similar to before. She had chest oppression, nausea, dry mouth, foul breath, dry stool, yellowish or reddish urine, and a reddish complexion. She could not stop groaning. The right wrist, external malleolus and big toe were red, swollen, hot and painful. The nodules on her left big toe and external malleolus were as big as pigeon eggs with ulcerative perforation that secreted a white fluid and refused pressure. She had a dark red tongue with thin white coating and a wiry, slightly rapid, and forceful pulse. Blood fasting sugar: 7.3 mmol/L; blood uric acid level: 1.08 mmol/L.

【Pattern Differentiation】

Binding constraint of damp-heat; stasis obstruction of the channels.

【Treatment Principle】

Clear heat, drain dampness, invigorate blood, transform stasis, unblock the collaterals, and relieve pain.

【Prescription】

Modified *Líng Xī Gǔ Pí Yǐn* (羚犀骨皮饮)

【Ingredients】

羚羊骨	líng yáng gǔ	15g	Os Saigae Tataricae (decocted first)
水牛角	shuǐ niú jiǎo	30g	Cornu Bubali (decocted first)
地骨皮	dì gǔ pí	30g	Cortex Lycii
生石膏	shēng shí gāo	30g	Gypsum Fibrosum (raw)
桑枝	sāng zhī	24g	Ramulus Mori
白茅根	bái máo gēn	18g	Rhizoma Imperatae
薏苡仁	yì yǐ rén	30g	Semen Coicis
茯苓皮	fú líng pí	30g	Cutis Poriae
威灵仙	wēi líng xiān	30g	Radix et Rhizoma Clematidis
蜈蚣	wú gōng	3g	Scolopendra
红花	hóng huā	9g	Flos Carthami
大黄	dà huáng	15g	Radix et Rhizoma Rhei (decocted later)

Decocted with 500ml of water until reduced to 200ml. The medicinals were repeatedly decocted. Take warm, 1 batch a day.

【External Treatment】

Huí Chūn Săn (回春散): The ingredients listed below were ground into powder and mixed together, then applied to the affected parts of the body.

田七	tián qī	15g	Radix et Rhizoma Notoginseng
大黄	dà huáng	9g	Radix et Rhizoma Rhei
荜茇	bì bá	6g	Fructus Piperis Longi
红条紫草	hóng tiáo zĭ căo	12g	Radix Lithospermi
僵蚕	jiāng cán	6g	Bombyx Batryticatus
玄明粉	xuán míng fĕn	9g	Natrii Sulfas Exsiccatus
半夏	bàn xià	6g	Rhizoma Pinelliae
紫花地丁	zĭ huā dì dīng	6g	Herba Violae
生南星	shēng nán xīng	6g	Rhizoma Arisaematis
血竭	xuè jié	6g	Sanguis Draconis
蟾酥	chán sū	1g	Venenum Bufonis

【Usage】

The powder was mixed with water in the proportion of 1:40 and decocted for 15 minutes. When the water cooled down to 38-40°C, the mixture was applied to the affected parts of the body for 2 hours and then covered with antiseptic gauze, twice a day.

【Second Visit】

Follow-up exam on April 23rd: After five batches of internal and external medicine, the patient had bowel movements twice a day, which consisted of loose stool. The chest oppression and nausea had disappeared. The red, swollen, and painful joints were relieved. The ulcerative perforation of the nodules of the left big toe and external malleolus had improved. She could walk on her own. Her urine was yellow and her pulse was wiry and rapid. The improvement indicated that the formula was appropriate for her condition. *Dà huáng* (Radix et Rhizoma Rhei) was instructed to be decocted together with the other ingredients and *chǎo shān jiǎ* (dry-fried Manis Squama) (decocted first) 18g was added to strengthen the formula's effect of unblocking the collaterals. One batch was prescribed a day; the medicinals were repeatedly decocted and taken. The external treatment was the same as before.

【Third Visit】

April 30th, 1986: After seven batches of the internal formula combined with external treatment, the redness, swelling, and pain in the joints had improved a great deal, and she was able to walk to the hospital by herself. She was also able to do some house work. However, the color of the skin around the nodules of the left big toe and external malleolus were still somewhat dark red. She had a red tongue with scanty coating, and a thready and rapid pulse. Since there were symptoms of yin impairment, medicinals that nourish yin were added to the prescription. The external treatment was the same as before.

大黄	dà huáng	12g	Radix et Rhizoma Rhei
黄芪	huáng qí	18g	Radix Astragali
生地	shēng dì	24g	Radix Rehmanniae Recens
牡丹皮	mǔ dān pí	12g	Cortex Moutan
茯苓皮	fú líng pí	30g	Cutis Poriae
泽泻	zé xiè	15g	Rhizoma Alismatis
蜈蚣	wú gōng	3g	Scolopendra
炒山甲	chǎo shān jiǎ	18g	Squama Manis (dry-fried)
丹参	dān shēn	15g	Radix et Rhizoma Salviae Miltiorrhizae
羚羊骨	líng yáng gǔ	15g	Os Saigae Tataricae(decocted first)

【Fourth Visit】

May 6th 1986: After taking seven batches of internal medicinals combined with external treatment, the redness, swelling, and pain of the joints disappeared. Most of the nodules of the left big toe and external malleolus disappeared. The ulceration was reduced significantly. The color of the skin returned to normal. Blood uric acid was 0.48 mmol/L. Using the previous formula as the base, the dosages of *líng yáng gǔ* (Os Saigae Tataricae) and *huáng qí* (Radix Astragali) were reduced, while *shān yú ròu* (Fructus Corni) 12g was added to nourish yin. The external treatment was the same as before, and administered once every two days.

【Fifth Visit】

July, 2nd 1986: After the patient took 26 batches of the prescribed formula, the nodules of the left big toe and external malleolus had completely vanished. The ulceration was cured. Lab test revealed a normal blood uric acid level. The patient was advised to take two batches of the previously prescribed formula every week for one month to consolidate the curative effect. The patient did not have any recurrent attacks for one year.

【Comments】

The patient had a good appetite but did not like to exercise; hence, she was fat and had damp-heat accumulation, which affected her organs and collaterals. Blood and qi flow were inhibited, and the resulting obstruction in the collaterals causes red, swollen and painful joints. Over time, the qi stagnation led to the formation of nodules. The main pathology of this disease was wind, damp and heat obstructing the qi, blood, channels and collaterals. The key point of the treatment was to dispel evils, invigorate blood, move qi, and course and unblock the collaterals.

Since the joint pain, dry mouth with bitter taste, foul breath, yellowish or reddish urine, dry stool, dark red tongue with white greasy coating, and thready, rapid, and forceful pulse were all caused by damp-heat, it was appropriate to use *Líng Xī Gǔ Pí Yǐn* (羚犀骨皮饮) to clear heat, drain dampness, invigorate blood, transform stasis, unblock the collaterals, and relieve pain. *Líng yáng gŭ* (Os Saigae Tataricae), *shuĭ niú gŭ* (Os Bubali), and *dì gŭ pí* (Cortex Lycii) deeply enter the sinews and bones to clear heat from the bones, drain fire, and extinguish wind; hence, their pain-relieving effect is quick. *Yì yĭ rén* (Semen Coicis), *fú líng pí* (Cutis Poriae), *bái máo gēn* (Rhizoma Imperatae), and *lăo sāng zhī* (Ramulus Mori) are great for clearing dampness and fire. *Wú gōng* (Scolopendra) and *wēi líng xiān* (Radix et Rhizoma Clematidis), because of their mobile nature, guide the strength of the medicinals directly to the disease location, unblocking the channels and collaterals. *Shēng shí gāo* (raw Gypsum Fibrosum) clears heat and relieves pain. *Hóng huā* (Flos Carthami) and *dān shēn* (Radix et Rhizoma Salviae Miltiorrhizae) invigorate blood and transform stasis. *Dān pí* (Cortex Moutan) clears the latent heat within the blood. For hard gouty tophi (nodules), a large dosage of *chuān shān jiă* (Squama Manis) was prescribed to dissipate the masses. *Dà huáng* (Radix et Rhizoma Rhei) was used to flush out the damp-turbidity in the *zang-fu* organs [if a patient complains of sloppy stool, decocting *dà huáng* (Radix et Rhizoma Rhei) together with the other medicinals would clear dampness and transform turbidity without causing diarrhea]. The externally used formula, *Huí Chūn Săn* (回 春 散), clear heat, resolves toxins, invigorates blood, unblocks the collaterals, drains dampness, and disperses swelling. In addition, it has a powerful effect of removing hard nodules and lumps.

The patient had a constitution of yang excess and yin deficiency as a result of a history of diabetes mellitus and hypertension. Hence, in the advanced stage of the disease, she had a red tongue with scanty coating and a thready and rapid pulse. Medicinals that enrich yin and subdue yang were prescribed to consolidate the effect of the treatment.

[Huang Zhen-ming, Huang Yong-yuan. *The Sequelae of Odd, Difficult and Complex Diseases* (奇难杂症续集). *Guangzhou: Guangdong Technology Press* (广东科技出版社). 1993: 119]

Discussions

1. Zhu Liang-chun on Discharging Turbidity and Transforming Stasis to Treat Gout

The important clinical manifestations of gout are:

- Prevalence increases gradually with age.
- The disease often has a family history.
- It often occurs in people who are overweight, those with alcohol addictions, and/or those that consume fatty, sweet, and greasy foods.
- The attacks of joint pain usually occur at night and mostly involve the lower extremities.

Eventually, there will also be formation of gouty tophi or ulceration and turbid resinosis. Other accompanying symptoms may include stone strangury with lumbar pain and bloody urination. In severe cases, there may be frequent vomiting, dysuria, and intense beating of the carotid and radial pulses.

Dr. Zhu believes that gout (痛风, *tòng fēng*) is caused by stagnation of turbid toxins. The Chinese name of the disease includes the word "wind" but in actuality it is not due to wind evil. The symptoms resemble wind but the disease itself is not caused by the invasion of wind evil. The turbid toxins stagnate and remain in the blood and are unable to be discharged. At first, the condition is mild, hence there is no pain. However, as time goes by, the accumulation gradually increases and may combine with external pathogens until it eventually leads to stasis and binds or obstruction in the channels and collaterals. Consequently, there will be sudden and severe bone and joint pain that may be complicated by the formation of gouty tophi (nodules) due to congealing phlegm. Over time, the phlegm turbidity and stasis will give rise to ulceration and turbid resinosis. If the phlegm-stasis solidifies, it will lead to joint stiffness, swelling, and deformity. Since constraint and blockage have a high tendency to transform into heat, the syndrome will often include signs and symptoms of heat. For instance, damp-turbidity brews into heat; the heat boils up the urine and causes stone strangury with bloody urine. If the turbid toxins linger, they will damage the spleen and kidney. When cold and heat mix together, they cause congestion in the *san jiao*, hence the dangerous signs and symptoms of "block and repulsion"(关格 , *guān gé*), i.e., frequent vomiting, dysuria, and intense beating of the carotid and radial pulses. All of these signs and symptoms are caused by turbid toxins and stasis accumulation, not the invasion of wind evil.

In gout, the turbid toxins are produced within the body itself and not contracted from without. However, the common pre-existing conditions for the development of gout include either a congenital insufficiency or a gradual debilitation of *zang* qi due to old age. In addition, dietary irregularities, prolonged excessive consumption of alcohol, and indulgence in sweet, fatty and rich foods (fatty meat, fine grain, strong flavors) can lead to the dysfunction of the *zang-fu* organs, particularly the spleen-kidney's metabolism of the clear and the turbid. Failure of the spleen to transform and transport impairs the ascent of the clear and the descent of the turbid. Failure of the kidney's transformative ability leads to a disturbance in the separation of the clear and the turbid. Consequently, food and water cannot be properly transformed; turbid toxins are thus produced and stagnate within the blood, giving rise to stasis bind.

Once the diagnosis of gout is confirmed, the treatment principles of discharging turbidity and transforming stasis should be applied, with modifications as necessary according to the varied signs and symptoms. Gradually discharging turbidity and transforming stasis will result in the continuous drop of blood uric acid levels, and eventually the goal of restoring the *zang-fu*'s metabolism of the clear and the turbid will be reached. The treatment effect cannot be guaranteed if one fails to stick to the main treatment principles, modify the formula too soon, or discontinue the treatment because of impatience with seeing only slight improvement. Straying from the recommended treatment plan will cause the patient's condition to fluctuate, and over time the condition will only get worse.

Zhu uses *tǔ fú líng* (Rhizoma Smilacis Glabrae), *bì xiè* (Rhizoma Dioscoreae Hypoglaucae), *shēng yì yǐ rén* (raw Semen Coicis), *zé lán* (Herba Lycopi), *zé xiè* (Rhizoma Alismatis), *quán dāng guī* (whole Radix Angelicae Sinensis), *táo rén* (Semen Persicae), and *hóng huā* (Flos Carthami) as the base formula combined with other medicinals that downbear and discharge turbid toxins, invigorate blood, and transform stasis. The formula as a whole enhances the treatment effect by promoting the discharge and transformation of turbid toxins, removing stasis bind, and doing away with the old while engendering the new. Commonly added medicinals include *xī xiān cǎo* (Herba Siegesbeckiae), *xú cháng qīng* (Radix Cynanchi Paniculati), *wēi líng xiān* (Radix et Rhizoma Clematidis), *lǎo guàn cǎo* (Herba Erodii; Herba Geranii), *jī xuè téng* (Caulis Spatholobi), *wū shāo shé* (Zaocys), and *dì lóng* (Pheretima). Medicinals that treat wind can also overcome damp-turbidity, unblock the collaterals and facilitate the transformation of stasis, which make them especially effective in the treatment of gout with pain of the bones and joints.

【Modifications】

- For pronounced turbid dampness, add *cāng zhú* (Rhizoma Atractylodis), *cán shā* (Faeces Bombycis), and *chē qián zǐ* (Semen Plantago).
- For severe blood stasis, add *chì sháo* (Radix Paeoniae Rubra), *dì biē chóng* (Eupolyphaga seu Steleophaga), and *dān shēn* (Radix et Rhizoma Salviae Miltiorrhizae).
- For damp turbidity brewing into heat, add *Sān Miào Wán* (三妙丸), *hàn fáng jǐ* (Stephania tetrandra), and *qín jiāo* (Radix Gentianae

Macrophyllae).

➢ For severe *bi* and violent pain, add *quán xiē* (Scorpio), *wú gōng* (Scolopendra), *chǎo xuán hú* (dry-fried Rhizoma Corydalis), and *liù zhóu zǐ* (Rhododendri Mollis Fructus).

➢ For cases complicated by congealing phlegm manifesting as diffuse joint swelling and soft nodules, add *jiāng cán* (Bombyx Batryticatus), *bái jiè zǐ* (Semen Sinapis), and *chén dǎn xīng* (Arisaema cum Bile) to transform phlegm-stasis.

Zhu explains that the formula can rapidly eliminate joint pain if the appropriate phlegm-transforming medicinals are added; the modified formula will also have the effects of assisting the rapid alleviation of joint swelling and pain and lowering the concentration of blood uric acid. If the phlegm and stasis combine to invade the bones and joints, there will be joint swelling and deformity with hard nodules; *páo shān jiǎ* (blast-fried Squama Manis), *qiāng láng chóng* (Catharsius Molossus), *jiāng cán* (Bombyx Batryticatus), *fēng fáng* (Nidus Vespae) should be added to break the nodules, transform stasis, disperse phlegm, and soften hardness.

Gǔ suì bǔ (Rhizoma Drynariae), *shú dì* (Radix Rehmanniae Praeparata), *bǔ gǔ zhī* (Fructus Psoraleae), and *ròu cōng róng* (Herba Cistanches) can be added to tonify the kidney, strengthen the bones and replenish marrow, which is indicated for the chronic or interval stages of gout.

During acute episodes of gout, the dosages of *tǔ fú líng* (Rhizoma Smilacis Glabrae) and *bì xiè* (Rhizoma Dioscoreae Hypoglaucae) should be increased with the addition of a large number of insect medicinals to track down and scrape away the pathogens, remove obstruction, and relieve pain. If it is a heat pattern, add *hán shuǐ shí* (Glauberitum), *dà shēng dì* (Radix Rehmanniae Recens), *zhī mǔ* (Rhizoma Anemarrhenae), *hǔ zhàng* (Rhizoma Polygoni Cuspidati), *rěn dōng téng* (Caulis Lonicerae Japonicae), *shuǐ niú jiǎo* (Cornu Bubali), and *lǜ cǎo* (Humulus Scandens) to clear heat and unblock the collaterals. If it is a cold pattern, add *zhì chuān wū* (Radix Aconiti Praeparata), *cǎo wū* (Radix Aconiti Kusnezoffii), *zhì fù zǐ* (Radix Aconiti Lateralis Praeparata), *chuān guì zhī* (Ramulus Cinnamomi), *xì xīn* (Radix et Rhizoma Asari), *xiān líng pí* (Herba Epimedii), and *dà shú dì* (Radix Rehmanniae Praeparata) to warm the channels and disperse cold.

For gout with urinary calculi or gouty nephropathy, the treatment principles of discharging turbidity and transforming stasis should be strengthened. The former refers to promoting urination to expel stones, and the latter refers to boosting qi and tonifying the kidney.

As for the selection of medicinals that downbear and discharge turbid toxins, Zhu prefers *tǔ fú líng* (Rhizoma Smilacis Glabrae) and *bì xiè* (Rhizoma Dioscoreae Hypoglaucae), which are included in all of his formulas. The dosage of *tǔ fú líng* (Rhizoma Smilacis Glabrae) is 30-120g a day, while that of *bì xiè* (Rhizoma Dioscoreae Hypoglaucae) is 15-45g a day. *Tǔ fú líng* (Rhizoma Smilacis Glabrae) is sweet, bland, and neutral in property, enters the spleen and stomach channels, and assists in upbearing the clear and downbearing the turbid. *Bì xiè* (Rhizoma Dioscoreae Hypoglaucae) is bitter, sweet, and neutral in property, enters the kidney and bladder channels, and separates the clear and turbid. Both medicinals have the effect of eliminating dampness, resolving toxins, and disinhibiting the joints. The ancient Chinese often used them to treat syphilis, urinary difficulty, beriberi, scrofula, furuncles and carbuncles, and spasmodic pain of the muscles and bones. Since gout is caused by turbid toxins and blood stasis, these two medicinals are chosen to downbear the turbid toxins while benefiting the joints. They not only lower blood uric acid, but also relieve joint swelling and pain. In addition, Zhu emphasizes the effect of dietary factors, lifestyle, and emotions on the disease. He advises patients to avoid alcohol and cigarettes while undergoing treatment, and to refrain from eating purine-rich foods such as animal organs, clam, crab, and certain seafoods. He also recommends that patients drink more water.

[Wu Da-zhen, Qiao Mo. *The Unique Skill of Modern Famous Doctors of Chinese Medicine* (现代名中医内科绝技). Beijing: Scientific and Technological Literature Press. 1993: 228]

2. Wang Lü-qiu Uses *Wŭ Jī Săn* (五积散) to Treat Gout

Wang believes that gout falls under the category of *bi* syndromes in Chinese Medicine. *Bi* syndromes are wind, cold, dampness, and heat invasion of the muscles and bones, resulting in obstruction of the collaterals and impaired flow of qi and blood. When dealing with gout, one should differentiate between primary and secondary, mild and severe, and yin and yang. Violent joint pain of fixed location is caused by cold evil congealing and leading to severe obstruction and blockage of qi and blood flow. *Yellow Emperor's Inner Classic: Basic Questions, Treatise on Bi* Syndrome (黄帝内经素问 · 痹论, *Huáng Dì Nèi Jīng Sù Wèn: Bì Lùn*) mentions: "Prevalence of cold qi causes painful *bi*." (寒气胜者为痛痹。) Abnormally high concentration of uric acid that is unable to be excreted out of the body accumulates in the joints, resulting in local soreness. This is accumulation of substantial phlegm and damp-turbidity. Outbreaks of gout are thought to be caused by wind, while the local distending pain is attributed to qi stagnation. Most importantly, damp-cold congeals and stagnates within the joints and persists throughout the entire duration of the disease. When the six qi (pathogenic influences) are divided into categories of yin and yang, dampness and cold fall under the yin category, and thus this disease is considered a yin disease. This fact should be emphasized during clinical practice.

In gout, the redness, swelling, and pain of the joints are carefully differentiated as either yin fire or yang fire. Wang points out that although in yin fire there is joint swelling and pain with elevated local skin temperature (and sensation of heat), the color is dark and the burning pain is not pronounced, which is a manifestation of long-term constraint of cold-damp pathogen transforming into heat. This type of heat is different from both heat *bi* and shank erysipelas. During acute episodes, two to three out of ten patients exhibit yang fire, the manifestations of which include local redness and swelling, hot skin of scorching bright red color, and strong fever with aversion to cold. However, these are only the signs and symptoms of a brief stage in the course of gout. After the yang fire has subsided, once again we will see signs of yin cold congealing and stagnating. *Collected Treatises of Zhang Jing-yue*: Wind *Bi* (景岳全书 · 风痹 , *Jǐng Yuè Quán Shū: Fēng Bì*) states: "Excessive heat is a yang pattern; absence of heat is a yin pattern. As *bi* syndrome is often caused by yin pathogens, it manifests mostly as cold with occasional heat." (多热者是阳证，无热者便是阴证，然痹本阴邪，故惟寒者多而热者少也 .)

Wang treats gout by warming and dispersing with medicinals that are mobile and penetrating while protecting the right qi. A modification of *Wŭ Jī Săn* (五积散) is often used. *Wŭ Jī Săn* was created during the Song dynasty and was first mentioned in *Formulary of the Bureau of Medicines of the Taiping Era* (太平惠民和剂局方 , *Tài Píng Huì Mín Hé Jì Jú Fāng*). Its main ingredients are listed in the table below. Later, *Investigations of Medical Formulas* (医方考 , *Yī Fāng Kǎo*), *Medical Formulas Collected and Analyzed* (医方集解 , *Yī Fāng Jí Jiě*), *Effective Use of Established Formulas* (成方切用 , *Chéng Fāng Qiè Yòng*) also mentioned this formula, indicating that *Wŭ Jī Săn* was widely used during Song and Yuan dynasties. Wang An explained in his book, *Medical Formulas Collected and Analyzed* (医方集解 , *Yī Fāng Jí Jiě*), that "this formula disperses cold accumulation, food accumulation, qi accumulation, blood accumulation, and phlegm accumulation; hence it is named Five Accumulations Powder." (本方能散寒积、食积、气积、血积、痰积，故名五积。) He also analyzed the cause of the five accumulations: "They are all caused by cold-damp." Xie Guan mentioned in *Chinese Medicine Dictionary* (中国医学大辞典) that *Wŭ Jī*

Săn treats soreness of the lumbus and foot caused by cold-damp invading the channels and collaterals.

苍术	cāng zhú	Rhizoma Atractylodis
麻黄	má huáng	Herba Ephedrae
厚朴	hòu pò	Cortex Magnoliae Officinalis
白芷	bái zhǐ	Radix Angelicae Dahuricae
川芎	chuān xiōng	Rhizoma Chuanxiong
枳壳	zhǐ qiào	Fructus Aurantii
桔梗	jié gěng	Radix Platycodi
芍药	sháo yào	Radix Paeoniae Alba
肉桂	ròu guì	Cortex Cinnamomi
当归	dāng guī	Radix Angelicae Sinensis
茯苓	fú líng	Poria
半夏	bàn xià	Rhizoma Pinelliae
陈皮	chén pí	Pericarpium Citri Reticulatae
干姜	gān jiāng	Rhizoma Zingiberis
甘草	gān căo	Radix et Rhizoma Glycyrrhizae

Wang uses the first nine ingredients of *Wŭ Jī Săn* (五积散), replacing *ròu guì* (Cortex Cinnamomi) with *guì zhī* (Ramulus Cinnamomi), as a formula to treat gout.

苍术	cāng zhú	Rhizoma Atractylodis
麻黄	má huáng	Herba Ephedrae
厚朴	hòu pò	Cortex Magnoliae Officinalis
白芷	bái zhǐ	Radix Angelicae Dahuricae
川芎	chuān xiōng	Rhizoma Chuanxiong
枳壳	zhǐ qiào	Fructus Aurantii
桔梗	jié gěng	Radix Platycodi
芍药	sháo yào	Radix Paeoniae Alba
桂枝	guì zhī	Ramulus Cinnamomi

There are three characteristics of this formula in clinical practice:

(1) The specific formula to treat the specific disease: Wang said that diagnostic knowledge should consist of Chinese and Western medicine

to make up for each other's deficiencies and improve the therapeutic effect. On syndrome differentiation, once there is joint soreness with elevated blood uric acid in accordance with chronic or acute gout in biomedical principle, Wang uses *Wŭ Jī Săn* (五积散) with modification to disperse cold and dampness and clear away turbid pathogen to remove obstruction. This is a specific formula for a specific disease.

(2) Emphasize the effect of *cāng zhú* (Rhizoma Atractylodis) and *má huáng* (Herba Ephedrae): Wang points out that *cāng zhú* (Rhizoma Atractylodis) and *má huáng* (Herba Ephedrae) are the principal medicinals combined together to disperse cold and dampness. Of the original formula, *Wŭ Jī Săn* (五积散), the dosage of *cāng zhú* (Rhizoma Atractylodis) is 720g, which is two to six times that of other medicinals. *Cāng zhú* (Rhizoma Atractylodis) is acrid, bitter and aromatic. It disperses the turbid pathogens. According to the experience of the ancients, *cāng zhú* (Rhizoma Atractylodis) is the most effective at treating external dampness. Zhu strongly insists that *cāng zhú* (Rhizoma Atractylodis) is an essential medicinal for the treatment of gout and is included in his formula *Shàng Zhōng Xià Tōng Yòng Tòng Fēng Fāng* (上中下通用痛风方). Wang uses *má huáng* (Herba Ephedrae) in large dosages to treat gout, up to 10-15g. Even in the hot summer he uses it without side effects. For acute attacks of gout with yang fire, a large amount of *má huáng* (Herba Ephedrae) should also be used. Wang said, in the formulae composed by Zhang Zhong-jing to treat *bi* syndromes such as *Má Huáng Jiā Zhú Tāng* (麻黄加术汤), *Má Xìng Shí Gān Tāng* (麻杏石甘汤), *Yuè Bì Jiā Zhú Tāng* (越婢加术汤), *má huáng* (Herba Ephedrae) is the main ingredient. As recorded in *Discussion of Medicinal Properties* (药性论 , *Yào Xìng Lùn*) that "*má huáng* (Herba Ephedrae) can treat toxic wind and obstinate *bi* syndromes of the body", it is necessary to use *má huáng* (Herba Ephedrae) as one of the chief medicinals in the treatment of gout.

(3) Modification according to symptoms: Wang prefers specific formulas for specific patterns when treating gout. However, he also modifies his formulas according to symptoms.

1) For yang fire symptoms, *zǐ huā dì dīng* (Herba Violae), *pǔ gōng yīng* (Herba Taraxaci), *lián qiáo* (Fructus Forsythiae), and *huáng bǎi* (Cortex Phellodendri Chinensis) were added. For dampness and heat in the lower body, modified *Sì Miào Sǎn* (四妙散) is added.

2) For obstruction in the collaterals, branch and vine medicinals were added, i.e., *hǎi fēng téng* (Caulis Piperis Kadsurae), *luò shí téng* (Caulis Trachelospermi), *qīng fēng téng* (Caulis Sinomenii), *tiān xiān téng* (Herba Aristolochiae), and *yín huā téng* (Lonicerae Caulis). Insect medicinals such as *quān xiē* (Scorpio), *fēng fáng* (Nidus Vespae), and *wú gōng* (Scolopendra) were added to invigorate blood, remove stasis and dispel wind pathogen from the collaterals.

3) For chronically ill, weak patients, *huáng qí* (Radix Astragali), *dǎng shēn* (Radix Codonopsis), and *bái zhú* (Rhizoma Atractylodis Macrocephalae) were added to fortify the spleen and nourish the kidney.

[Li Ning, Sun Jian-xi. Wang Lü-qiu's Experience in the Treatment of Gout (汪履秋治疗痛风经验撷萃). *Anhui Clinical Journal of Chinese Medicine* (安徽中医临床杂志). 1998, 10 (1): 32]

3. Lü Cheng-quan on Three Methods of Treating Gout

Based on years of clinical experience, Lü summarizes three principle methods of treating gout:

(1) Regulating the spleen and kidney.

(2) Clearing heat and draining dampness.

(3) Transforming stasis to unblock the collaterals.

These three methods were clinically tested and produced fairly good results. Lü points out that although there are three principle methods for treating this disease, in clinical practice, spleen and kidney deficiency, damp-turbidity brewing internally, and obstruction of the channels, collaterals, and joints are commonly seen together, and often present as a deficiency-excess complex pattern. Consequently, one should not be confined to one treatment method, but should adjust the treatment approach according to the pulse manifestation and symptoms.

Lü believes gout can be attributed to kidney insufficiency, qi and blood depletion, impaired qi transformation, or spleen and stomach deficiency and excessive consumption of fatty and greasy foods leading to phlegm-damp brewing internally, which finally result in the generation of damp-turbidity. Although damp-turbidity is a yin evil, if one drinks alcohol when exposed to wind, goes into water when sweating, or has undigested food accumulating in the body, the damp-turbidity can transform into heat and give rise to damp-heat brewing and steaming. This damp-heat will obstruct the channels, collaterals, and joints, manifesting as fever and unremitting joint swelling and pain that is worse at night. To treat this disease, it is necessary to clear heat and drain dampness, assisted by medicinals that invigorate blood and unblock the collaterals.

Those who have chronic, persistent gout with recurrent attacks exhibit gouty tophi nodules around the joints of the limbs or on the auricles. They are as hard as stone and can lead to joint deformity. Gouty tophi are most common found on the articular bones of the big toe. The gouty tophi can sometimes rupture, releasing a yellow, thick and sticky fluid, which in severe cases, forms pus and becomes chronic and difficult to treat. Lü believes this condition is caused by spleen and kidney deficiency, phlegm-damp turbidity pouring into the channels, collaterals, and joints, and qi and blood stasis obstruction; thus he advocates the use of medicinals that break stasis, dissipate nodules, and unblock the channels and collaterals, such as *chuān shān jiă* (Squama Manis), *yù jīn* (Radix Curcumae), *táo rén* (Semen Persicae), *hóng huā* (Flos Carthami), *dān shēn* (Radix et Rhizoma Salviae Miltiorrhizae), *chì sháo*

(Radix Paeoniae Rubra), *chuān niú xī* (Radix Cyathulae), *jī xuè téng* (Caulis Spatholobi), and *luò shí téng* (Caulis Trachelospermi), in addition to heat-clearing and damp-draining medicinals, such as *yì yǐ rén* (Semen Coicis), *tǔ fú líng* (Rhizoma Smilacis Glabrae), *zhū líng* (Polyporus), and *zé xiè* (Rhizoma Alismatis).

In chronic gout, the functions of the internal organs are impaired, and the most commonly seen pattern is spleen and kidney deficiency. The kidney governs the bones, controls water [metabolism], and stores essence; it is the foundation of congenital constitution. The spleen governs transportation and transformation, and controls the rotting and ripening of the essence of water and grain; it is the foundation of acquired constitution. Dual deficiency of the spleen and kidney is the main cause of the generation of damp-turbidity. Dual deficiency of the spleen and kidney also causes the bones to be deprived of nourishment. When the kidney fails to seal and store, yin-essence is exhausted, and one complains of frequent and copious night urination and soreness of the lumbus and knees. During treatment, it is necessary to regulate the functions of the kidney and the spleen. *Chǎo dù zhòng* (dry-fried Cortex Eucommiae), *bā jǐ tiān* (Radix Morindae Officinalis), *ròu cōng róng* (Herba Cistanches), *shú dì* (Radix Rehmanniae Praeparata), *chǎo bái zhú* (dry-fried Rhizoma Atractylodis Macrocephalae), and *chǎo cāng zhú* (dry-fried Rhizoma Atractylodis) are used to regulate the spleen and kidney and support the right while dispelling the evil.

Furthermore, Lü emphasizes that fatty and greasy foods, meat, fish, and spinach should be avoided. The patient's compliance combined with proper treatment can assure the normal functioning of the spleen and kidney, thereby gradually eliminating damp-turbidity and unblocking the channels and collaterals.

[Lü Hong-sheng and Peng Bo. A Summary of Lü Cheng-quan's Experience in the Treatment of Gout (吕承全治疗痛风经验总结). *Henan*

Journal of Chinese Medicine (河南中医药学刊). 1994, 9(2): 32]

4. Huang Chun-lin on Pattern Differentiation and Differential Diagnosis in the Treatment of Gout

Huang considers the origin of gout to be dysfunction of the spleen and kidney. According to traditional pattern differentiation, the disease can be divided into the following types:

(1) Damp-heat *Bi*

Symptoms include red, hot, swollen, and painful muscles or joints, difficulty in walking, fever, thirst but no desire to drink, vexation and restlessness, cloudy yellow urine, a red tongue with yellow greasy coating, and a soggy rapid or slippery rapid pulse. The treatment principle is to clear heat, drain dampness, and unblock the collaterals. The representative formula is modified *Sān Miào Tāng* (三妙汤).

(2) Blood Stasis *Bi*

Symptoms include severe, sharp, and fixed pain of the muscles and joints that refuses pressure, local swelling with hard nodules, and stasis macules. There is possible darkening and dryness of the skin, thirst but no desire to drink, a dark purple tongue with stasis macules, and a deep, thready and rough pulse. The treatment principle is to invigorate blood, transform stasis, unblock the collaterals, and relieve pain. The representative formula is modified *Shēn Tòng Zhú Yū Tāng* (身痛逐瘀汤).

(3) Kidney Deficiency with Damp-heat

Symptoms include frequent urination with scorching hot pain, yellowish-red urine, urgent but incomplete urination, soreness of the lumbus and knees, a yellow greasy tongue coating, and a slippery rapid pulse. The treatment principle is to enrich yin, tonify the kidney, clear heat, and drain dampness. The representative formula is modified *Zhī Bǎi*

Bā Wèi Tāng (知柏八味汤).

(4) Kidney Deficiency Stone Strangury

Symptoms include urinary stones, difficult urination or sudden interruption of urine flow, sharp pain of the urethra, lesser abdominal tenderness, bloody urine (in severe cases), soreness of the lumbus and knees, a pale tongue with yellow coating, and a thready pulse. The treatment principle is to enrich the kidney, drain dampness, free strangury, and expel stones. The representative formula is a modified combination of *Liù Wèi Dì Huáng Tāng* (六味地黄汤) plus *Shí Wěi Săn* (石苇散).

(5) Kidney Yin and Yang Deficiency

Symptoms include a long disease course, extreme lack of strength, a withered-yellow facial complexion, fatigue, poor appetite, nausea and vomiting, soreness and weakness of the lumbus and knees, a pale enlarged tooth-marked tongue with white greasy coating, and a thready pulse. The treatment principle is to tonify yin and yang. The representative formula is modified *Shèn Qì Wán* (肾气丸).

【Modifications】

➢ For joint rigidity and deformity, add medicinals that unblock the collaterals and transform stasis, e.g., *wú gōng* (Scolopendra), *wū shāo shé* (Zaocys), *chuān shān jiă* (Squama Manis), *táo rén* (Semen Persicae), *hóng huā* (Flos Carthami), *luò shí téng* (Caulis Trachelospermi), and *jī xuè téng* (Caulis Spatholobi).

➢ For ruptured and ulcerated gouty tophi, add *fă bàn xià* (Rhizoma Pinelliae Praeparatum), *māo zhuă căo* (Radix Ranunculi Ternati), *chuān pò shí* (Radix Cudraniae), *hăi zăo* (Sargassum), *shān cí gū* (Pseudobulbus Cremastrae seu Pleiones) to dispel phlegm, soften hardness, dissipate nodules, and unblock the collaterals.

➢ For severe pain, externally apply *Sì Huáng Shuĭ Mì* (四黄水蜜) to the local area to clear heat and disperse swelling.

➢ In cases of elevated blood uric acid level or during the remission stage, patients show the signs of spleen and kidney insufficiency and internal exuberance of damp-turbidity. The treatment principle is to fortify the spleen, tonify the kidney, and downbear turbidity.

For the treatment of hyperuricemia, gout, and gouty nephropathy, Huang advocates the following approaches:

(1) Treat the primary disease and eliminate the factors that cause or aggravate the disease:

In the case of secondary hyperuricemia, one needs to find the cause as soon as possible. As for blood disorders, renal disease, and drug-induced disease, treating the original disease will control the hyperuricemia. Cold, emotional stress, infections, a high purine diet, or incorrect medication can all induce or aggravate gout. As in the case of chemotherapy or radiotherapy for secondary myeloproliferative disease, the rapid cell division and breakdown of nucleic acid can lead to a sudden increase in uric acid. The accumulation of uric acid crystals within the collecting duct, renal pelvis, and renal calices can cause acute obstructive nephropathy. The prophylactic use of *dà huáng* (Radix et Rhizoma Rhei), *qín pí* (Cortex Fraxini), *chē qián cǎo* (Herba Plantaginis), and *tǔ fú líng* (Rhizoma Smilacis Glabrae) can prevent this condition.

(2) Treatment of hyperuricemia:

Endogenous uric acid accounts for 80 percent, while exogenous occupies 20 percent. One-third of the uric acid is excreted through the gastrointestinal tract and two-third is eliminated through the kidneys. Hyperuricemia can be resolved in two ways:

1) Limit the amount of uric acid production: Reducing the intake of protein purine-rich foods helps to reduce the amount of uric acid in the body. The genkwanin and pelargidenon found in *yuán huā* (Flos Genkwa) and the emodin contained in *dà huáng* (Radix et Rhizoma

Rhei) powerfully suppress xanthine oxidase, thereby reducing uric acid production.

2) Promote uric acid excretion: *qín pí* (Cortex Fraxini), *chē qián cǎo* (Herba Plantaginis), *tǔ fú líng* (Rhizoma Smilacis Glabrae), and *cāng zhú* (Rhizoma Atractylodis) facilitate the excretion of uric acid through the stool.

(3) Treatment of acute attacks of gout and gouty nephropathy:

Acute attacks of gout and gouty nephropathy are usually managed with NSAIDs. Most Chinese medicinals that dispel wind and eliminate dampness also belong to this category of medicine. Acute gouty arthritis manifests as heat *bi*, hence Chinese medicinals that clear heat and eliminate inflammation are chosen, e.g., *huáng bǎi* (Cortex Phellodendri Chinensis), *fáng jǐ* (Radix Stephaniae Tetrandrae), and *rěn dōng téng* (Caulis Lonicerae Japonicae). However, in those who live in cold regions or those attacked by wind and cold, there may be manifestations of interior heat with exterior cold. Medicinals that disperse cold and unblock *bi* can be used, e.g., *qiāng huó* (Rhizoma et Radix Notopterygii), *dú huó* (Radix Angelicae Pubescentis), *qín jiāo* (Radix Gentianae Macrophyllae), and *xiāng fù* (Rhizoma Cyperi). *Bǎi hé* (Bulbus Lilii) and *shān cí gū* (Pseudobulbus Cremastrae seu Pleiones) have colchicine-like effects, which means that they inhibit the movement of white blood cells, thereby relieving the inflammation of gouty arthritis.

[Li Fang, Xu Da-ji. Professor Huang Chun-lin's Experience in the Treatment of Gout and Gouty Nephropathy (名中医黄春林教授治疗痛风及痛风性肾病之经验). *Chinese Medicine Research* (中医药研究). 1999, 15(3):1]

5. Peng Jie-shou on Gout as Patterns of "Leg Qi"

In Chinese medicine, gout is called *tòng fēng* (痛风, which translates literally as "pain wind"). Peng points out that *tòng fēng* was first mentioned during the Song and Yuan dynasties, and there have been discussions of this disease in numerous medical works ever since. Since the disease is thought to be caused by invasion of wind cold damp pathogen in nearly all medical texts, *tòng fēng* is considered a type of *bi* syndrome or an alternate name for *bi* syndrome. In accordance with the opinion of medical experts, the Ministry of Public Health advocated *Guidelines for Research on the Treatment of Bi Syndromes with New Chinese Medicinals* (中药新药治疗痹病的临床研究指导原则). The definition of *bi* syndromes in the guidelines is as follows: *Bi* syndromes are caused by the invasion of the channels and collaterals by external evils. Symptoms include joint pain, numbness, and inhibited movement. In severe cases, there may be physical disability and lack of strength. It is similar to autoimmune diseases in modern medicine, e.g., rheumatoid arthritis, rheumatic arthritis, ankylosing spondylitis, and osteoarthritis (particularly rheumatoid arthritis and rheumatic arthritis). The clinical manifestations include pain of the joint, muscles, bones, and skin, swelling, rigidity, numbness, inhibited movement, and joint deformity. The disease responds to changes in weather, and is most prevalent among young adults (particularly females). Lab tests show elevation of O-antigen, an elevated ESR, and/or positive rheumatoid factors. X-ray may reveal bone destruction. Through analyzing and studying ancient texts, Peng has found that some discussions on "leg qi" in post-Tang classical texts bear a resemblance to gout in modern medicine, though there are some significant differences.

(1) On the Disease Name

The term "leg qi (脚气, *jiăo qì*)" originated in the Jin dynasty. By the Tang dynasty, there were a lot of discussions on "leg qi" in medical texts, some of which included the modern medical concept of gout. Sun Si-miao wrote in his book, *Important Formulas Worth a Thousand Gold Pieces - Discussion on Leg Qi* (千金要方 · 脚气论 , *Qiān Jīn Yào Fāng - Jiǎo Qì Lùn*): "Since the Tang dynasty has expanded the country, there is no place that does not fall within its boundaries. Soldiers wore heavy uniforms and wielded weapons to guard the borders; since they could not adapt to the environment of the new lands, all of them fell ill. Recently, although some high-ranking officials do not go south, they also acquired this disease. This is because the wind of the different parts of the country are mixed together, making the environment similar all throughout the country. Since the disease affects the feet first, causing swelling in the legs, the people of that era called it leg qi." (此病自圣唐开辟六合，外无南极之地，襟带是重，爪牙之寄，作镇于彼，不袭水土，往者皆遭。近来中国士大夫，虽不涉江表，亦有居然而患之者，良由今代天下风气混同，物类齐等所致之耳，然此病初得，即先从脚起，因即胫肿，时人号为脚气。) Thus it is apparent that in ancient texts, "leg qi" (equivalent to beriberi in modern medicine) not only refers to Vitamin B_1 deficiency, but also includes gout as described in modern medicine. Not only those who live in remote areas and live on dairy and meat are prone to this disease, but those who live in developed regions, including high-ranking officials, are susceptible as well.

(2) Etiology and Pathogenesis

The disease is primarily caused by endogenous factors. As for the cause of beriberi, Li Dong-yuan said: "The condition is quite dry, there is no dampness, and those who are strong are resistant to this disease. It is hard to understand how one catches this disease. One possible cause is excessive consumption of dairy and alcohol, combined with a rich diet which leads to dampness and stagnation. The dampness flows down to the feet. The long-term accumulation causes swollen, painful feet."(今观此方爽垲，而无卑湿之地，况腠理致密，外邪难侵，而有此者，何也？盖

多饮乳酪醇酒水湿之属也，加以奉养过度，以滋其湿水之润下，气不能煦之，故下注于足，积久而作肿满疼痛，此饮之下流之气所致也。) [*Elucidation of Medicine – Leg Qi* (医学发明 · 脚气 , *Yī Xué FāMíng – Jiāo Qì*)] .

Dan-bo Yuan-jian gave a more in-depth description of the causes and risk factors of this disease. He said: "Eighty to ninety percent of all cases are caused by endogenous factors; twenty to thirty percent are caused by exogenous factors. Fifty to sixty percent are coupled with other diseases. Senior officials who ride in carriages and live in luxurious homes seldom have their feet touch the ground, but many of them catch this disease because they eat excessively and drink too much alcohol. "(大抵由内因者十之八九，由外因者十之二三，与诸病并发者，十之五六。夫王侯贵官，出则肥马华轿，入则高堂大厦，足未常履地，其多患此者，无他。膏腴过分，酒食越度，因以致之) [*Jiǎo Qì Gōu Yào - Xù* (脚气钩要 · 序)]

Dampness evil brewing internally and causing the stagnation of qi and blood is the main pathogenesis of the disease. Peng holds that the theory of dampness evil congestion is the best possible explanation for the cause of gout. *Collected Treatises of Zhang Jing-yue - Leg Qi* (景岳全书 · 脚气 , *Jǐng Yuè Quán Shū - Jiǎo Qì*) stated: "In leg qi, there is excess evil. Where there is congestion, swelling, pain, blockages and binds, or distending fullness, the appropriate main treatment principle is to course, guide, and free blockages..." (脚气有实邪，凡壅盛肿痛而为闭结或为胀满者，治宜以疏导通利为主) *Extensive Summary of Miscellaneous Diseases - Leg Qi* (杂病广要 · 脚气 , *Zá Bìng Guǎng Yào - Jiǎo Qì*) mentioned: "All those with leg qi disease die because of qi excess. Not one died from deficiency caused by medication." ("凡脚气之疾皆由气实而死，终无一人以服药致虚而殂……")

The characteristics of leg qi are found in the two discussions regarding gout. Firstly, leg qi often coincides with other diseases. Zhang Jing-yue explained in *Collected Treatises of Zhang Jing-yue - Leg Qi* (景岳

全书 · 脚气 , *Jǐng Yuè Quán Shū - Jiǎo Qì*): "Leg qi is not restricted to one disease or one channel. It is often mixed with other diseases, so it is difficult to differentiate. To treat this condition, it is necessary to seek out the yin and yang of the channels and collaterals, and then check to see if the pulse is excessive or deficient..." (脚气不专一气，亦不专在一经，兼有杂生诸病，未易分别，须寻经络之阴阳，再察脉息之虚实，以为治也……) Secondly, the clinical manifestations during the onset of the disease are quite mild and can easily be overlooked. *Arcane Essentials from the Imperial Library - Leg Qi* (外台秘要 · 脚气 , *Wài Tái Mì Yào - Jiǎo Qì*): "Those who acquire this disease are often unaware of the fact; those who ignore their congenital predisposition for the disease later acquire it; some acquire the disease after suffering from many other diseases. The disease is mild at first, so most people eat, drink, and carry on as usual. Only with careful observation can the disease be detected." (得此病者多不即觉，或先天它病而忽得之，或因众病后得之，初甚微，饮食嬉戏气力如常，当熟察之。)

(3) Clinical Signs and Symptoms

In the description of the clinical characteristics of beriberi in ancient medical texts, there are a lot of similarities to the clinical symptoms and signs of gout in modern medical texts. For instance:

The Orthodox Tradition of Medicine - Leg Qi (医学正传 · 脚气 , *Yī Xué Zhèng Zhuàn - Jiǎo Qì*): "…it starts with hidden lumps and pain at LV 3 (*tài chōng*) and red swollen shins, or aversion to cold with dragging pain and contraction of the sinews; these are the signs and symptoms. Ten days or half a month later, the same symptoms return, and gradually lead to swelling of the sinews of the feet that resemble gourds." (……是以先从太冲穴隐核痛起，及两足胫红肿，或恶寒筋挛掣痛，是其候也，或一旬，或半月复作如故，渐渐而致足筋肿大如瓜瓢者，多有之矣。)

The characteristics of disease onset:

1) Acute Attacks with Severe Pain

Zhu Shi's Collection of Empirical Formulas - Leg Qi (类编朱氏集验方 · 脚气 , *Lèi Biān Zhū Shì Jí Yàn Fāng - Jiǎo Qì*): "In the middle of the night, leg qi reaches its peak (夜半脚气病绝)". "The disease is hard to bear. Hanging the patients cannot stop him from yelling. Their sinews and vessels are swollen and enlarged." (病不可忍，用索悬吊，叫声不绝，筋脉肿大。)

Extensive Summary of Miscellaneous Diseases - Leg Qi (杂病广要 · 脚气 , *Zá Bìng Guǎng Yào - Jiǎo Qì*): "Some patients feel as if the arch of the foot has been shot by an arrow." (有忽患脚心如中箭。)

2) Recurrent Attacks

Extensive Summary of Miscellaneous Diseases - Leg Qi (杂病广要 · 脚气 , *Zá Bìng Guǎng Yào - Jiǎo Qì*) reveals that the disease "comes and goes sporadically (发歇不时)".

Arcane Essentials from the Imperial Library - Leg Qi (外台秘要 · 脚气 , *Wài Tái Mì Yào - Jiǎo Qì*): "Leg qi often comes on during spring (before summer). It is caused by steaming of heat and emotional stress. It gets worse in the summer and is relieved in the autumn. Most cases are like this with some exceptions." (凡脚气病，多以春末夏初发动得之，皆因热蒸，情地忧愦，春发如轻，夏发更重，入秋少轻，至秋自歇，大约如此，亦时有异于此候者。)

The Orthodox Tradition of Medicine - Leg Qi (医学正传 · 脚气 , *Yī Xué Zhèng Zhuàn - Jiǎo Qì*): "Ten days, or half a month later, the condition comes back. Slowly the muscles of the feet swell like gourds." (或一旬，或半月复作如故，渐渐而致足筋肿大如瓜瓤者).

3) Local Characteristics

a. Skin and Muscle

Extensive Summary of Miscellaneous Diseases - Leg Qi (杂病广要 · 脚气 , *Zá Bìng Guǎng Yào - Jiǎo Qì*): "Redness and swelling like the shape of clouds, or a faint red color; the area feels hot to the touch and there is pain upon palpation." (红肿如云痕，或隐见红色，按之热且痛者是也。)

b. Leg Qi Forms Leakage

Extensive Summary of Miscellaneous Diseases - Leg Qi (杂病广要 · 脚气 , *Zá Bìng Guǎng Yào - Jiǎo Qì*): "Leg qi concentrates in one spot, at the depth of approximately one and a half inches beneath the skin. Every latter half of the day there is severe pain. This is known as leg qi pouring and leaking." (脚气，跟注一孔，深寸半许，每下半日疼异常，此乃脚气注成漏。)

(4) Prognosis and Prevention

Arcane Essentials from the Imperial Library - Leg Qi (外台秘要 · 脚气 , *Wài Tái Mì Yào - Jiǎo Qì*), written by Wang Tao in the Tang dynasty, explains that leg qi cannot be fully cured and that the disease would attack again in the following spring and summer. Because of its incurability, there is a lot of information on how to avoid or reduce its recurrence. For instance, *Extensive Summary of Miscellaneous Diseases - Leg Qi* (杂病广要 · 脚气 , *Zá Bìng Guǎng Yào - Jiǎo Qì*) reveals: "Patients who suffer from leg qi should not eat crucian carp." (患脚气病人，不可吃鲫鱼。) The text also divulges: "Ginger and garlic can be eaten, but flour, lamb, radishes, and chives should be avoided. Excessive consumption of alcohol before sexual intercourse, standing for long periods of time in cold and damp environments, exposure to dampness from boat rides, living in a house that is hot and damp during the summer months, fatigue, excessive crying, and emotional stress can all induce the onset of this disease." (生姜蒜鼓当食大佳，不宜食面及羊肉萝卜蔓菁韭。酒醉房室，久立冷湿，船行水气，夏月屋中湿气热气，劳剧哭泣忧愦，如此等类，好使气发也。) Sun Si-miao was quoted saying: "Those who suffer from leg qi should be cautious of sexual activities and refrain from eating lamb, beef, fish, garlic, houttuynia, Chinese cabbage, vitex, sweet gourd, alcohol, flour, butter, milk, gruel, pork, chicken, goose, and duck. Recipes that contain crucian carp head should be avoided. Intense anger should also be avoided." (患脚气之病，极须慎房室，羊肉、牛肉、鱼、蒜、蕺菜、菘菜、蔓青、瓠子、酒面、酥油、乳糜、猪鸡鹅鸭。有方用鲫鱼头，此等并联切禁，不得犯之，并忌大怒。)

(5) Treatment

Many discussions on the treatment of leg qi in ancient times are quite similar to that of gout. For instance, *Arcane Essentials from the Imperial Library - Leg Qi* (外台秘要 · 脚气 , *Wài Tái Mì Yào - Jiǎo Qì*) explains: "Leg qi patients should avoid the frequent intake of medicinal tonics. The tonics often make the swelling more intense and difficult to treat." (夫脚气病不可常服补药，补药多令鼓胀紧实难救也。) It also said that: "Leg qi and edema of the legs are caused by congestion; both require coursing and precipitation." (脚气病胫肿，是为壅疾，皆当疏下。) *Sagacious Benevolence Formulary* (圣惠方 , *Shèng Huì Fāng*) declares: "To treat leg qi, prevent its onset in the spring and summer; the formula *Shū Fēng Tiáo Qì Bīng Láng Sǎn Fāng* (疏风调气槟榔散方) is suitable for this purpose." (治脚气春夏防发，宜服此疏风调气槟榔散方。) *Extensive Summary of Miscellaneous Diseases - Leg Qi* (杂病广要 · 脚气 , *Zá Bìng Guǎng Yào - Jiǎo Qì*) reveals: "All those with leg qi disease die because of qi excess. Not one died from deficiency caused by medication. Thus, leg qi patients should not receive major supplementation or major drainage." (凡脚气之疾，皆由气实而死，终无一人以服药致虚而殂，故脚气之人，皆不得大补，亦不可大泻。) Although Zhang Jing-yue opposes the idea that leg qi does not require supplementation, for those with excess, he still holds that the treatment principle should be primarily to course, guide, and disinhibit the joints. In *Collected Treatises of Zhang Jing-yue - Leg Qi* (景岳全书 · 脚气 , *Jǐng Yuè Quán Shū - Jiǎo Qì*), he emphasized: "In leg qi, there is excess evil. Where there is congestion, swelling, pain, blockages and binds, or distending fullness, the appropriate primary treatment principle is to course, guide, and free blockages…" (脚气有实邪，凡壅盛肿痛而为闭结

或为胀满者，治宜以疏导通利为主……）.

Based on the knowledge of the ancients and the analysis of personal clinical experience, Peng applies the treatment principles of warming, diffusing, and downbearing turbidity, moving qi and resolving congestion. He treated several thousands of patients with acute gouty arthritis using these methods. Symptom relief was achieved quickly and without any side effects. Peng created *Tòng Fēng No. 1 Hé Jì* (痛风 I 号合剂) and *Tòng Fēng Níng Kǒu Fú Yè* (痛风宁口服液), whose therapeutic effect proved to be reliable and rapid through years of clinical application in the treatment of acute and chronic gouty arthritis. The patent formulas can even relieve acute symptoms such as redness, swelling, heat, and pain within 12-72 hours without any marked side effects. They effectively lower blood uric acid levels and prevent the recurrence of acute gouty arthritis. Clinical results show that the main treatment effect of the formulas is the same in patients of varying ages, severity of disease, and symptoms.

[Peng Jie-shou , He Guo-jian. Chinese Medical Differential Diagnosis of Gout (痛风病中医辨病之我见). *Journal of Chengdu University of Chinese Medicine* (成都中医药大学学报). 1996, 19 (3): 1]

PERSPECTIVES OF INTEGRATIVE MEDICINE

Challenges and Solutions

In gout, if the kidney is not affected, the prognosis is good, provided that the disease is treated effectively. If not treated properly, the acute attacks will not only cause the patient great pain, but will also lead to the development of chronic gout, giving rise to joint rigidity and deformity, gouty tophi, fistulas, kidney stones, and impairment of renal function. Thus, the prevention of gout, the reduction of its recurrence, the rapid alleviation of acute attacks, and the prevention of renal insufficiency have become challenges for the health care practitioner.

Challenge 1: Preventing Onset and Reducing Recurrence

Primary gout is a type of hereditary disease caused by the congenital dysfunction of purine metabolism, and thus its onset is closely related to constitution and diet.

(1) Family History

The prevalence of gout is higher in some families due to hereditary factors, and thus it is necessary to inquire about the patient's family history to reveal those with asymptomatic hyperuricemia. For those with a blood uric acid level above 0.42 mmol/L, Chinese medicinals or Western pharmaceuticals that facilitate the excretion of uric acid or suppress its production should be prescribed to bring the blood uric acid level back down to the normal range, thereby preventing the onset of gout. For patients who already have gout, routine blood tests to monitor the blood uric acid level are required to prevent its recurrence.

(2) Dietary Guidelines

Gout patients should avoid foods that are high in purine content. Animal organs, bone marrow, seafood, shrimp, and crab contain the highest level of purine. Fish, meat, peas, and spinach also contain a certain amount of purine, while vegetables, fruit, milk, and eggs do not contain any.

Gout is often accompanied by hypertension, hyperlipidemia, arteriosclerosis, coronary heart disease, and diabetes mellitus type II. It is believed that gout has no direct relationship with the aforementioned diseases but it is closely related to obesity, dietary irregularities, and alcohol consumption, which happen to be common factors of these diseases. Watching the diet can help reduce weight to control hyperuricemia, diabetes mellitus, hypertension, and hyperlipemia.

In addition to the guidelines mentioned above, patients should avoid factors such as overtiredness, nervousness, alcohol, cold, dampness, and joint injury. They should also drink more water to facilitate the excretion of uric acid. These are all important measures to help prevent the occurrence of gout.

(3) Treatment of Hyperuricemia

Hyperuricemia is an important sign of gout, but hyperuricemia does not always indicate gout. Controlling hyperuricemia is the key to preventing and treating gout. The early stages of gout manifest as symptoms in the extremities and joints, and then progress on to affect the sinews and bones and damage the *zang-fu* organs. It is noteworthy to point out that before the symptoms arise, there are manifestations of congenital liver and kidney deficiency and failure of the spleen to transform and transport, which should not be overlooked. Thus, medicinals that regulate the functions of the liver and kidney as well as those that lower uric acid should be prescribed, i.e., *tǔ fú líng* (Rhizoma Smilacis Glabrae), *bì xiè* (Rhizoma Dioscoreae Hypoglaucae), *cán shā* (Faeces Bombycis), *yì yǐ rén* (Semen Coicis), *chē qián zǐ* (Semen Plantaginis), *jīn qián cǎo* (Herba Lysimachiae), *qín pí* (Cortex Fraxini), *qín jiāo* (Radix Gentianae Macrophyllae), *wēi líng xiān* (Radix et Rhizoma Clematidis), *xī xiān cǎo* (Herba Siegesbeckiae), *dì lóng* (Pheretima), *yín yáng huò* (Herba Epimedii), and *shān cí gū* (Pseudobulbus Cremastrae seu Pleiones). With these approaches, the severity of the disease can be controlled to a certain degree.

(4) Avoiding Drugs that Inhibit Uric Acid Excretion

Hydrochlorothiazide, ethacrynic acid, furosemide, aldinamide, and small doses of aspirin can all impair the elimination of uric acid and thus lead to hyperuricemia. Avoiding the clinical use of these drugs can help to prevent gout.

Challenge 2: Preventing Kidney Damage

Gout-induced kidney damage includes gouty nephropathy, acute renal failure, and urinary calculi. The major cause of gouty nephropathy is urinary retention as a result of obstruction of the urinary tract due to the deposition of uric acid crystal in the renal tubules and renal interstitium and the resulting inflammation; or the deposition of uric acid crystals in the collecting duct, renal pelvis, or ureters.

To prevent the deposition of uric acid crystals in the kidney from causing renal impairment, the key is to control hyperuricemia. Among chronic gout patients, one-third of them have renal impairment; therefore, when dealing with gout (especially in long-term gout patients), careful measures must be adopted to prevent the development of gouty nephropathy. Treatment during the interval and chronic stages of gout should be emphasized, and focus should be placed on lowering the blood uric acid level, alkalinizing the urine to lower the urine uric acid level, preventing the recurrence of gout, and preventing kidney damage. In addition to strictly adhering to dietary guidelines and increasing the patient's daily water consumption to alkalinize the urine, one should also strengthen the effects of clearing heat, promoting urination, freeing strangury, and dissolving stones to assist the dispersal of the inflammation caused by uric acid deposits in the renal tubules and renal interstitium as well as the removal of urinary obstruction caused by uric acid crystals. *Jīn qián cǎo* (Herba Lysimachiae), *hǎi jīn shā* (Spora Lygodii), *jī nèi jīn* (Endothelium Corneum Gigeriae Galli), *shí wěi* (Folium Pyrrosiae), *qú mài* (Herba Dianthi), *shēng yì yǐ rén* (raw Semen Coicis), *chē qián zǐ* (Semen Plantaginis), *mù tōng* (Caulis Akebiae), *dà huáng* (Radix et Rhizoma Rhei), *zé xiè* (Rhizoma Alismatis), and *huá shí* (Talcum) are commonly selected. Furthermore, decocting *chē qián cǎo* (Herba Plantaginis), *yù mǐ xū* (stigmata maydis), and *shēng yì yǐ rén* (raw

Semen Coicis) in water to be taken frequently as a beverage in place of tea can also promote uric acid excretion. Since gout is mainly caused by congenital deficiency and dysfunction of the spleen and kidney, it belongs to the pattern of root deficiency and branch excess. Thus, in the chronic stage, emphasis is placed on the use of tonics to restore the patient's health. Long-term nourishment and regulation of the liver, spleen, and kidney is essential; the treatment principle includes nourishing the liver and kidney, warming the kidney and fortifying the spleen, or fortifying the spleen to boost qi. Modifications of *Dú Huó Jì Shēng Tāng* (独活寄生汤), *Zuǒ Guī Yǐn* (左归饮), *Yòu Guī Wán* (右归丸), and *Shēn Líng Bái Zhú Sǎn* (参苓白术散) are commonly used. Clinical experience has proven that it is necessary to add medicinals that lower uric acid.

Insight from Empirical Wisdom

1. Strengthen Recognition of the Disease to Avoid Misdiagnosis

The prevalence of gout has a tendency to increase year by year. There was once a low incidence of gout in China, with only 25 cases of gout reported in 1958. As dietary habits change due to the continuing improvement of living conditions, the incidence of gout has increased considerably.

It is important to know how to recognize this disease. Gout involves the bones and joints and tends to affect the kidney, the blood vessels, and the heart. It is a type of metabolic disease which can be severely damaging to the health. There is little known about this disease. The course of this disease is long and it occurs mostly during old age. It is also commonly complicated by many other illnesses, hence the patient complains of different symptoms during different stages. If a detailed history is overlooked or the blood uric acid level is not checked in time, the condition can often be misdiagnosed as erysipelas, synovitis, rheumatoid arthritis, rheumatic arthritis, erythema of the finger or toes, or bone tumor. If treatment is delayed, the consequence can be severe and can possibly lead to amputation. It is also a mistake to base a diagnosis of gout solely on arthritis and an elevated blood uric acid level. Differential diagnosis should be made carefully to avoid an erroneous diagnosis. For patients with joint swelling and pain, especially intermittent pain of the big toe and metatarsal joints, emphasis should be placed on checking for signs of gout and acquiring the blood uric acid level. If necessary, experimental treatment with colchicine can be given to assist in the diagnosis.

Clinically, the diagnosis of gout is based on the three diagnostic criteria set forth by the American Rheumatism Association in 1977. Increasing disease recognition will facilitate the correct diagnosis of gout.

2. Gout is a Type of *Bi* Syndrome with Unique Features

From the Chinese medical viewpoint, whether the main clinical manifestation of gout is acute or chronic arthritis, it still belongs to the category of *bi* syndromes. However, gout is not entirely the same as the common phrase that states: "The mixture of wind, cold, and damp qi becomes *bi*." Gout has its own characteristics. *Teachings of Zhu Dan-xi* (丹溪心法, *Dān Xī Xīn Fǎ*) mentions: "Bone and joint pain of the entire body that is calm during the day but becomes violent at night and is likened to a tiger's bite is called white tiger joint-running wind." (遍身骨节疼痛，昼静夜剧，如虎噬之状，名曰白虎历节风。) This description illustrates that the pain of gout is as unbearable as the pain of a tiger's bite, and thus during acute episodes it is imperative that we relieve pain as quickly as possible to ease the patient's suffering. At this time, the combination of internal and external treatment can be employed on the basis of pattern differentiation. For wind-damp-heat *bi*, use *Bái Hǔ Guì Zhī Tāng* (白虎桂枝汤), *Sì Miào Wán* (四妙丸), or *Lóng Dǎn Xiè Gān Tāng* (龙胆泻肝汤)

with modifications to clear heat, unblock the collaterals, dispel wind, and remove dampness. For wind-cold-damp *bi*, use modified *Yì Yǐ Rén Tāng* (薏苡仁汤) to dispel wind, disperse cold, eliminate dampness, and unblock the collaterals. Externally used formulas include *Sì Huáng Shuǐ Mì* (四黄水蜜) or *Fú Huáng Gāo* (芙黄膏) applied topically, and *Fēng Shī Xǐ Jì* (风湿洗剂) used as a wash. These external applications directly effect the location of the disease and enhance the treatment effect.

Attacks of gout often occur at night, hence the saying: "The pain is calm during the day but becomes violent at night." Gong Ting-xian holds that "a great number of diseases…are increasingly violent at night but quiet during the day. This is due to superabundance of yin disease, hence the blood is affected but not the qi." (百病……夜则增剧，昼则安静。是阴病有余，乃血病而气不病。) This concept emphasizes the close connection between the formation of gout and the congealing and stagnation of blood stasis and turbid evils within the channels and vessels. Simply dispelling wind, clearing heat, eliminating dampness, unblocking the collaterals, and relieving pain is not enough. On the basis of pattern differentiation, one must also incorporate transforming stasis and discharging turbidity into the treatment plan. Use large dosages of *máo dōng qīng* (Ilex Pubescens), *zé lán* (Herba Lycopi), *dāng guī* (Radix Angelicae Sinensis), *tǔ fú líng* (Rhizoma Smilacis Glabrae), *bì xiè* (Rhizoma Dioscoreae Hypoglaucae), and *shēng yì rén* (raw Semen Coicis) to facilitate the excretion of blood uric acid.

Furthermore, gout is due to root deficiency and branch excess. Liver, spleen, and kidney deficiency exists throughout the entire course of gout. Even before the appearance of gout symptoms, there are manifestations of liver, spleen, and kidney deficiency, which are in accordance with the fact that the disease is more common among middle-aged to old adults. Therefore, special focus should be placed on regulating and tonifying the liver, spleen, and kidney in the treatment of gout.

3. Chronic Stage Tonification Without Neglecting to Disperse

Gout is due to root deficiency and branch excess. During the chronic stage, treat the root by tonifying deficiency. Over time, the circulation of qi and blood is no longer smooth, and eventually leads to the following situations: (1) "enduring illness enters the collaterals," (2) "enduring illness invariably gives rise to stasis," and (3) "when blood stops [flowing], there is stasis; when dampness congeals, there is phlegm." *Systematized Patterns with Clear-cut Treatments - Bi Syndromes* (类证治裁·痹证, *Lèi Zhèng Zhì Cái - Bì Zhèng*) clearly points out that in the case of chronic *bi* syndromes, "there will inevitably be damp-phlegm, vanquished blood, and stasis and stagnation in the channels and collaterals." (必有湿痰败血瘀滞经络。) Phlegm and stasis bind together to obstruct and block the channels and collaterals, pour into the bones and joints, and form phlegm nodules that are as hard as stone; phlegm and stasis coagulate and cause to joint stiffness, swelling, and deformity; chronic depletion of the spleen and kidney causes the inability to transform water-dampness which accumulates and turns into heat; the heat consumes the body fluids and causes urinary strangury. Thus, during the chronic stage of gout, it is necessary to combine the treatment principles of dispelling stasis, clearing phlegm, dissolving stones, and freeing strangury in order to remove phlegm turbidity and static blood accumulation. This method of treatment is known as "tonifying without forgetting to disperse."

(1) Dispelling Stasis and Clearing Phlegm

During the chronic stage of gout, there is inflammation and recurrent episodes of mild joint swelling and pain. Gouty tophi form and give rise to subcutaneous nodules, which are immobile and dark-colored, and in severe cases, accompanied by joint stiffness and deformity. This is due to phlegm turbidity and static blood lingering and stagnating in the channels, joints, and flesh. It is necessary to strongly invigorate blood, transform stasis, clear phlegm, unblock the collaterals, soften hardness, and dissipate nodules in addition to tonifying and boosting the liver, spleen, and kidney. *Táo Hóng Yǐn* (桃红饮) and *Èr Chén Tāng* (二陈汤) are often selected. When the disease has progressed to this stage, the evil enters deep inside the body while phlegm and static blood bind together. Ordinary medicinals are unable to penetrate and reach the disease location; only insect medicinals that have the power to strongly track down wind and scrape the collaterals can treat the condition.

(2) Freeing Strangury and Dissolving Stones

Spleen and kidney deficiency leads to the failure of dampness to be transformed; over time, the dampness accumulates and transforms into heat that consumes the body fluids, giving rise to stone strangury. According to statistics, about 20%-25% of primary gout patients have urinary calculi. Thus, urinary calculus is an important clinical symptom in chronic gout; treatment requires medicinals that tonify deficiency, promote urination, free strangury, and dissolve stones.

4. Understanding the Use of Medicinals

Gout belongs to the category of "*bi* syndromes" in Chinese medicine; therefore, it is appropriate to treat it with medicinals according to the characteristic of *bi* syndromes.

Bi refers to obstruction and blockage; thus, during treatment it is necessary to unblock the channels, quicken the collaterals, and remove obstruction. In the clinic, we often use acrid and warm medicinals with sweet and cold medicinals that unblock the collaterals. In addition, we employ the treatment principles of dispelling wind and stasis, transforming phlegm, unblocking the collaterals, moving qi, and invigorating blood.

Common Chinese medicinals that unblock the channels and quicken the collaterals to remove obstruction include *jiāng huáng* (Rhizoma Curcumae Longae), *sōng jié* (Lignum Pini Nodi), *wēi líng xiān* (Radix et Rhizoma Clematidis), *hǎi fēng téng* (Caulis Piperis Kadsurae), *mù guā* (Fructus Chaenomelis), *qiān nián jiàn* (Rhizoma Homalomenae), *rǔ xiāng* (Olibanum), *mò yào* (Myrrha) and *wú gōng* (Scolopendra). Medicinals that cool and unblock include *qín jiāo* (Radix Gentianae Macrophyllae), *xī xiān cǎo* (Herba Siegesbeckiae), *luò shí téng* (Caulis Trachelospermi), *rěn dōng téng* (Caulis Lonicerae Japonicae), *huáng yào zǐ* (Rhizoma Dioscoreae Bulbiferae), and *dì lóng* (Pheretima). Blood-invigorating, vines and insects medicinals often used to unblock the collaterals and relieve pain. In addition to the treatment principles specific to the various stages of gout, one may also add medicinals that unblock the channels, quicken the collaterals, and remove obstruction; this will help improve the symptoms and increase the curative effect.

In patients with chronic gout, there may be deformity, stiffness and severe pain of the joints and formation of tophi, which are attributed to evil lingering and penetrating the joints and bones. Insect medicinals can track down wind and remove evil. According to the symptoms and signs, treat the condition with the following medicinals: for wind-damp-heat *bi*, use *dì lóng* (Pheretima), *fēng fáng* (Nidus Vespae), *jiāng cán* (Bombyx Batryticatus), and *cán shā* (Faeces Bombycis); for wind-cold-damp *bi*, use *quán xiē* (Scorpio), *wú gōng* (Scolopendra), and *bái huā shé* (Agkistrodon); for stasis *bi*, use *tǔ biē chóng* (Eupolyphaga seu Steleophaga) and *chuān shān jiǎ* (Squama Manis); for all types of *bi* syndromes, *wū shāo shé* (Zaocys) and *qí shé* (Agkistrodon) can be used.

Vine medicinals excel at unblocking the channels, and can act as an envoy to guide the effects of the medicinals to the disease location (i.e., limbs). For instance, *luò shí téng* (Caulis Trachelospermi) unblocks the collaterals, dispels wind, and removes stagnation in the channels. it is very suitable for the pattern of deficiency of liver and kidney. Both *qīng fēng téng* (Caulis Sinomenii) and *hǎi fēng téng* (Caulis Piperis Kadsurae) can dispel wind-damp and unblock the channels and collaterals, making them suitable for treating gout due to wind-damp evil. The former is better for relieve pain and itching while the latter excels at dispelling wind in the channels to relieve wandering pain. *Rěn dōng téng* (Caulis Lonicerae Japonicae) can clear heat and resolve toxins, especially toxic heat in the channels; it can effectively treat swelling and pain caused by heat *bi*. *Jī xuè téng* (Caulis Spatholobi) unblocks the collaterals, soothes the sinews, invigorates and nourishes blood, and has the special function of freeing blood stasis in the collaterals, making it most suitable for women with blood deficiency. *Shēn jīn téng* (Caulis Lycopodii) soothes the sinews, quickens the collaterals, clears heat, and drains dampness; it can treat tendon and bone pain caused by wind-damp. *Tiān xiān téng* (Herba Aristolochiae) expels wind-damp, unblocks the channels and collaterals, transforms water-damp, disperses swelling, and relieves pain; it is most suitable for wind-damp *bi* pain with swelling. *Sī guā luò* (Retinervus Luffae Fructus) unblocks the collaterals and dispels dampness, especially dampness in the collaterals. *Sāng zhī* (Ramulus Mori) unblocks the collaterals, clears heat, soothes the sinews, and frees the joints; it is also an envoy to the limbs.

Summary

Gouty arthritis is a type of inflammatory reaction caused by dysfunction of purine metabolism resulting in uric acid deposits in the joints and surrounding tissue. Excessive purine in the diet can induce and aggravate the progression of the disease. Gout crystals deposit in the kidney and can lead to kidney damage (gouty nephropathy). Therefore, during treatment one must control the diet to promote the excretion of uric acid.

Gout falls within the scope of "*bi* syndromes" in Chinese medicine.

It is known as "white tiger joint-running wind (白虎历节风 ; *bái hŭ lì jié fēng*)," a name that reflects the severity and fierce onset of the pain. The pain is felt in the bones and joints of the whole body, is worse at night, and is likened to a tiger's bite. Gout belongs to the pattern of root deficiency and branch excess since chronic, recurrent disease invariably leads to deficiency and stasis. Thus, during treatment, emphasis should be placed on regulating and tonifying the liver and kidney; because of the branch excess it is also important to tonify without forgetting to disperse, which means that one should employ medicinals that dispel stasis, flush out phlegm, free strangury, dissolve stones, unblock the collaterals, and relieve pain.

SELECTED QUOTES FROM CLASSICAL TEXTS

Essentials from the Golden Cabinet - The Pulse, Patterns, and Treatment of Wind Strike and Joint-running Disease (金匮要略 · 中风历节病脉证治 , *Jīn Guì Yào Lüè - Zhòng Fēng Lì Jié Bìng Mài Zhèng Zhì*):

"病历节不可屈伸疼痛，乌头汤主之。"

"In joint-running disease, when there is pain with inability to bend and stretch, *Wū Tóu Tāng* (乌头汤) is indicated."

Skilled Prescriptions of Universal Benefit (普济本事方 , *Pŭ Jì Bĕn Shì Fāng*):

"麝香丸，治白虎历节诸风疼痛，游走无定，壮如虫啮，昼静夜剧，及一切手足不测疼痛。……如绿豆大，每服七丸，甚者十丸。夜卧令膈空，温酒下，微出冷汗一身，便差。予得此方，凡是历节及不测疼痛，一二服便差。"

"*Shè Xiāng Wán* (麝香丸) treats the pain of white tiger joint-running [wind], which is wandering in nature, resembles the gnawing of worms, and is calm during the day but violent at night. This pill can also treat all types of pain in the hands and feet…It is the size of a mung bean, and one dose is seven to ten pills. Before bed, on an empty stomach, take the pills with warm wine; breaking out in a mild cold sweat indicates that there will be recovery. After one or two doses, all kinds of joint pain will be cured."

Sagacious Benevolence Formulary (圣惠方 , *Shèng Huì Fāng*):

"夫白虎风痛者，是风、寒、暑、湿之毒，因虚而起，将摄失理，受此风邪，经脉结滞，血气不行，蓄于滑节之间，或在四肢，肉色不变，其疾昼静而夜发，夜发即彻骨髓酸疼，其痛如虎之噬，故名曰虎风病也。"

"White tiger wind pain is caused by wind, cold, summer heat, and dampness toxins, and is triggered by deficiency. Exposure to wind evil leads to binding stagnation in the channels and vessels, qi and blood stagnation, and amassment in the joint spaces or in the four limbs with discoloration of the flesh. The illness is calm during the day but emerges at night. During the night, the aching radiates to the bone marrow and the pain is like the bite of a tiger, hence it is called tiger wind disease."

Simple Formulary (直指方 , *Zhí Zhǐ Fāng*):

"历节风之状，短气自汗，头晕欲吐，手指挛曲，身体魁羸，其肿如脱，渐至推落，其痛如掣，不能屈伸……遍身走痒，彻骨疼痛，昼静夜剧，发如虫啮。"

"The symptoms of joint-running wind are shortness of breath with spontaneous sweating, dizziness with the desire to vomit, twisted fingers, a plump but weak body, swelling that resembles dislocation, and pain that is like a pulling sensation, and inability to bend and stretch… wandering itch all over the body, aching that radiates to the bones, [symptoms that are] calm during the day but violent at night, and flare-ups that resemble the gnawing of worms."

Teachings of Zhu Dan-xi (丹溪心法 , *Dān Xī Xīn Fǎ*):

“痛风者，四肢百节走痛；方书谓之白虎历节证是也。”

“Gout is wandering pain in the hundred joints of the four limbs; it is what is known as white tiger joint-running [wind] pattern in the formula books.”

Teachings of Zhu Dan-xi (丹溪心法 , *Dān Xī Xīn Fǎ*):

“遍身骨节疼痛，昼静夜剧，如虎噬之状，名曰白虎历节风。”

“Bone and joint pain of the entire body that is calm during the day but becomes violent at night and is likened to a tiger's bite is called white tiger joint-running wind.”

Further Treatises on the Properties of Things - Treatise on Gout (格至余论 · 痛风论 , *Gé Zhì Yú Lùn - Tòng Fēng Lùn*):

“痛风者，大率因血受热已自沸腾；其后或涉冷水，或立湿地，或扇取凉，或卧当风，寒凉外搏，热血得寒，污浊凝涩，所以作痛，夜则痛甚，行于阴也，治法以辛热之剂，流散寒湿，开发腠理，其血得行，与气相合，其病自安。”

“Gout is generally due to exposure of blood to heat, after which [the person] wades in cold water, is exposed to fanning to keep cool, or is exposed to wind during sleep. The blood heat combines with the cold and congeals with filthy turbidity; hence there is pain which worsens at night, the time of yin. Treatment requires acrid and hot formulas to dissipate cold-damp, open the interstices, and allow the blood to move in conformity with qi, thereby leading to recovery.”

Yong Lei Seal Formulary (永类钤方 , *Yǒng Lèi Qián Fāng*):

“体虚之人，受风寒湿毒之气，使血气筋脉凝滞，使于骨节四肢间，肉色不变，骨如虎噬之痛，昼静夜剧。”

“Exposure to wind, cold, and damp qi in those with constitutional deficiency will result in the congealing of qi and blood in the sinews, vessels, bones, and joints of the four limbs; no discoloration of the flesh;

bone pain that resembles a tiger's bite; and [symptoms that are] calm during the day but violent at night."

Essential Rhymes for Patterns and Treatment (证治要诀 , *Zhèng Zhì Yào Jué*):

"遍身骨节疼痛，昼静夜剧，如虎之噬，名白虎历节风。并宜加减地仙丹，或青龙丹、乳香丸等。"

"Bone and joint pain of the entire body that is calm during the day but becomes violent at night and is likened to a tiger's bite is called white tiger joint-running wind. Modified *Dì Xiān Dān* (地仙丹), *Qīng Lóng Dān* (青龙丹), or *Rǔ Xiāng Wán* (乳香丸) is the appropriate treatment."

Precepts for Physicians (医门法律 , *Yī Mén Fǎ Lǜ*):

"痛风一名白虎历节风，实即痛痹也。……独千金犀角汤一方，深有合于经意，特表之为例。"

"One of the names for gout is white tiger joint-running wind, which is painful *bi*…according to the classics, only *Qiān Jīn Xī Jiǎo Tāng* (千金犀角汤) is the suitable formula."

MODERN RESEARCH

Clinical Research

1. Pattern Differentiation and Corresponding Treatment

(1) Liu Ming-hui holds that gout falls within the scope of *bi* syndromes, which are primarily caused by excess wind evil. Wind evil combines with damp-heat or cold-damp, and invades the sinews and vessels, resulting in this disease.

Gout can be divided into heat *bi* and wind-cold-damp *bi*. Liu uses a self-composed formula, *Tòng Fēng Tāng* (痛风汤), which consists of the following ingredients:

五加皮	wǔ jiā pí	30g	Cortex Acanthopanacis
半枫荷	bàn fēng hé	30g	Pterospermum heterophyllum Hance
薏苡仁	yì yǐ rén	30g	Semen Coicis
木瓜	mù guā	30g	Fructus Chaenomelis
防己	fáng jǐ	15g	Radix Stephaniae Tetrandrae
牛膝	niú xī	15g	Radix Achyranthis Bidentatae
甘草	gān cǎo	5g	Radix et Rhizoma Glycyrrhizae

- For heat *bi*, add *qín jiāo* (Radix Gentianae Macrophyllae), *xī xiān cǎo* (Herba Siegesbeckiae), and *kuān jīn téng* (Caulis Tinosporae Sinensis).
- For wind-cold-damp *bi*, add *hǎi fēng téng* (Caulis Piperis Kadsurae), *qiān jīn bá* (Moghania Philippinensis), and *bái huā shé shé cǎo* (Herba Hedyotis).
- For severe joint pain, add *rù dì jīn niú* (Radix Zanthoxyli Nitidi).
- For fever, add *gōu téng* (Ramulus Uncariae Cum Uncis) and *qīng tiān kuí* (Nervilia Fordii).

The control group was administered allopurinol and vitamin B_1. The total efficacy rate of the treatment group was 94.9%, while that of the control group was 77.4%. Comparing the results of the two groups, the difference is significant ($P<0.01$). [1]

(2) Liu Zai-peng believes that the pathogenesis of gout involves congenital deficiency of spleen qi or acquired spleen damage due to an excessively rich and greasy diet.

In the initial stages of this disease, typical damp-heat symptoms include acute redness, swelling and pain of the joints. Over time, dampness transforms into turbid phlegm and accumulates, which appear as nodules surrounding the joints of sizes ranging from peas to ping-pong balls. Liu divided gout into five patterns: damp-heat pouring downward, stasis heat obstruction, spleen qi deficiency, and liver and kidney depletion. He often uses his own self-drafted formula, *Tòng Fēng Dìng Tòng Tāng* (痛风定痛汤), with modifications.

金钱草	jīn qián cǎo	Herba Lysimachiae
海金沙	hǎi jīn shā	Spora Lygodii
土茯苓	tǔ fú líng	Rhizoma Smilacis Glabrae
汉防己	hàn fáng jǐ	Radix Stephaniae Tetrandrae
车前子	chē qián zǐ	Semen Plantaginis
盐黄柏	yán huáng bǎi	Cortex Phellodendri Chinensis (salted)
泽泻	zé xiè	Rhizoma Alismatis
知母	zhī mǔ	Rhizoma Anemarrhenae
生地	shēng dì	Radix Rehmanniae Recens
生石膏	shēng shí gāo	Gypsum Fibrosum (raw)
广地龙	guǎng dì lóng	Pheretima
伸筋草	shēn jīn cǎo	Herba Lycopodii

➢ For redness, swelling, and burning pain of the joints, add *shēng shí gāo* (Gypsum Fibrosum).

➢ For obstruction due to blood stasis and heat manifesting as dark purple skin with sharp pain, add *huái niú xī* (Radix Achyranthis Bidentatae), *shēn jīn cǎo* (Herba Lycopodii), and *zé lán* (Herba Lycopi).

➢ For obstruction due to phlegm turbidity manifesting as nodules, add *shān cí gū* (Pseudobulbus Cremastrae seu Pleiones), *jiāng nán xīng* (Rhizoma Arisaematis), *jiāng cán* (Bombyx Batryticatus), and *cāng zhú* (Rhizoma Atractylodis) to transform phlegm and disperse nodules. Remove *shēng dì* (Radix Rehmanniae Recens), *shí gāo* (Gypsum Fibrosum), and *zhī mǔ* (Rhizoma Anemarrhenae).

➢ For spleen deficiency, add *dǎng shēn* (Radix Codonopsis) and *bái zhú* (Rhizoma Atractylodis Macrocephalae).[2]

(3) Huang Xiu-zhen, et al. explains that gout is caused by an excessively rich and greasy diet or excessive consumption of alcohol, all of which give rise to damp-heat, spleen-stomach damage, spleen and kidney deficiency, and dysfunction of the *zang-fu*.

The pathogenesis of gout involves failure of the spleen to transform and transport and failure of the kidney to control qi transformation, which cause the internal generation of water-dampness. The dampness collects to form phlegm, and the phlegm and damp-heat bind together and linger in the vessels to impair blood circulation, then pour into the joints to damage the sinews and corrode bones. This disease can be divided into the following three patterns: damp-heat brewing and binding, phlegm-stasis obstruction, and chronic *bi* giving rise to right qi deficiency. The following prescription is used as a base formula:

土茯苓	tǔ fú líng	10-30g	Rhizoma Smilacis Glabrae
车前子	chē qián zǐ	10-30g	Semen Plantaginis
萆薢	bì xiè	10-20g	Rhizoma Dioscoreae Hypoglaucae
黄精	huáng jīng	10-30g	Rhizoma Polygonati
丹参	dān shēn	15g	Radix et Rhizoma Salviae Miltiorrhizae
地龙	dì lóng	10g	Pheretima

➢ For damp-heat accumulation, add *huáng bǎi* (Cortex Phellodendri Chinensis) 15g, *cāng zhú* (Rhizoma Atractylodis) 10g, *chuān niú xī* (Radix Cyathulae) 15g, *yì yǐ rén* (Semen Coicis) 15g, *rěn dōng téng* (Caulis Lonicerae Japonicae) 30g, *shān cí gū* (Pseudobulbus Cremastrae seu Pleiones) 10g, *xī xiān cǎo* (Herba Siegesbeckiae) 30g, *hǔ zhàng* (Rhizoma Polygoni Cuspidati) 15g, *wēi líng xiān* (Radix et Rhizoma Clematidis) 15g, and *gān cǎo* (Radix et Rhizoma Glycyrrhizae) 5g.

➢ For phlegm-stasis obstruction, add *dāng guī* (Radix Angelicae Sinensis) 15g, *chuān xiōng* (Rhizoma Chuanxiong) 5g, *táo rén* (Semen Persicae) 10g, *hóng huā* (Flos Carthami) 5g, *wēi líng xiān* (Radix et Rhizoma Clematidis) 10g, *bái jiè zǐ* (Semen Sinapis) 10g, *zhì nán xīng* (Rhizoma Arisaematis Praeparatum) 10g, *bái sháo* (Radix Paeoniae Alba) 10g, *xī xiān cǎo* (Herba Siegesbeckiae) 30g, and *gān cǎo* (Radix et Rhizoma Glycyrrhizae) 5g.

➢ For chronic *bi* giving rise to right qi deficiency, add *dāng guī* (Radix Angelicae Sinensis) 10g, *bái sháo* (Radix Paeoniae Alba) 10g, *bái zhú* (Rhizoma Atractylodis Macrocephalae) 10g, *sāng jì shēng* (Herba Taxilli)

15g, *dù zhòng* (Cortex Eucommiae) 10g, *gǒu qǐ* (Fructus Lycii) 15g, *huáng qí* (Radix Astragali) 20g, *jī xuè téng* (Caulis Spatholobi) 20g, and *wū shāo shé* (Zaocys) 15g.

The control group consisted of 52 patients who were given ibuprofen and allopurinol. The total efficacy rate of the treatment group (which consisted of 56 patients) was 94.64%, while that of the control group was 78.85%. The difference of two groups was significant ($P<0.01$).[3]

(4) Fang Ce and Yu Zhi-qiang believe that gout belongs to the categories of heat *bi* or wind-damp-heat *bi*. They treat this disease according to the pathogenesis as determined by the signs and symptoms.

1) Damp-heat Brewing and Binding

Treatment is focused on clearing heat, draining dampness, invigorating blood, dissipating binds, and resolving toxins. *Sì Miào Sǎn* (四妙散) is often prescribed, with modifications.

苍术	cāng zhú	15g	Rhizoma Atractylodis
黄柏	huáng bǎi	15g	Cortex Phellodendri Chinensis
萆薢	bì xiè	15g	Rhizoma Dioscoreae Hypoglaucae
牛膝	niú xī	15g	Radix Achyranthis Bidentatae
薏苡仁	yì yǐ rén	20g	Semen Coicis
当归	dāng guī	15g	Radix Angelicae Sinensis
金银花	jīn yín huā	15g	Flos Lonicerae Japonicae
木通	mù tōng	15g	Caulis Akebiae
山慈菇	shān cí gū	20g	Pseudobulbus Cremastrae seu Pleiones

2) Obstruction of Stasis Heat

Treatment is aimed at clearing heat, dispersing stasis, unblocking the collaterals, and relieving pain. *Zhī Téng Tāng* (枝藤汤) is often prescribed, with modifications.

桑枝	sāng zhī	30g	Ramulus Mori
忍冬藤	rěn dōng téng	30g	Caulis Lonicerae Japonicae
牛膝	niú xī	10g	Radix Achyranthis Bidentatae

生地	shēng dì	15g	Radix Rehmanniae Recens
丹皮	dān pí	10g	Cortex Moutan
白芍	bái sháo	15g	Radix Paeoniae Alba
乳香	rǔ xiāng	15g	Olibanum
没药	mò yào	15g	Myrrha
红花	hóng huā	15g	Flos Carthami

3) Phlegm-turbidity Obstruction

Treatment involves clearing phlegm, transforming turbidity, dispersing stasis, and discharging heat. *Dí Tán Tāng* (涤痰汤) is often prescribed, with modifications.

半夏	bàn xià	20g	Rhizoma Pinelliae
陈皮	chén pí	15g	Pericarpium Citri Reticulatae
竹茹	zhú rú	15g	Caulis Bambusae in Taenia
木通	mù tōng	15g	Caulis Akebiae
枳壳	zhǐ qiào	15g	Fructus Aurantii
牛膝	niú xī	10g	Radix Achyranthis Bidentatae
丹参	dān shēn	10g	Radix et Rhizoma Salviae Miltiorrhizae
红花	hóng huā	10g	Flos Carthami
赤芍	chì sháo	15g	Radix Paeoniae Rubra

4) Liver and Kidney Yin Deficiency

Treatment requires enriching the liver and tonifying the kidney. The selected formula is *Liù Wèi Dì Huáng Tāng* (六味地黄汤) with modifications. Decoct the medicinals with water to 100 ml and take three times a day. The efficacy rate is 94.6%. [4]

山药	shān yào	15g	Rhizoma Dioscoreae
山茱萸	shān zhū yú	15g	Fructus Corni
熟地	shú dì	15g	Radix Rehmanniae Praeparata
茯苓	fú líng	20g	Poria
丹皮	dān pí	10g	Cortex Moutan
黄柏	huáng bǎi	15g	Cortex Phellodendri Chinensis
知母	zhī mǔ	10g	Rhizoma Anemarrhenae

枸杞子	gǒu qǐ zǐ	20g	Fructus Lycii
女贞子	nǚ zhēn zǐ	20g	Fructus Ligustri Lucidi
牛膝	niú xī	10g	Radix Achyranthis Bidentatae
苍术	cāng zhú	15g	Rhizoma Atractylodis

(5) Zhang Chun-hua believes that gout is caused by the internal accumulation of damp-heat due to excessive consumption of fatty and sweet foods. The damp-heat seeps into the flesh and joints and may be complicated by contraction of external evils that invade the channels and collaterals, resulting in a phlegm-stasis complex. In the initial stage, the disease is located in the channels and the evil excess dominates, manifesting as damp-heat and phlegm-stasis obstruction. In the chronic stage of gout, there is liver, spleen, and kidney deficiency and damp-phlegm stasis obstruction as the disease enters the sinews and bones, the *zang-fu*, and the collaterals. Clinical treatment is based on pathogenesis as determined by differentiation of signs and symptoms:

1) Damp-heat and Stasis Binding

Clear heat, drain dampness, transform stasis, and relieve pain. Modified *Sì Miào Sǎn* (四妙散) plus *Bái Hǔ Jiā Guì Zhī Tāng* (白虎加桂枝汤) can be prescribed. The dregs can be used to administer a foot bath.

苍术	cāng zhú	10g	Rhizoma Atractylodis
黄柏	huáng bǎi	10g	Cortex Phellodendri Chinensis
知母	zhī mǔ	10g	Rhizoma Anemarrhenae
桂枝	guì zhī	10g	Ramulus Cinnamomi
生石膏	shēng shí gāo	30g	Gypsum Fibrosum (raw)
薏米仁	yì mǐ rén	30g	Semen Coicis
牛膝	niú xī	15g	Radix Achyranthis Bidentatae
元胡	yuán hú	15g	Rhizoma Corydalis
木瓜	mù guā	15g	Fructus Chaenomelis
甘草	gān cǎo	6g	Radix et Rhizoma Glycyrrhizae

2) Liver, Spleen, and Kidney Deficiency with Phlegm, Dampness and Stasis Obstruction

Enrich and tonify the liver and kidney, fortify the spleen and drain dampness, invigorate blood, and relieve pain. Use a modified version of *Liù Wèi Dì Huáng Tāng* (六味地黄汤). The dregs can be redecocted and used to wash the affected area.

熟地	shú dì	24g	Radix Rehmanniae Praeparata
山药	shān yào	12g	Rhizoma Dioscoreae
山萸肉	shān yú ròu	12g	Fructus Corni
丹皮	dān pí	10g	Cortex Moutan
茯苓	fú líng	10g	Poria
泽泻	zé xiè	10g	Rhizoma Alismatis
木瓜	mù guā	15g	Fructus Chaenomelis
牛膝	niú xī	15g	Radix Achyranthis Bidentatae
元胡	yuán hú	15g	Rhizoma Corydalis
秦艽	qín jiāo	30g	Radix Gentianae Macrophyllae
薏米仁	yì mǐ rén	30g	Semen Coicis
蜈蚣	wú gōng	2	Scolopendra
甘草	gān cǎo	6g	Radix et Rhizoma Glycyrrhizae

Based on clinical observation, Chinese medicinals can effectively improve symptoms and relieve pain. The internal medicinals combined with using the redecocted dregs as an external wash can achieve the effects of warming and unblocking the channels and collaterals to relieve pain. [5]

2. Treatment According to Stages

Most scholars divide gout into acute, interval, and chronic stages.

Yu Li believes that in acute conditions, one should treat the branch. In gout, the main pathogenesis of the acute stage is damp-heat evil, thus treatment should emphasize clearing heat, draining dampness, resolving toxins, and unblocking the collaterals. Use modified *Sān Miào Săn* (三妙散). In moderate conditions, one should treat the root. During the remission stage of gout, the root is spleen deficiency, while the branch is damp-turbidity transforming into heat; treat by fortifying spleen qi using modified *Shēn Líng Bái Zhú Sǎn* (参苓白术散).[6]

Cao Yong-xiang, et al. believe that in the acute stage of gout, red, swollen, hot, and painful joints should be identified as damp-heat *bi*; the chronic stage is often attributed to cold-damp *bi*; if recurrent attacks cause joint deformity, treat the condition as lame *bi* (尪痹 , *wāng bì*); in the late stage, uric acid crystals deposit in renal interstitium and renal tubules and cause pathological changes to the renal tubules and renal interstitium, a characteristic of gouty nephropathy. According to the main clinical manifestations, gouty nephropathy can be attributed to "water swelling" and "deficiency taxation." This disease can be divided into four stages: acute stage, interval stage, chronic arthritis stage, and gouty nephropathy stage.

1) Treat the acute stage by clearing heat, resolving toxins, draining dampness, and dispersing swelling. Use a modified combination of *Sì Miào Sǎn* (四妙散) plus *Wǔ Wèi Xiāo Dú Yǐn* (五味消毒饮).

黄柏	huáng bǎi	12g	Cortex Phellodendri Chinensis
苍术	cāng zhú	12g	Rhizoma Atractylodis
栀子	zhī zǐ	12g	Fructus Gardeniae
赤芍	chì sháo	12g	Radix Paeoniae Rubra
薏苡仁	yì yǐ rén	15g	Semen Coicis
威灵仙	wēi líng xiān	15g	Radix et Rhizoma Clematidis
天葵	tiān kuí	15g	Radix Semiaquilegiae
茵陈	yīn chén	18g	Herba Artemisiae Scopariae
络石藤	luò shí téng	30g	Caulis Trachelospermi
地丁草	dì dīng cǎo	30g	Herba Corydalis Bungeanae
蒲公英	pú gōng yīng	30g	Herba Taraxaci

2) The interval stage is the period of symptom relief after attacks subside. It is often identified as spleen deficiency with damp encumbrance;

treat by fortifying the spleen to transform dampness. A modified combination of *Sān Rén Tāng* (三仁汤) plus *Shēn Líng Bái Zhú Sǎn* (参苓白术散) is often used.

杏仁	xìng rén	12g	Semen Armeniacae Amarum
蔻仁	kòu rén	12g	Fructus Amomi Rotundus
滑石	huá shí	12g	Talcum
苍术	cāng zhú	12g	Rhizoma Atractylodis
黄柏	huáng bǎi	12g	Cortex Phellodendri Chinensis
防己	fáng jǐ	12g	Radix Stephaniae Tetrandrae
白术	bái zhú	12g	Rhizoma Atractylodis Macrocephalae
人参	rén shēn	18g	Radix Ginseng
法半夏	fǎ bàn xià	15g	Rhizoma Pinelliae Praeparatum
苡仁	yǐ rén	15g	Semen Coicis
茯苓	fú líng	15g	Poria

3) Chronic arthritis stage often manifests with bone erosion; fibrosis of the surrounding tissue; joint stiffness, deformity, and pain; emaciation of the body; a pale red tongue, and a thready pulse. The symptoms and signs of this stage can be differentiated as liver and kidney depletion or phlegm-stasis obstructing the collaterals. Treat by invigorating blood, transforming stasis, and tonifying and boosting the liver and kidney. A modified combination of *Dú Huó Jì Shēng Tāng* (独活寄生汤) plus *Sì Miào Sǎn* (四妙散) is commonly used.

独活	dú huó	12g	Radix Angelicae Pubescentis
防风	fáng fēng	12g	Radix Saposhnikoviae
苍术	cāng zhú	12g	Rhizoma Atractylodis
桃仁	táo rén	12g	Semen Persicae
红花	hóng huā	12g	Flos Carthami
陈皮	chén pí	12g	Pericarpium Citri Reticulatae
寄生	jì shēng	15g	Herba Taxilli
威灵仙	wēi líng xiān	15g	Radix et Rhizoma Clematidis
牛膝	niú xī	15g	Radix Achyranthis Bidentatae

法半夏	fǎ bàn xià	15g	Rhizoma Pinelliae Praeparatum
苡仁	yǐ rén	30g	Semen Coicis
鸡血藤	jī xuè téng	30g	Caulis Spatholobi

4) During gouty nephropathy stage, the differentiation of symptoms and signs should be based on the principles of yin and yang. For liver and kidney yin deficiency, use modified *Guī Sháo Dì Huáng Tāng* (归芍地黄汤); for dual deficiency of qi and yin, prescribe modified *Shēn Qí Dì Huáng Tāng* (参芪地黄汤); for spleen and kidney yang deficiency, use modified *Bǎo Yuán Tāng* (保元汤).[7]

Wu Qi-fu, et al. divided gout into the following patterns: spleen deficiency with phlegm turbidity (elevated blood uric acid stage), damp-heat (acute episode stage), and kidney deficiency with phlegm-stasis (prolonged active stage). *Tòng Qīng No. 2 Chōng Jì* (痛清2号冲剂) was made into granules and used to treat 60 cases of acute gouty arthritis.

黄柏	huáng bǎi	Cortex Phellodendri Chinensis
大黄	dà huáng	Radix et Rhizoma Rhei
苦参	kǔ shēn	Radix Sophorae Flavescentis
丹皮	dān pí	Cortex Moutan
虎杖	hǔ zhàng	Rhizoma Polygoni Cuspidati
金银花	jīn yín huā	Flos Lonicerae Japonicae
乳香	rǔ xiāng	Olibanum
没药	mò yào	Myrrha
制附子	zhì fù zǐ	Radix Aconiti Lateralis Praeparata

The control group consisted of 60 patients that were administered colchicine plus a non-steroidal anti-inflammatory drug (NSAID). After the symptoms were controlled, the patients were administered probenecid or allopurinol. Ten days equaled a course of treatment. After two treatment courses, the therapeutic effects were evaluated: The relief of red, swollen, hot, and painful joints and the decrease in the blood uric acid and blood lipid levels in the experimental group far surpassed those in the control group (P<0.01).[8]

Chen Jin-ye believes that most gout patients consume too much alcohol and foods that are high in fat and protein, making them susceptible to the development of damp-heat in their bodies. The damp-heat lingers in the spleen and stomach and travels along the spleen channel of foot taiyin and the stomach channel of foot yangming, resulting in redness, swelling, and burning pain of the big toe. Dr. Chen uses a self-composed formula, *Yùn Pí Lì Niào Liáng Xuè Fāng* (运脾利尿凉血方), to fortify the spleen, transform dampness, promote urination to discharge turbidity, clear heat, and cool blood.

土茯苓	tǔ fú líng	20g	Rhizoma Smilacis Glabrae
川萆薢	chuān bì xiè	20g	Rhizoma Dioscoreae Hypoglaucae
焦山楂	jiāo shān zhā	20g	Fructus Crataegi (scorch-fried)
猪苓	zhū líng	15g	Polyporus
瞿麦	qú mài	15g	Herba Dianthi
萹蓄	biǎn xù	15g	Herba Polygoni Avicularis
车前子	chē qián zǐ	15g	Semen Plantaginis
玄参	xuán shēn	15g	Radix Scrophulariae
黄柏	huáng bǎi	15g	Cortex Phellodendri Chinensis
生薏仁	shēng yǐ rén	30g	Semen Coicis (raw)
清风藤	qīng fēng téng	30g	Caulis Sinomenii
白术	bái zhú	10g	Rhizoma Atractylodis Macrocephalae
丹皮	dān pí	10g	Cortex Moutan

➢ In the acute stage, *shēng shí gāo* (raw Gypsum Fibrosum) 60g, *cāng zhú* (Rhizoma Atractylodis) 10g, and *zhī mǔ* (Rhizoma Anemarrhenae) 10g can be added.

➢ In the chronic stage, *dāng guī* (Radix Angelicae Sinensis) 10g, *zé xiè* (Rhizoma Alismatis) 10g, and *zào jiǎo cì* (Spina Gleditsiae) 10g can be added.

➢ For patients with urinary calculi, the dosage of *xuán shēn* (Radix Scrophulariae) may be reduced, and *shí wěi* (Folium Pyrrosiae) 20g and *jīn qián cǎo* (Herba Lysimachiae) 20g can be added.

Decoct the ingredients in water; take one batch per day. Fifteen days equals a course of treatment. Usually, 2 to 3 treatment courses are required, with a one-week interval between each course. In the late stage, the patient may take the decoction every other day.

55 patients were administered 1-3 courses of treatment, of which 49 were cured, 4 showed improvement, and 2 received no effect. The total efficacy rate was 96.4%. [9]

Chen Xiang-jun regards the root of gout as spleen deficiency and the branch as damp-turbidity. Over time, the disease enters the collaterals and combines with phlegm-stasis to cause obstruction. Treat the acute stage by clearing heat, discharging turbidity, and unblocking the collaterals in conjunction with fortifying the spleen. Treat the chronic stage by fortifying the spleen, boosting the kidney, and transforming turbidity.

1) For the acute stage, the base formula is modified *Sān Miào Wán* (三妙丸):

苍术	cāng zhú	12g	Rhizoma Atractylodis
知母	zhī mǔ	12g	Rhizoma Anemarrhenae
黄柏	huáng bǎi	12g	Cortex Phellodendri Chinensis
牛膝	niú xī	15g	Radix Achyranthis Bidentatae
土茯苓	tǔ fú líng	30g	Rhizoma Smilacis Glabrae
山慈菇	shān cí gū	15g	Pseudobulbus Cremastrae seu Pleiones
虎杖	hǔ zhàng	30g	Rhizoma Polygoni Cuspidati
忍冬藤	rěn dōng téng	30g	Caulis Lonicerae Japonicae
制大黄	zhì dà huáng	15g	Radix et Rhizoma Rhei (prepared)
野木瓜	yě mù guā	15g	Fructus Chaenomelis
蚕沙	cán shā	15g	Faeces Bombycis
茯苓	fú líng	15g	Poria
白术	bái zhú	12g	Rhizoma Atractylodis Macrocephalae
露蜂房	lù fēng fáng	12g	Nidus Vespae
地鳖虫	dì biē chóng	12g	Eupolyphaga seu Steleophaga

Sān Miào Wán plus *tǔ fú líng* (Rhizoma Smilacis Glabrae), *shān cí gū* (Pseudobulbus Cremastrae seu Pleiones), *hǔ zhàng* (Rhizoma Polygoni Cuspidati), *yě mù guā* (Fructus Chaenomelis), *cán shā* (Faeces Bombycis), *zhì dà huáng* (Radix et Rhizoma Rhei) to clear away heat and turbidity, expel damp-heat in the lower *jiao*; *fú líng* (Poria) and *bái zhú* (Rhizoma Atractylodis Macrocephalae) to invigorate spleen and eliminate dampness; *lù fēng fáng* (Nidus Vespae), *rěn dōng téng* (Caulis Lonicerae Japonicae) and *dì biē chóng* (Eupolyphaga seu Steleophaga) to unblock the channels and collaterals and disperse stasis; all of the medicinals have the function of clearing heat, draining turbidity and unblocking collaterals.

2) For the chronic stage, use the following formula to invigorate the blood and unblock the collaterals, which is in accordance with the theory that chronic disease will invariably lead to stasis and enter the collaterals.[10]

生白术	shēng bái zhú	12g	Rhizoma Atractylodis Macrocephalae (raw)
生黄芪	shēng huáng qí	30g	Radix Astragali (raw)
茯苓	fú líng	15g	Poria
杜仲	dù zhòng	12g	Cortex Eucommiae
补骨脂	bǔ gǔ zhī	15g	Fructus Psoraleae
牛膝	niú xī	15g	Radix Achyranthis Bidentatae
土茯苓	tǔ fú líng	30g	Rhizoma Smilacis Glabrae
山慈菇	shān cí gū	15g	Pseudobulbus Cremastrae seu Pleiones
野木瓜	yě mù guā	15g	Fructus Chaenomelis
鸡血藤	jī xuè téng	30g	Caulis Spatholobi
川芎	chuān xiōng	30g	Rhizoma Chuanxiong

Xu Xiao-fang and Zhu Rong feel that the root of gout is attributed to dual deficiency of the spleen and kidney, qi and blood deficiency, and yang insufficiency, while the branch is attributed to dampness, stasis, and cold. Internal exuberance of damp-turbidity is the main pathomechanism of gout; the main treatment principles include tonifying deficiency, fortifying the spleen, boosting the kidney, and transforming dampness.

Use *Sì Jūn Zǐ Tāng* (四君子汤) with the addition of medicinals that fortify the spleen and transform dampness, and those that invigorate blood and unblock the collaterals. In the acute stage, slightly reduce the number of tonifying medicinals that are cloying, and add agents that clear heat and transform dampness. Beware of overusing cold medicinals after most of the symptoms have been alleviated. During the chronic stage, there is kidney yang insufficiency complicated by varying proportions of stasis and cold; use a formula that warms the kidney, frees yang, dispels stasis, and dissipates cold.

1) Acute episodes:

A. For damp-heat pattern, fortify the spleen, transform dampness, and clear heat; prescribe *Sì Miào Sǎn* (四妙散) plus medicinals that fortify the spleen and transform dampness, in addition to external application of medicinals.

B. For cold-damp pattern, treat by dispelling wind, overcoming dampness, warming the channels, and dissipating cold; prescribe modified *Guì Zhī Sháo Yào Zhī Mǔ Tāng* (桂枝芍药知母汤) in conjunction with external application of medicinals.

2) The chronic stage mostly involves the spleen and the kidney:

A. For weakness of qi due to spleen deficiency, fortify the spleen, transform dampness, and warm and unblock the channels and collaterals; use *Sì Jūn Zǐ Tāng* (四君子汤) with modifications.

B. For deficiency cold in the middle *jiao*, fortify the spleen, transform dampness, and warm and unblock the channels and collaterals; use *Lǐ Zhōng Wán* (理中丸) with modifications.

C. For spleen and kidney yang deficiency, fortify the spleen, warm the kidney, discharge turbidity, and invigorate blood; use *Lǐ Zhōng Wán* (理中丸) plus *Jīn Guì Shèn Qì Wán* (金匮肾气丸) or modified *Yòu Guī Wán* (右归丸).[11]

3. Specific Formulas

(1) Research on Traditional Formulas

A. ***Jiā Wèi Shàng, Zhōng, Xià Tōng Yòng Tòng Fēng Wán [Tāng]*** **(加味上、中、下通用痛风丸[汤])**

黄柏	huáng bǎi	10g	Cortex Phellodendri Chinensis
苍术	cāng zhú	10g	Rhizoma Atractylodis
南星	nán xīng	10g	Rhizoma Arisaematis
神曲	shén qū	10g	Massa Medicata Fermentata
川芎	chuān xiōng	10g	Rhizoma Chuanxiong
桃仁	táo rén	10g	Semen Persicae
龙胆草	lóng dǎn cǎo	10g	Radix et Rhizoma Gentianae
防己	fáng jǐ	10g	Radix Stephaniae Tetrandrae
白芷	bái zhǐ	10g	Radix Angelicae Dahuricae
羌活	qiāng huó	10g	Rhizoma et Radix Notopterygii
威灵仙	wēi líng xiān	10g	Radix et Rhizoma Clematidis
桂皮	guì pí	10g	Cortex Cinnamomi
红花	hóng huā	10g	Flos Carthami

➢ For spleen deficiency with damp-turbidity, add *dǎng shēn* (Radix Codonopsis), *huáng qí* (Radix Astragali), *yì yǐ rén* (Semen Coicis), and *jiǔ jié chāng pǔ* (Rhizoma Acori Tatarinowii).

➢ For damp-heat brewing and binding, add *tǔ fú líng* (Rhizoma Smilacis Glabrae), *bàn zhī lián* (Herba Scutellariae Barbatae), and *luò shí téng* (Caulis Trachelospermi).

➢ For phlegm-stasis obstruction, add *hǔ zhàng* (Rhizoma Polygoni Cuspidati), *bèi mǔ* (Bulbus Fritillaria), and *tiān zhú huáng* (Concretio Silicea Bambusae).

➢ For liver and kidney yin deficiency, add *shēng dì* (Radix Rehmanniae Recens), *shān yú ròu* (Fructus Corni), and *biē jiǎ* (Carapax Trionycis).

86 patients of primary gout were randomly divided into treatment and control groups. The treatment group consisted of 48 patients while the control group consisted of 38. Patients in the control group were given

Huá Tuó Zài Zào Wán (华佗再造丸) orally to invigorate blood, transform stasis, transform phlegm, and unblock the collaterals. The treatment group was treated with the above formula and modifications. In the treatment group, 29 were cured, 15 showed excellent improvement, and 4 had no effect; the total efficacy rate was 91.66%. In the control group, 10 were cured, 16 had excellent improvement, and 12 had no effect; the total efficacy rate was 68.42%. Statistically, the therapeutic results of the treatment group was better than that of the control group ($P<0.05$). [12]

Chen Zu-hong treated gout with the following formula:

苍术	cāng zhú	15g	Rhizoma Atractylodis
黄柏	huáng bǎi	15g	Cortex Phellodendri Chinensis
防己	fáng jǐ	15g	Radix Stephaniae Tetrandrae
威灵仙	wēi líng xiān	15g	Radix et Rhizoma Clematidis
制南星	zhì nán xīng	15g	Rhizoma Arisaematis Praeparatum
泽泻	zé xiè	15g	Rhizoma Alismatis
车前子	chē qián zǐ	15g	Semen Plantaginis
川芎	chuān xiōng	10g	Rhizoma Chuanxiong
桃仁	táo rén	10g	Semen Persicae
红花	hóng huā	10g	Flos Carthami
羌活	qiāng huó	10g	Rhizoma et Radix Notopterygii
桂枝	guì zhī	10g	Ramulus Cinnamomi
土茯苓	tǔ fú líng	25g	Rhizoma Smilacis Glabrae
萆薢	bì xiè	20g	Rhizoma Dioscoreae Hypoglaucae

➢ For exuberant damp-heat manifesting as red, swollen, and hot joints, constipation, scanty reddish urine, a yellow greasy tongue coating, and a slippery rapid pulse, reduce the dosage of *nán xīng* (Rhizoma Arisaematis) and *guì zhī* (Ramulus Cinnamomi), increase *tǔ fú líng* (Rhizoma Smilacis Glabrae) to 45g, and add *bì xiè* (Rhizoma Dioscoreae Hypoglaucae) to 35g, *dà huáng* (Radix et Rhizoma Rhei) 12g (decocted later), *rěn dōng téng* (Caulis Lonicerae Japonicae) 15g, and *xī xiān cǎo* (Herba Siegesbeckiae) 15g.

➢ For exuberant cold-damp manifesting as severe joint pain with mild swelling that is aggravated by cold, a white tongue coating, and a deep wiry pulse, add *zhì fù zǐ* (Radix Aconiti Lateralis Praeparata), *zhì chuān wū* (Radix Aconiti Praeparata), *zhì cǎo wū* (Radix Aconiti Kusnezoffii Praeparata), *xì xīn* (Radix et Rhizoma Asari) and *hǎi fēng téng* (Caulis Piperis Kadsurae). Adjust dosages according to the symptoms.

➢ For chronic, elderly patients with recurrent attacks accompanied by soreness and weakness of the lumbus and knees, frequent nocturia, and sloppy stool, add *jī xuè téng* (Caulis Spatholobi) 30g, *sāng jì shēng* (Herba Taxilli) 30g, *dù zhòng* (Cortex Eucommiae) 15g, *wǔ jiā pí* (Cortex Acanthopanacis) 15g, *wū shāo shé* (Zaocys) 15g, and *quán xiē* (Scorpio) 8g.

➢ During periods of pain relief, add *Dú Huó Jì Shēng Tāng* (独活寄生汤) with modifications.

Of 55 cases treated with the above formula and appropriate modifications, 44 were cured (80%), 4 showed excellent improvement, 5 showed some improvement, and 2 showed no effect. The total efficacy rate was 96.4%. [13]

B. Modified *Sì Miào Wán* (四妙丸):

苍术	cāng zhú	12g	Rhizoma Atractylodis
黄柏	huáng bǎi	12g	Cortex Phellodendri Chinensis
薏苡仁	yì yǐ rén	30g	Semen Coicis
牛膝	niú xī	30g	Radix Achyranthis Bidentatae
忍冬藤	rěn dōng téng	30g	Caulis Lonicerae Japonicae
伸筋草	shēn jīn cǎo	30g	Herba Lycopodii
土茯苓	tǔ fú líng	30g	Rhizoma Smilacis Glabrae
鸡血藤	jī xuè téng	30g	Caulis Spatholobi
萆薢	bì xiè	30g	Rhizoma Dioscoreae Hypoglaucae
苏木	sū mù	15g	Lignum Sappan
刘寄奴	liú jì nú	15g	Herba Artemisiae Anomalae
蜂房	fēng fáng	12g	Nidus Vespae
血竭	xuè jié	6g	Sanguis Draconis
车前子	chē qián zǐ	20g	Semen Plantaginis
山慈菇	shān cí gū	15g	Pseudobulbus Cremastrae seu Pleiones

➢ For severe pain, add *zhì nán xīng* (Rhizoma Arisaematis Praeparatum) 30g and *qín jiāo* (Radix Gentianae Macrophyllae) 12g.

➢ For severe redness and swelling, add *shuǐ niú jiǎo* (Cornu Bubali) 30g and *shí gāo* (Gypsum Fibrosum) 30g.

➢ For constipation, add *dà huáng* (Radix et Rhizoma Rhei) 6g.

One batch per day; decocted in water until reduced to 300ml; divided into three portions and taken warm.. Ten days equaled a course of treatment. Of 24 cases, 9 were cured, 13 showed excellent improvement, and 2 received no effect. The total efficacy rate was 91.67%. [14]

Yin Lian treated acute gouty arthritis with modified *Sì Miào Wán* (四妙丸). In 45 reports on 1 500 patients of acute gouty arthritis, the total efficacy rate was above 90%, with a significant reduction in uric acid levels and low recurrence rate. [15]

C. *Dāng Guī Niān Tòng Tāng* (当归拈痛汤):

当归	dāng guī	12g	Radix Angelicae Sinensis
茵陈	yīn chén	12g	Herba Artemisiae Scopariae
川芎	chuān xiōng	12g	Rhizoma Chuanxiong
羌活	qiāng huó	10g	Rhizoma et Radix Notopterygii
防风	fáng fēng	10g	Radix Saposhnikoviae
葛根	gé gēn	10g	Radix Puerariae Lobatae
知母	zhī mǔ	10g	Rhizoma Anemarrhenae
秦艽	qín jiāo	15g	Radix Gentianae Macrophyllae
猪苓	zhū líng	15g	Polyporus
泽泻	zé xiè	15g	Rhizoma Alismatis
苍术	cāng zhú	15g	Rhizoma Atractylodis
茯苓	fú líng	30g	Poria
白术	bái zhú	30g	Rhizoma Atractylodis Macrocephalae
甘草	gān cǎo	6g	Radix et Rhizoma Glycyrrhizae

After controlling the redness, swelling, and pain, modify the formula according to the symptoms:

➢ For spleen and kidney deficiency, tonify and boost the spleen and kidney with medicinals such as *shān yào* (Rhizoma Dioscoreae) 30g and *yín yáng huò* (Herba Epimedii) 30g.

➢ For dampness stagnating in the channels and collaterals resulting in soreness, distention, and heaviness, and inhibited bending and stretching, add *yì yǐ rén* (Semen Coicis) 15g and *bì xiè* (Rhizoma Dioscoreae Hypoglaucae) 15g.

Wén Hé Gāo (蚊合膏) was added for external application :

五倍子	wǔ bèi zǐ	30g	Galla Chinensis
大黄	dà huáng	15g	Radix et Rhizoma Rhei
黄柏	huáng bǎi	15g	Cortex Phellodendri Chinensis
冰片	bīng piàn	5g	Borneolum Syntheticum
米醋	mǐ cù		rice vinegar

The ingredients were made into a paste with rice vinegar and used as an external application. Of 42 patients, 37 achieved a clinical cure, 4 showed marked improvement, 1 showed some improvement. The total efficacy rate was 100%. [16]

D. *Fù Fāng Chèn Tòng Sǎn* (复方趁痛散)

制川乌	zhì chuān wū	10g	Radix Aconiti Praeparata
桑枝	sāng zhī	30g	Ramulus Mori
萆薢	bì xiè	15g	Rhizoma Dioscoreae Hypoglaucae
金钱草	jīn qián cǎo	15g	Herba Lysimachiae
牵牛子	qiān niú zǐ	15g	Semen Pharbitidis
田七	tián qī	5g	Radix et Rhizoma Notoginseng
海马	hǎi mǎ	5g	Hippocampus
白芍	bái sháo	15g	Radix Paeoniae Alba
益母草	yì mǔ cǎo	15g	Herba Leonuri
刺五加	cì wǔ jiā	15g	Radix et Rhizoma seu Caulis Acanthopanacis Senticosi
甘草	gān cǎo	6g	Radix et Rhizoma Glycyrrhizae

Of 42 cases, 31 showed marked improvement, 9 showed some improvement, and 2 had no effect. The total efficacy rate was 95.22%. [17]

E. Modified *Mù Fáng Jǐ Tāng* (木防己汤):

防己	fáng jǐ	30g	Radix Stephaniae Tetrandrae
滑石	huá shí	20g	Talcum
苡仁	yǐ rén	20g	Semen Coicis
石膏	shí gāo	30g	Gypsum Fibrosum
桂枝	guì zhī	10g	Ramulus Cinnamomi
通草	tōng cǎo	10g	Medulla Tetrapanacis
杏仁	xìng rén	12g	Semen Armeniacae Amarum

- For severe pain, add *jiāng huáng* (Rhizoma Curcumae Longae) and *hǎi tóng pí* (Cortex Erythrinae).
- For pronounced heat, add *zhī mǔ* (Rhizoma Anemarrhenae) and *sāng zhī* (Ramulus Mori).
- For marked swelling, add *bì xiè* (Rhizoma Dioscoreae Hypoglaucae), *cāng zhú* (Rhizoma Atractylodis), and *jiǎ zhū* (Squama Manis).
- For absence of sweating, add *qiāng huó* (Rhizoma et Radix Notopterygii) and *xì xīn* (Radix et Rhizoma Asari).
- For excessive sweating, add *huáng qí* (Radix Astragali) and *zhì gān cǎo* (Radix Glycyrrhizae Praeparata cum Melle).
- For phlegm-rheum, add *bàn xià* (Rhizoma Pinelliae), *hòu pò* (Cortex Magnoliae Officinalis), and *guǎng chén pí* (Pericarpium Citri Reticulatae).

Decocted in water for oral intake, one batch per day, divided into three portions a day. Seven days equaled a course of treatment, and 2-3 courses were given consecutively. The total efficacy rate of 55 cases treated with the above formula and modifications was 96.36%. [18]

G. *Guì Zhī Sháo Yào Zhī Mǔ Tāng* (桂枝芍药知母汤):

炙桂枝	zhì guì zhī	Ramulus Cinnamomi (liquid-fried)
赤芍	chì sháo	Radix Paeoniae Rubra
白芍	bái sháo	Radix Paeoniae Alba
知母	zhī mǔ	Rhizoma Anemarrhenae
生麻黄	shēng má huáng	Herba Ephedrae (raw)

熟附子	shú fù zĭ	Radix Aconiti Lateralis Praeparata
白术	bái zhú	Rhizoma Atractylodis Macrocephalae
炙甘草	zhì gān căo	Radix Glycyrrhizae Praeparata cum Melle
汉防己	hàn fáng jĭ	Radix Stephaniae Tetrandrae

Xu Tian-jing, et al. treated acute gout with the above formula, modified according to symptoms. One batch was prescribed daily. The dregs were used as an external application on the affected areas. The total efficacy rate was 95.56%. [19]

H. *Xuè Fŭ Zhú Yū Tāng* (血府逐瘀汤):

当归	dāng guī	Radix Angelicae Sinensis
桃仁	táo rén	Semen Persicae
红花	hóng huā	Flos Carthami
川牛膝	chuān niú xī	Radix Cyathulae
生地	shēng dì	Radix Rehmanniae Recens
枳壳	zhĭ qiào	Fructus Aurantii
赤芍	chì sháo	Radix Paeoniae Rubra
川芎	chuān xiōng	Rhizoma Chuanxiong
柴胡	chái hú	Radix Bupleuri
桔梗	jié gěng	Radix Platycodi
土茯苓	tŭ fú líng	Rhizoma Smilacis Glabrae
生甘草	shēng gān căo	Radix et Rhizoma Glycyrrhizae (raw)
川萆薢	chuān bì xiè	Rhizoma Dioscoreae Hypoglaucae
车前子	chē qián zĭ	Semen Plantaginis

Zhao Dong-ying treated gout with the above formula, modified according to symptoms. The therapeutic results were satisfactory.

I. Modified *Xuān Bì Tāng* (宣痹汤):

汉防己	hàn fáng jĭ	Radix Stephaniae Tetrandrae
赤小豆	chì xiăo dòu	Semen Phaseoli
杏仁	xìng rén	Semen Armeniacae Amarum
滑石	huá shí	Talcum

连翘	lián qiào	Fructus Forsythiae
地龙	dì lóng	Pheretima
栀子	zhī zǐ	Fructus Gardeniae
苡仁	yǐ rén	Semen Coicis
半夏	bàn xià	Rhizoma Pinelliae
蚕沙	cán shā	Faeces Bombycis
石膏	shí gāo	Gypsum Fibrosum
制马钱子	zhì mǎ qián zǐ	Semen Strychni (prepared)

Yao Gui-rong, et al. treated primary gout with the above formula. Total efficacy rate: 95.66%. [21]

(2) Research on Empirical Formulas

A. Jiao Shu-de uses *Bǔ Shèn Qīng Rè Zhì Wāng Tāng* (补肾清热治尪汤):

生地	shēng dì	20g	Radix Rehmanniae Recens
骨碎补	gǔ suì bǔ	15g	Rhizoma Drynariae
桑枝	sāng zhī	20g	Ramulus Mori
桑寄生	sāng jì shēng	20g	Herba Taxilli
地骨皮	dì gǔ pí	10g	Cortex Lycii
知母	zhī mǔ	12g	Rhizoma Anemarrhenae
白芍	bái sháo	15g	Radix Paeoniae Alba
威灵仙	wēi líng xiān	15g	Radix et Rhizoma Clematidis
忍冬藤	rěn dōng téng	30g	Caulis Lonicerae Japonicae
羌活	qiāng huó	9g	Rhizoma et Radix Notopterygii
独活	dú huó	9g	Radix Angelicae Pubescentis
络石藤	luò shí téng	20g	Caulis Trachelospermi
桂枝	guì zhī	9g	Ramulus Cinnamomi
红花	hóng huā	9g	Flos Carthami
穿山甲	chuān shān jiǎ	9g	Squama Manis
制乳香	zhì rǔ xiāng	6g	Olibanum (prepared)
制没药	zhì mò yào	6g	Myrrha (prepared)
萆薢	bì xiè	10g	Rhizoma Dioscoreae Hypoglaucae
黄柏	huáng bǎi	12g	Cortex Phellodendri Chinensis

苍术	cāng zhú	10g	Rhizoma Atractylodis
牛膝	niú xī	20g	Radix Achyranthis Bidentatae

Decocted in water, one batch prescribed per day, divided into two portions to be taken warm. Ten days equaled a course of treatment. Of 42 cases treated with the above formula, 15 were cured, 24 showed marked improvement, and 3 showed no change. The total efficacy rate was 94.3%.[22]

B. *Tòng Fēng Fāng* (痛风方), a self-drafted formula:

生石膏	shēng shí gāo	40g	Gypsum Fibrosum (raw) (decocted first)
知母	zhī mŭ	10g	Rhizoma Anemarrhenae
黄柏	huáng băi	10g	Cortex Phellodendri Chinensis
生地	shēng dì	15g	Radix Rehmanniae Recens
丹皮	dān pí	10g	Cortex Moutan
赤芍	chì sháo	10g	Radix Paeoniae Rubra
茅根	máo gēn	10g	Rhizoma Imperatae
二花藤	èr huā téng	20g	Caulis Lonicerae
全虫	quán chóng	10g	Bombyx Batryticatus
桑寄生	sāng jì shēng	10g	Herba Taxilli
滑石	huá shí	15g	Talcum
淡竹叶	dàn zhú yè	10g	Herba Lophatheri
车前草	chē qián căo	15g	Herba Plantaginis
灯芯草	dēng xīn căo	4g	Medulla Junci
黄连	huáng lián	6g	Rhizoma Coptidis
甘草	gān căo	6g	Radix et Rhizoma Glycyrrhizae

One batch a day. Each batch is decocted in water and divided into three portions. One month equals a course of treatment. Generally, 2 courses are given. Of 68 patients treated with the above formula, 24 were cured, 40 showed marked improvement, 4 received no effect. The total efficacy rate was 94.12%. [23]

C. Huang Li-ping treats gout caused by damp-heat with stasis obstruction by discharging turbidity, transforming stasis using a formula created by Zhu Liang-chun, a contemporary *bi* syndrome specialist.

土茯苓	tǔ fú líng	30g	Rhizoma Smilacis Glabrae
生薏苡仁	shēng yì yǐ rén	30g	Semen Coicis (raw)
萆薢	bì xiè	30g	Rhizoma Dioscoreae Hypoglaucae
金钱草	jīn qián cǎo	30g	Herba Lysimachiae
威灵仙	wēi líng xiān	15g	Radix et Rhizoma Clematidis
泽兰	zé lán	15g	Herba Lycopi
虎杖	hǔ zhàng	15g	Rhizoma Polygoni Cuspidati
蚕沙	cán shā	15g	Faeces Bombycis
川牛膝	chuān niú xī	15g	Radix Cyathulae
骨碎补	gǔ suì bǔ	15g	Rhizoma Drynariae
当归	dāng guī	10g	Radix Angelicae Sinensis
地龙	dì lóng	10g	Pheretima
桃仁	táo rén	10g	Semen Persicae
红花	hóng huā	10g	Flos Carthami

One batch a day, decocted in water.

➢ For fever and thirst, add *zhī mǔ* (Rhizoma Anemarrhenae) 15g, *shēng shí gāo* (Gypsum Fibrosum) 30g, and *shān zhī zǐ* (Fructus Gardeniae) 10g.

➢ For swollen joints, add *jiāng huáng* (Rhizoma Curcumae Longae) 10g and *wēi líng xiān* (Radix et Rhizoma Clematidis) 15g.

➢ For low-grade fever, dry mouth, and burning sensation of the five centers caused by heat scorching the yin, add *qīng hāo* (Herba Artemisiae Annuae) 10g and *qín jiāo* (Radix Gentianae Macrophyllae) 15g.

➢ For pronounced dampness, add *chē qián cǎo* (Herba Plantaginis) 15g and *fáng jǐ* (Radix Stephaniae Tetrandrae) 10g.

➢ For severe joint pain, add *yán hú suǒ* (Rhizoma Corydalis) 10g and *dì lóng* (Pheretima) 15g.

32 patients were effectively treated with the above formula and appropriate modifications. The efficacy rate of the treatment group was

93.75%. The patients in the control group were administered allopurinol orally, with an efficacy rate of 74.99%. The effects in the treatment group were better than that in the control group ($P<0.05$).[24]

D. Gai Guo-zhong uses a self-composed formula, *Tòng Fēng Tāng* (痛风汤), to treat acute gouty arthritis effectively.

土茯苓	tǔ fú líng	Rhizoma Smilacis Glabrae
山慈菇	shān cí gū	Pseudobulbus Cremastrae seu Pleiones
益智仁	yì zhì rén	Fructus Alpiniae Oxyphyllae
秦皮	qín pí	Cortex Fraxini
槐角	huái jiǎo	Fructus Sophorae

One batch a day, decocted in water until reduced to 200ml. Divided into two portions to be taken in the morning and evening.

- For severe pain, add *yán hú suǒ* (Rhizoma Corydalis), *luò shí téng* (Caulis Trachelospermi), and *rěn dōng téng* (Caulis Lonicerae Japonicae).
- For urinary calculi, add *jīn qián cǎo* (Herba Lysimachiae) and *jī nèi jīn* (Endothelium Corneum Gigeriae Galli).
- For severe swelling of the joints, add *bì xiè* (Rhizoma Dioscoreae Hypoglaucae) and *fáng jǐ* (Radix Stephaniae Tetrandrae).
- For gouty tophi, add *chuān shān jiǎ* (Squama Manis) and *dì lóng* (Pheretima).
- For constipation, add *dà huáng* (Radix et Rhizoma Rhei).
- For blood stasis, add *dān shēn* (Radix et Rhizoma Salviae Miltiorrhizae) and *chì sháo* (Radix Paeoniae Rubra).[25]

E. He Ze-min randomly divided 80 patients of gouty arthritis into two groups. The treatment group, which consisted of 40 patients, were given *Zhèn Tòng Xī Fēng Tāng* (镇痛息风汤).

制马钱子	zhì mǎ qián zǐ	0.5g	Semen Strychni (prepared)
光慈菇片	guāng cí gū piàn	8g	Tulipae Edulis Tuber

细辛	xì xīn	6g	Radix et Rhizoma Asari
怀牛膝	huái niú xī	20g	Radix Achyranthis Bidentatae
赤芍	chì sháo	15g	Radix Paeoniae Rubra
木瓜	mù guā	15g	Fructus Chaenomelis
牡丹皮	mŭ dān pí	15g	Cortex Moutan
石膏	shí gāo	20g	Gypsum Fibrosum (decocted first)
黄柏	huáng băi	12g	Cortex Phellodendri Chinensis
知母	zhī mŭ	10g	Rhizoma Anemarrhenae
萆薢	bì xiè	15g	Rhizoma Dioscoreae Hypoglaucae
薏米	yì mĭ	20g	Semen Coicis
苍术	cāng zhú	15g	Rhizoma Atractylodis
桂枝	guì zhī	15g	Ramulus Cinnamomi
淫羊藿	yín yáng huò	10g	Herba Epimedii
肉苁蓉	ròu cōng róng	15g	Herba Cistanches

➢ The differences in synthetic curative effect, blood uric acid concentration, and one-year recurrence rate between the two groups were significant ($P<0.05$). The curative effect of *Zhèn Tòng Xī Fēng Tāng* (镇痛息风汤) is better than biomedicine in the treatment of acute gouty arthritis.[26]

F. *Yán Hú Dìng Tòng Tāng* (延胡定痛汤):

延胡索	yán hú suŏ	10g	Rhizoma Corydalis
金钱草	jīn qián căo	30g	Herba Lysimachiae
车前子	chē qián zĭ	10g	Semen Plantaginis (wrapped)
泽泻	zé xiè	10g	Rhizoma Alismatis
防己	fáng jĭ	10g	Radix Stephaniae Tetrandrae
黄柏	huáng băi	10g	Cortex Phellodendri Chinensis
萆薢	bì xiè	10g	Rhizoma Dioscoreae Hypoglaucae
生薏仁	shēng yĭ rén	30g	Semen Coicis (raw)
虎杖	hŭ zhàng	10g	Rhizoma Polygoni Cuspidati
银花藤	yín huā téng	10g	Caulis Lonicerae
光慈菇	guāng cí gū	10g	Tulipae Edulis Tuber
赤芍	chì sháo	10g	Radix Paeoniae Rubra

One batch a day, decocted twice.

- For fever, add *shēng shí gāo* (Gypsum Fibrosum) 30g.
- For joint pain of the upper limbs, add *sāng zhī* (Ramulus Mori) 10g.
- For joint pain of the lower limbs, add *niú xī* (Radix Achyranthis Bidentatae) 10g.
- For inhibited bending and stretching, add *shēn jīn cǎo* (Herba Lycopodii) 10g.
- For a prolonged disease course, add *hǎi zǎo* (Sargassum) 10g.

Of 50 cases, 45 were cured (90%), and 5 were improved (10%). The total efficacy rate was 100%. [27]

(3) Research on Chinese Patent Medicine

A. Ji Wei, Tan Wen-feng, Lu Yan, et al. consider the internal factors of gout to be failure of the spleen to transform and transport and dietary irregularities, and the external factor to be damp-turbidity pouring into the joints. Treatment requires discharging turbidity and clearing heat with *Rè Bì Xiāo* (热痹消), a Chinese patent formula based on *Medical Insights* (医学心悟, *Yī Xué Xīn Wù*)'s modified *Bì Xiè Fēn Qīng Yǐn* (萆薢分清饮). A treatment group of 60 patients were treated with the above patent, resulting in a clinical cure rate of 26.7% and an improvement rate of 68.3%. The total efficacy rate was 95%, which was only slightly higher than that of the control group ($P>0.05$). However, the treatment group's rate of symptom improvement was much higher than the control group's ($P<0.05$). *Rè Bì Xiāo* acts rapidly, making it a suitable formula for treating acute conditions. Blood uric acid levels were markedly reduced in the treatment group, which when compared with the control group is a significant deviation ($P<0.05$). [28]

B. Song Ping treated 40 patients of acute gouty arthritis with Cao Ke-guang's empirical formula, *Tòng Fēng Jiāo Náng* (痛风胶囊):

土茯苓	tǔ fú líng	60g	Rhizoma Smilacis Glabrae
萆薢	bì xiè	15g	Rhizoma Dioscoreae Hypoglaucae

山慈菇	shān cí gū	10g	Pseudobulbus Cremastrae seu Pleiones
延胡索	yán hú suǒ	10g	Rhizoma Corydalis

Four pills, three times one day. Four weeks equaled a course of treatment. Clinical improvement rate: 50.0%. Total efficacy rate: 62.5%. The 30 patients in the control group were administered *Tòng Fēng Dìng Jiāo Náng* (痛风定胶囊) orally (3 pills, three times a day), resulting in an improvement rate of 30.0% and a total efficacy rate of 63.3%. The difference in total efficacy rate between the two groups was insignificant, while the improvement rate of the treatment group was notably higher than that of the control group. The difference in blood uric acid levels of the patients in the treatment group before and after taking the medicine was significant ($P<0.05$). *Tòng Fēng Capsule* (痛风胶囊) can not only remove heat and relieve swelling, but also lower the blood uric acid level without producing adverse effects.[29]

C. Cao Xiao-tian, et al. used *Xī Tòng Níng Jiāo Náng* (息痛宁胶囊) to treat gouty arthritis. The results of pharmacodynamic tests showed that there was no significant difference in the anti-inflammatory and analgesic effects between the Chinese medicine group and the indomethacin group ($P>0.05$). There was no significant difference in the anti-inflammatory, swelling-reducing and blood uric acid lowering effects between the Chinese medicine group and the allopurinol group ($P>0.05$). Since this patent formula has few adverse effects and is well tolerated by patients, it can be administered orally over a long period of time. [30]

D. Yan Qun-chao and Mo Mu-shun observed the curative effects of *Tòng Fēng Níng Piàn* (痛风宁片) on acute and chronic gouty arthritis. Researchers randomly divided 160 patients into a treatment group (100 patients) and a control group (60 patients). The former was given *Tòng Fēng Níng Piàn* while the latter was given *Zhōng Huì Tòng*

Fēng Dìng Jiāo Náng (中汇痛风定胶囊). The total efficacy rate of the treatment group was 92%, and that of the control group was 81.67% (P<0.05). [31]

E. Wen Shao-dun observed the treatment of 107 patients with hyperuricemia accompanied by hyperlipidemia. The patients in the treatment group were given *Suān Zhǐ Qīng Jiāo Náng* (酸脂清胶囊) while those in the control group (106 patients) were given *Tòng Fēng Shū Jiāo Náng* (痛风舒胶囊). The difference of the results between the two groups were significant (P<0.01). *Suān Zhǐ Qīng Jiāo Náng* (酸脂清胶囊) can effectively treat gout hyperuricacidemia, and can regulate blood lipid levels.[32]

大黄	dà huáng	40%	Radix et Rhizoma Rhei
姜黄	jiāng huáng	33%	Rhizoma Curcumae Longae
土茯苓	tǔ fú líng	27%	Rhizoma Smilacis Glabrae

F. Zhao Wei and Zhang Long-ji observed the treatment of 18 patients of gouty arthritis with *Xīn Huáng Piàn* (新癀片). 12 showed marked improvement, 5 showed some improvement, and 1 had no effect. Total efficacy rate: 94.44%.

九节茶	jiǔ jié chá	Sarcandra glabra
三七	sān qī	Radix et Rhizoma Notoginseng
牛黄	niú huáng	Calculus Bovis
珍珠粉	zhēn zhū fěn	Margarita (powdered)

Xīn Huáng Piàn has the effects of clearing heat, dispelling wind, draining dampness, invigorating blood, dispersing swelling, and relieving pain. It can treat gouty arthritis with few adverse effects. The therapeutic effects of this patent are better than those of nonsteroidal pain-killers or colchicin, making it widely accepted. [33]

4. Acupuncture and Moxibustion

(1) Acupuncture Therapy

A. Zhang Hai-jiang, et al. used local collateral bloodletting to release thick blood that contains uric acid crystals, thereby lowering the tension in the blood vessels, improving capillary resistance, and reducing local inflammation. This method comes from *Yellow Emperor's Inner Classic-Divine Pivot: The Nine Needles and Twelve Sources* (内经·灵枢·九针十二原, *Líng Shū - Jiǔ Zhēn Shí Èr Yuán*), which states: "Stasis should be eliminated (菀陈则除之)", and "prevent disease before it occurs; once disease has taken form, prevent its transformation (未病先防，既病防变)." The total efficacy rate was 100%.

Treatment method:

1) Acupuncture: Bleed the engorged, cyanosed or dilated collaterals of the affected limbs, the corresponding adjacent points, or the points along the corresponding channel pathways.

2) Standard of bloodletting: Determined by local pathological changes such as redness, swelling, pain, and blood uric acid level. In mild cases, squeeze out 10ml of blood; in severe cases, squeeze out 30-50ml. Generally, approximately 20ml is sufficient.

3) Timing of bloodletting: Decided by the severity of the pathological changes and the condition of the affected joints. In severe cases, bleed once a day; in mild cases, once a week. Generally, once every four days is sufficient, and three sessions equal a course of treatment.

4) Auxiliary treatment: External application using medicinals that clear heat, resolve toxins, cool blood, and disperse swelling, or internal administration of medicinals that clear heat, resolve toxins, promote water flow, and unblock the stool.[34]

B. Li Zhao-wen, Lin Shi-ming, Lin Jun-shan, et al. observed and compared the curative effects of point bloodletting of different volumes of blood with those of Western pharmaceutical drugs. 90 patients of acute gouty arthritis were randomly divided into A, B and C groups. Groups A and B were administered bloodletting to release 5ml and 10ml of blood, respectively, while group C were given oral indomethacin and allopurinol. Acupoints selected: LV 2 (*xíng jiān*), LV 3 (*tài chōng*), SP 3 (*tài bái*), and ST 43 (*xiàn gǔ*) of the affected side.

LV 2	xíng jiān	行间
LV 3	tài chōng	太冲
SP 3	tài bái	太白
ST 43	xiàn gǔ	陷谷

The findings indicated that the analgesic effects of group B's treatment were the strongest; the difference in blood uric acid reduction of groups B and C when compared to that of group A was considerable ($P<0.01$), but the difference between groups B and C was unremarkable ($P>0.05$). Point bloodletting was effective in treating acute gouty arthritis, with the efficacy being related to the volume of blood released. Point bloodletting therapy represses blood uric acid synthesis and promotes uric acid excretion. [35]

C. Wen Shao-dun divided 630 patients of acute gouty arthritis into groups A, B and C according to the order in which they came. Fire needles were quickly inserted and withdrawn to cause bleeding, and 20ml, 40ml, and 60ml of blood were released, respectively. The main points chosen are listed as follows, with the addition of *ashi* points, most of which were in middle of the dorsum of the foot (metatarsophalangeal joints):

LV 2	xíng jiān	行间
LV 3	tài chōng	太冲
ST 44	nèi tíng	内庭
ST 43	xiàn gǔ	陷谷

2-3 points were bled on the affected side for each session; one session was administered every three days, for a maximum of three sessions. The efficacy rates were 88.1%, 92.8%, and 97.6%, respectively. The difference between groups C and A was significant ($P<0.05$). Bloodletting effectively treated acute gouty arthritis of the foot, and the level of efficacy depended on the volume of blood released (the more the blood, the better the effect). [36]

D. Liu Xin randomly divided 93 gout patients into two groups: warming-needle moxibustion group and colchicin group. The following points were chosen for warming-needle moxibustion:

ST 36	zú sān lǐ	足三里
SP 4	gōng sūn	公孙
SP 6	sān yīn jiāo	三阴交
SP 9	yīn líng quán	阴陵泉
EX-LE 10	bā fēng	八风

SP 4 (*gōng sūn*), SP 6 (*sān yīn jiāo*), and SP 9 (*yīn líng quán*) were needled first, and then ST 36 (*zú sān lǐ*). After the arrival of qi, 2-3 cones of moxa were applied to ST 36 (*zú sān lǐ*), and the needles were withdrawn 30 minutes later. EX-LE 10 (*bā fēng*) was drained. Treatment was given once a day, with seven days equalling a course of treatment. The patients in the control group took colchicin orally. The initial dose was 1.0mg, then 0.5mg was given every hour. On the second day, each dose was 0.5mg, twice a day for seven days. After seven days of therapy, the results of the two groups were compared. The analgesic and therapeutic effects of the warming-needle moxibustion group were basically the same as those of the colchicin group ($P>0.05$), but the former did not have any adverse reactions from the treatment while the latter did ($P<0.01$). Warming needle moxibustion can not only clear and drain damp-heat, invigorate blood, dispel stasis, and course and unblock the channels and collaterals, but it can also fortify the spleen to treat the root, as well as promote the dissolution of blood uric acid and facilitate its excretion through the kidney.

E. Zhang Shu-ying treated gout with acupuncture. The following points are chosen for their regulatory functions: ST 36 (*zú sān lǐ*), SP 9 (*yīn líng quán*), BL 20 (*pǐ shù*), SP 6 (*sān yīn jiāo*), DU 14 (*dà zhuī*), ST 25 (*tiān shū*), ST 40 (*fēng lóng*).

Local points: SP 3 (*tài bái*) and LV 3 (*tài chōng*) for swelling and pain of the metatarsophalangeal joints; SP 5 (*shāng qiū*), ST 42 (*chōng yáng*), and ST 44 (*nèi tíng*) for swelling and pain of the metatarsal joints; GB 40 (*qiū xū*), KI 3 (*tài xī*), and SP 5 (*shāng qiū*) for swelling and pain of the ankle joints; *nèi xī yǎn* (EX-LE4), *xī yǎn* (EX-LE5) and *hè dǐng* (EX-LE2) for swelling and pain of the knee joints.

Method: ST 36 (*zú sān lǐ*) with warming-needle moxibustion; SP 9 (*yīn líng quán*), BL 20 (*pǐ shū*), and SP 6 (*sān yīn jiāo*) with needle rotation method of supplementation; DU 14 (*dà zhuī*) with collateral bloodletting; ST 40 (*fēng lóng*) and ST 25 (*tiān shū*) with lifting and thrusting method of drainage; local points with warming-needle moxibustion. Ten days equal a course of treatment. The total efficacy rate was 90.6%. Since 90% of all gout cases affect the metatarsophalangeal joints and the spleen, stomach and liver channels run through the big toe, Zhang Shu-ying believes that the pathological changes of gouty arthritis involve the spleen, stomach and liver channels, and that the pathogenic factors include an excessively rich and fatty diet which gives rise to the production of phlegm and dampness. Phlegm-dampness blocks the flow of blood; the phlegm, dampness, and static blood stagnate in the flesh and joints, obstructing the channels and collaterals. As a result, gout is formed.[37]

The treatment focus is on transforming dampness, downbearing turbidity, dispelling stasis, and unblocking the collaterals. Select the *he*-sea point of the foot yangming channel, ST 36 (*zú sān lǐ*) and the back-

shu point of the spleen, BL 20 (*pí shū*), to fortify the spleen and stomach in order to transport and transform water-damp. Select the *he*-sea point of the foot taiyin channel, SP 9 (*yīn líng quán*), and the intersecting point of the three yin channels of the foot, SP 6 (*sān yīn jiāo*), to fortify the spleen and drain dampness. Select the luo-connecting point of the foot yangming channel, ST 40 (*fēng lóng*) and the front-*mu* point of the large intestine, LI 25 (*tiān shū*), to transform phlegm, discharge turbidity, and unblock the stool. Prick to bleed DU 14 (*dà zhuī*) to drain heat and dispel stasis. [38]

F. Rao Guang-tao, et al. used a three-edged needle to bleed SP 1 (*yǐn bái*) and LV 1 (*dà dūn*) alternately, once a day, 4-6 drops of blood per point.

The following modifications were also applied:

➢ During the acute stage, SP 1 (*yǐn bái*), LV 1 (*dà dūn*), LV 3 (*tài chōng*), SP 6 (*sān yīn jiāo*), KI 3 (*tài xī*), KI 6 (*zhào hǎi*), and *ashi* points of the affected side were added.

➢ DU 14 (*dà zhuī*), LI 11 (*qū chí*), LI 4 (*hé gǔ*) were added for fever.

➢ GB 20 (*fēng chí*), and *tài yáng* (EX-HN5) were added for headache.

➢ RN 12 (*zhōng wǎn*) and ST 36 (*zú sān lǐ*) were added for obesity and loss of appetite.

➢ During the recovery phase, LV 3 (*tài chōng*), SP 6 (*sān yīn jiāo*), SP 3 (*tài bái*), KI 3 (*tài xī*), KI 6 (*zhào hǎi*), ST 36 (*zú sān lǐ*), BL 18 (*gān shù*), and BL 23 (*shèn shù*) were selected bilaterally, and 28-gauge filiform needles were used.

In the acute stage, the patients were given acupuncture with drainage, twice a day, seven days equalling a course of treatment. During the recovery stage, patients were treated with even supplementation and drainage, with ten days totalling a course. Of 61 cases, 48 showed excellent improvement, 11 showed some effect, and 2 showed no effect.[39]

G. Cheng Chun-kui selects acupoints according to the location of pain.

➢ For pain of the first metatarsophalangeal joint:

LV 3	tài chōng	太冲
SP 3	tài bái	太白
SP 6	sān yīn jiāo	三阴交
SP 2	dà dū	大都

- For pain of the ankle joint:

LV 4	zhōng fēng	中封
BL 60	kūn lún	昆仑
ST 41	jiě xī	解溪
GB 40	qiū xū	丘墟
BL 40	wěi zhōng	委中
GB 39	jué gŭ	绝骨

- For pain of the knee joint:

EX-LE 5	xī yǎn	膝眼
GB 34	yáng líng quán	阳陵泉
LV 8	qŭ quán	曲泉

- For pain of the wrist joint:[40]

SJ 4	yáng chí	阳池
SJ 5	wài guān	外关
LI 4	hé gŭ	合谷
LV 3	tài chōng	太冲

H. Wu Zi-li selected BL 27 (*xiāo cháng shū*) to treat 10 patients with gouty arthritis. This method is based on a Japanese acupuncturist's (Ze Tian-jian's) theory that "gout is caused by heat in the small intestine." The acupoint was shown to have good analgesic effects but no effect on blood uric acid.[41]

(2) Acupuncture Combined with Chinese Medicinals

Duan Wei-ping combined acupuncture and medicinal therapy to treat gouty arthritis and compared the therapeutic effects of this combined treatment with the separate administration of acupuncture and

Chinese medicinals.

The following points were chosen for the acupuncture group:

LI 11	qū chí	曲池
SP 10	xuè hǎi	血海
SP 6	sān yīn jiāo	三阴交
KI 3	tài xī	太溪

- LI 15 (*jiān yú*) and GB 21 (*jiān jǐn*) were added for shoulder pain.
- LI 10 (*shǒu sān lǐ*) was added for elbow pain.
- SJ 4 (*yáng chí*) and SJ 5 (*wài guān*) were added for wrist pain.
- *Xī yǎn* (EX-LE5) and GB 34 (*yáng líng quán*) were added for knee pain.
- GB 40 (*qiū xū*) and GB 39 (*xuán zhōng*) were added for ankle pain.
- LV 3 (*tài chōng*) and SP 2 (*dà dū*) were added for pain of the big toe.

Even supplementation and drainage was applied. After arrival of qi, the needles were retained for 30 minutes. Electro-acupuncture and TDP were also used when necessary. Treatment was administered once a day, with ten days equalling a course of treatment.

Patients in the Chinese medicinal group were given Duan's self-composed formula, *Fáng Fēng Wū Yǐ Xì Xīn Tāng* (防风乌苡细辛汤):

防风	fáng fēng	10g	Radix Saposhnikoviae
当归	dāng guī	10g	Radix Angelicae Sinensis
苡仁	yǐ rén	10g	Semen Coicis
茯苓	fú líng	10g	Poria
萆薢	bì xiè	10g	Rhizoma Dioscoreae Hypoglaucae
赤芍	chì sháo	10g	Radix Paeoniae Rubra
白芍	bái sháo	10g	Radix Paeoniae Alba
制川乌	zhì chuān wū	10g	Radix Aconiti Praeparata
制草乌	zhì cǎo wū	10g	Radix Aconiti Kusnezoffii Praeparata
威灵仙	wēi líng xiān	15g	Radix et Rhizoma Clematidis

忍冬藤	rěn dōng téng	15g	Caulis Lonicerae Japonicae
细辛	xì xīn	3g	Radix et Rhizoma Asari

➢ *Qiāng huó* (Rhizoma et Radix Notopterygii) 10g was added for pain of the upper limbs.

➢ *Dú huó* (Radix Angelicae Pubescentis) 10g was added for pain of the lower limbs.

The ingredients were decocted in water for oral administration. One batch a day was prescribed, and ten batches equaled a course of treatment.

In the combined acupuncture and Chinese medicinals group, the patients were given both of the above treatments, that is, a combination of the above-mentioned acupuncture therapy and the above-mentioned medicinal formula. Ten days counted as a course of treatment.

The total efficacy rates were as follows: The combined acupuncture and medicinal group: 95.83%; the acupuncture group: 86.67%; the medicinal group: 86.67%. [42]

In comparison, the curative effect of acupuncture and medicinals group was better than that of the other groups ($P<0.05$). Serum uric acid levels of the three groups all showed marked differences ($P<0.01$). [42]

Yang Jin-hong and Luo Yong-li treated 48 patients of acute gouty arthritis. The treatment group was administered acupuncture and local external application of *Tòng Fēng Hé Jì* (痛风合剂). The control group, which consisted of 31 patients, was given colchicine and fenbid orally.

Acupuncture points selected:

SP 6	sān yīn jiāo	三阴交
KI 13	tài xī	太溪
ST 36	zú sān lǐ	足三里

The acupoints on the affected side of the body were chosen. Even supplementation and drainage were applied. The needles were retained for 20 minutes, during which the needles were stimulated once every 5-10 minutes. Treatment was administered once a day for 10 days (one treatment course).

External application of medicinals: The ingredients of *Tòng Fēng Hé Jì* (listed below) were mixed with warm water and made into a paste and applied on the affected area. This was done once a day for ten days (one treatment course).

秦皮	qín pí	Cortex Fraxini
大黄	dà huáng	Radix et Rhizoma Rhei
黄柏	huáng bǎi	Cortex Phellodendri Chinensis
苍术	cāng zhú	Rhizoma Atractylodis
牛膝	niú xī	Radix Achyranthis Bidentatae
乳香	rǔ xiāng	Olibanum
没药	mò yào	Myrrha
丹皮	dān pí	Cortex Moutan

The results indicate that acupuncture combined with external application of Chinese medicinals can enhance the clinical cure rate and control recurrence. [43]

Jiang Xing-peng, et al. uses acupuncture and medicinal baths to treat gout:

With the patient in sitting or supine position, select the following points on the affected extremity and apply drainage.

LV 3	tài chōng	太冲
SP 2	dà dū	大都
SP 3	tài bái	太白
SP 4	gōng sūn	公孙
SP 6	sān yīn jiāo	三阴交

➢ For redness, swelling, heat, and pain, add ST 44 (*nèi tíng*), LI 11 (*qū chí*), and LI 4 (*hé gǔ*), with drainage. Perform bleeding and cupping to treat swollen joints.

➢ For a prolonged course of disease, add ST 36 (*zú sān lǐ*) with supplementation. Treat once a day. Seven days equal a course of treatment, with an interval of one or two days between courses.

Medicinal bath (for acute stage):

黄柏	huáng bǎi	30g	Cortex Phellodendri Chinensis
芒硝	máng xiāo	30g	Natrii Sulfas
大黄	dà huáng	30g	Radix et Rhizoma Rhei
制草乌	zhì cǎo wū	15g	Radix Aconiti Kusnezoffii Praeparata
制川乌	zhì chuān wū	15g	Radix Aconiti Praeparata
土茯苓	tǔ fú líng	30g	Rhizoma Smilacis Glabrae
路路通	lù lù tōng	30g	Fructus Liquidambaris
红藤	hóng téng	30g	Caulis Sargentodoxae
败酱草	bài jiàng cǎo	30g	Herba Patriniae
黄连	huáng lián	15g	Rhizoma Coptidis
明矾	míng fán	15g	Alumen
冰片	bīng piàn	5g	Borneolum Syntheticum

For a prolonged course of disease, use *Sì Shēng Sǎn* (四生散) [ingredients listed below] as a medicinal bath, twice a day, 30 minutes to 1 hour each time. One batch of medicinals can be redecocted and reused for up to 3-5 days. The total efficacy rate is 96%. [44]

生川乌	shēng chuān wū	Radix Aconiti (raw)
生草乌	shēng cǎo wū	Radix Aconiti Kusnezoffii (raw)
生南星	shēng nán xīng	Rhizoma Arisaematis (raw)
生半夏	shēng bàn xià	Rhizoma Pinelliae (raw)

(3) Acupuncture and Other Treatment Modalities

A. Acupuncture and Fire Cupping

Li Yang-zhen selects KI 6 (*zhào hǎi*), LV 3 (*tài chōng*), GB 40 (*qiū xū*), GB 42 (*dì wǔ huì*), GB 41 (*zú lín qì*), ST 41 (*jiě xī*), BL 40 (*wěi zhōng*), and *ashi* points on the dorsum of the foot that show apparent stasis in the collaterals. After routine sterilization, a three-edged needle is used to bleed the areas around the acupoints that have superficial vessels. 2-3 points are bled each time, to the depth of 1-2mm. Approximately 5-20ml of blood is released from each point. If the bleeding is less than 3ml, fire cupping can be performed and retained for 15 minutes. After each treatment session, the acupoints should be disinfected and covered with antiseptic gauze.

KI 6	zhào hǎi	照海
LV 3	tài chōng	太冲
GB 40	qiū xū	丘墟
GB 42	dì wǔ huì	地五会
GB 41	zú lín qì	足临泣
ST 41	jiě xī	解溪
BL 40	wěi zhōng	委中
ashi points	ā shì xuè	阿是穴

Collateral bloodletting can be performed once every 3 days, with 5 sessions equaling a course of treatment. If there is no improvement, administer another course of treatment after a rest period of one week. If the bleeding exceeds 30ml, press on the acupoint with a sterilized cotton ball. The efficacy rate is 96.9% after one course of treatment. Bleeding the above acupuncture points can drain heat, invigorate blood, disperse swelling, course and unblock the qi of the channels, collaterals, and *zang-fu* organs, and regulate qi and blood. The static blood and phlegm-turbidity are also expelled via this method, giving way to faster relief of the clinical symptoms.[45]

B. Acupuncture and Laser Therapy

Xu Hao and Mao Hong-rong uses acupuncture coupled with laser therapy to treat 38 patients of gouty arthritis. The selected acupoints are listed below.

SP 6	sān yīn jiāo	三阴交
SP 9	yīn líng quán	阴陵泉
ST 36	zú sān lǐ	足三里
KI 13	tài xī	太溪
ashi points	ā shì xuè	阿是穴

Manipulation: Drainage is applied to SP 9 (*yīn líng quán*), while even supplementation and drainage are applied to the other points. The needles are retained for 30 minutes, during which needle stimulation is performed every 10 minutes. Treatment is administered once a day. After each acupuncture session, a MDC-500 laser device is used to apply laser stimulation on the above acupoints with the output power of 250-350mW for 3 minutes each point. The total efficacy rate is 97.4%. [46]

(4) Research on Differential Diagnosis and Medication

A. Hyperuricemia

Zhao Fen believes that *tǔ fú líng* (Rhizoma Smilacis Glabrae) can dispel dampness, resolve toxins, and promote the excretion of uric acid. [47]

Jiang Xi, et al. use *tǔ fú líng* (Rhizoma Smilacis Glabrae) to discharge turbidity, resolve toxins, fortify the spleen, dry dampness, and disinhibit the joints. They use *bì xiè* (Rhizoma Dioscoreae Hypoglaucae) to separate the clear and turbid. Both of these medicinals are the chief ingredients of a formula that lowers blood uric acid. [48]

Chen Ma-huan uses *tǔ fú líng* (Rhizoma Smilacis Glabrae) to resolve toxins and eliminate dampness; *bì xiè* (Rhizoma Dioscoreae Hypoglaucae) to dispel wind-damp, disinhibit the joints, and separate the clear and turbid; and *cán shā* (Faeces Bombycis) to dispel wind, eliminate dampness, invigorate blood, and relieve pain. All of these medicinals can dispel wind, eliminate dampness, separate the clear and turbid, unblock the collaterals, lower blood uric acid and relieve pain. The dosage of the above three herbs should be large; the usual dosages are as follows: *tǔ fú líng* (Rhizoma Smilacis Glabrae) 50-100g, *chuān bì xiè* (Rhizoma Dioscoreae Hypoglaucae) 30-50g, *cán shā* (Faeces Bombycis) 30-50g. [49]

Zeng Xiang-yong divides the medicinals for treating gout into four groups to be used during different stages of gout:

- Medicinals that lower blood uric acid: *tǔ fú líng* (Rhizoma Smilacis Glabrae) 12g, *bì xiè* (Rhizoma Dioscoreae Hypoglaucae) 12g, and *cán shā* (Faeces Bombycis) 12g.
- Medicinals that dissolve and remove uric acid: *wēi líng xiān* (Radix et Rhizoma Clematidis) 15g and *qín jiāo* (Radix Gentianae Macrophyllae) 12g.
- Medicinals that promote the excretion of uric acid: *shēng yǐ rén* (Semen Coicis) 15g, *fú líng* (Poria) 15g, *zé xiè* (Rhizoma Alismatis) 12g, *chē qián zǐ* (Semen Plantaginis) 12g, and *dì lóng* (Pheretima) 12g.
- Medicinals that inhibit the synthesis of uric acid: *zé lán* (Herba Lycopi) 12g, *táo rén* (Semen Persicae) 12g, *dāng guī* (Radix Angelicae Sinensis) 12g, and *dì lóng* (Pheretima) 12g.[7]

Liu Meng-yuan holds that hyperuricacidemia is due to turbid dampness, phlegm, blood stasis, and toxins. Gouty arthritis is attributed to toxins and blood stasis which are caused by dampness blocking the joint, hence he suggests that the treatment of hyperuricemia requires herbs that drain dampness and discharge turbidity, e.g., *tǔ fú líng* (Rhizoma Smilacis Glabrae), *chuān bì xiè* (Rhizoma Dioscoreae Hypoglaucae), *jīn qián cǎo* (Herba Lysimachiae), *chē qián zǐ* (Semen Plantaginis), *zé xiè* (Rhizoma Alismatis), *cán shā* (Faeces Bombycis), and *dà huáng* (Radix et Rhizoma Rhei).[50]

Zheng Ping-dong created a formula to invigorate blood, unblock the collaterals, transform phlegm, discharge turbidity, and lower uric acid. The ingredients of the formula are listed below. One month equals a course of treatment; the recommended duration of treatment is three months. [51]

王不留行	wáng bù liú xíng	10g	Semen Vaccariae
白芥子	bái jiè zǐ	10g	Semen Sinapis
车前子	chē qián zǐ	15g	Semen Plantaginis (wrapped)
粉萆薢	fěn bì xiè	10g	Rhizoma Dioscoreae Hypoglaucae
生山楂	shēng shān zhā	10g	Fructus Crataegi (raw)
威灵仙	wēi líng xiān	15g	Radix et Rhizoma Clematidis
制大黄	zhì dà huáng	10g	Radix et Rhizoma Rhei (prepared)

B. For joint stiffness and deformity, gouty tophi, and a long disease course

Wang Fan-hong, et al. use *wēi líng xiān* (Radix et Rhizoma Clematidis), *wǔ jiā pí* (Cortex Acanthopanacis), *hǎi tóng pí* (Cortex Erythrinae), and *jiāng cán* (Bombyx Batryticatus). [52]

Xia Han, et al. use *hǎi fēng téng* (Caulis Piperis Kadsurae), *tiān xiān téng* (Herba Aristolochiae) and *wēi líng xiān* (Radix et Rhizoma Clematidis). [53]

Zhang Bo uses *shēn jīn cǎo* (Herba Lycopodii) and *lǎo guàn cǎo* (Herba Erodii; Herba Geranii). [54]

Jiang Xi, et al. suggest that joint stiffness and deformity and subcutaneous nodules are caused by turbidity complicated by dampness, stasis and phlegm. Deficiency-excess complexes are a common manifestation of this disease. Treatment requires insects and medicinals that transform phlegm and disperse stasis, i.e., *bái jiè zǐ* (Semen Sinapis), *zé lán* (Herba Lycopi), *shān jiǎ piàn* (Squama Manis), *tǔ biē chóng* (Eupolyphaga seu Steleophaga), and *jiāng cán* (Bombyx Batryticatus).[55]

For gouty nodules, Yang Jia-ren uses *xuán shēn* (Radix Scrophulariae), *zhè bèi* (Bulbus Fritillariae Thunbergii), *mǔ lì* (Concha Ostreae), *kūn bù* (Thallus Laminariae), and *hǎi zǎo* (Sargassum) to soften hardness and transform phlegm. [56]

For joint nodules, Luo Yu-tian often uses *tiān nán xīng* (Rhizoma

Arisaematis), *zhè bèi mǔ* (Bulbus Fritillariae Thunbergii), *fǎ bàn xià* (Rhizoma Pinelliae Praeparatum) and *xià kū cǎo* (Spica Prunellae) to dissipate phlegm and disperse binds. [57]

For joint swelling, pain, and deformity, Yan Dong-mei and Yan Xiao-ping use *nán xīng* (Rhizoma Arisaematis), *bái jiè zǐ* (Semen Sinapis), and *zhì shān jiǎ* (fried with liquid Squama Manis); for gouty tophi, they use *bèi mǔ* (Bulbus Fritillariae Thunbergii), *kūn bù* (Thallus Laminariae), and *shān cí gū* (Pseudobulbus Cremastrae seu Pleiones).[58]

Chen Li-ming uses *guì zhī* (Ramulus Cinnamomi), *qín jiāo* (Radix Gentianae Macrophyllae), *dú huó* (Radix Angelicae Pubescentis), *wēi líng xiān* (Radix et Rhizoma Clematidis), *bái fù zǐ* (Rhizoma Typhonii), and *dǎn nán xīng* (Arisaema cum Bile) to transform phlegm and invigorate blood in order to treat joint stiffness. [59]

Ren Da-ran believes that *Huà Zhuó Qū Yū Tòng Fēng Fāng* (化浊祛瘀痛风方), the ingredients of which are listed below, can treat gouty tophi.[60]

土茯苓	tǔ fú líng	30-60g	Rhizoma Smilacis Glabrae
虎杖	hǔ zhàng	30g	Rhizoma Polygoni Cuspidati
粉萆薢	fěn bì xiè	20g	Rhizoma Dioscoreae Hypoglaucae
忍冬藤	rěn dōng téng	30g	Caulis Lonicerae Japonicae
苡仁	yǐ rén	30-50g	Semen Coicis
威灵仙	wēi líng xiān	15g	Radix et Rhizoma Clematidis
黄柏	huáng bǎi	10g	Cortex Phellodendri Chinensis
川牛膝	chuān niú xī	10g	Radix Cyathulae
木瓜络	mù guā luò	10g	Fructus Chaenomelis
泽泻	zé xiè	10g	Rhizoma Alismatis
路路通	lù lù tōng	10g	Fructus Liquidambaris
制乳香	zhì rǔ xiāng	10g	Olibanum (prepared)
制没药	zhì mò yào	10g	Myrrha (prepared)
金钱草	jīn qián cǎo	30g	Herba Lysimachiae
海金沙	hǎi jīn shā	10g	Spora Lygodii (wrapped)
鱼脑石	yú nǎo shí	15-18g	Sagitta Pseudosciaenae

For joint stiffness, swelling, and deformity due to phlegm-stasis bind, Zhang Rui-bin uses *páo shān jiă* (blast-fried Squama Manis), *jiŭ xiāng chóng* (Aspongopus), *jiāng cán* (Bombyx Batryticatus), and *fēng fáng* (Nidus Vespae) to break binds, expel stasis, transform phlegm, and soften hardness. Zhang also uses *gŭ suì bŭ* (Rhizoma Drynariae), *shú dì huáng* (Radix Rehmanniae Praeparata), *bŭ gŭ zhī* (Fructus Psoraleae), and *ròu cōng róng* (Herba Cistanches) to tonify the kidney, strengthen the bones, and replenish marrow and essence. This is an effective treatment for the chronic or interval stages of gout.[61]

C. Urinary calculi

Chen Jin-yi, et al. use *shí wĕi* (Folium Pyrrosiae) and *jīn qián căo* (Herba Lysimachiae) to treat urinary calculi due to uric acid buildup. [62]

Yao Jie-ming uses *jīn qián căo* (Herba Lysimachiae), *jī nèi jīn* (Endothelium Corneum Gigeriae Galli), and *hăi jīn shā* (Spora Lygodii) to free strangury and expel stones. [63]

Before uric acid stones form, Fan Yi-shan uses *jīn qián căo* (Herba Lysimachiae) to promote urination and free strangury to prevent urinary calculi. [64]

Duan Hua-duan, et al. uses *jīn qián căo* (Herba Lysimachiae), *hăi jīn shā* (Spora Lygodii), *chē qián zĭ* (Semen Plantaginis), and *zé xiè* (Rhizoma Alismatis) to clear heat, promote urination, expel stones, promote the excretion of uric acid, and eliminate uric acid crystals, thereby preventing the formation of gouty tophi.[65]

(5) Additional Treatment Modalities

A. External Application of Medicinals

Huang Xuan-zhu employed the external application of *Shuāng Băi Gāo* (双柏膏) [ingredients listed below] mixed with peanut oil as an adjuvant treatment for acute gouty arthritis. 72 patients of acute gouty arthritis were divided into a treatment group and a control group, with each group consisting of 36 patients. The treatment group was administered colchicine and NSAIDs in conjunction with the external application of *Shuāng Bǎi Gāo* while the control group was administered only colchicine and NSAIDs. The difference between the total efficacy rates of both groups was insignificant (P>0.05). However, the time in which it took the pain relief to take effect in the treatment group was 4.1±1.2 hours, and lasted for 5.2±1.1 days; in the control group, it took 8.4 ±2.3 hours and lasted 9.44±2.0 days. The difference between these values is significant (P<0.05). Conclusion: The external application of *Shuāng Bǎi Gāo* as an adjuvant treatment for acute gouty arthritis is effective and can shorten the course of the disease considerably. [66]

黄柏	huáng bǎi	1g	Cortex Phellodendri Chinensis
侧柏	cè bǎi	1g	Cacumen Platycladi
大黄	dà huáng	1g	Radix et Rhizoma Rhei
泽兰	zé lán	1g	Herba Lycopi
冰片	bīng piàn	1g	Borneolum Syntheticum

Liu Guang-zhen uses *Juān Bì Xǐ Jì* (蠲痹洗剂) [ingredients listed below] to treat 32 patients with acute gouty arthritis. The ingredients were decocted in water for 40 minutes, and 800ml of liquid was filtered and separated from the dregs. The decoction was allowed to cool to 35°C, and then used to wash and steep the affected area for 1 hour each time, three times a day. 12 days equaled a course of treatment. Total efficacy rate: 93.75%. [67]

泽兰	zé lán	20g	Herba Lycopi
片姜黄	piàn jiāng huáng	20g	Rhizoma Wenyujin Concisum
当归	dāng guī	15g	Radix Angelicae Sinensis
防风	fáng fēng	15g	Radix Saposhnikoviae
五倍子	wǔ bèi zǐ	15g	Galla Chinensis
黄柏	huáng bǎi	15g	Cortex Phellodendri Chinensis
苦参	kǔ shēn	15g	Radix Sophorae Flavescentis

土茯苓	tǔ fú líng	15g	Rhizoma Smilacis Glabrae
白鲜皮	bái xiǎn pí	15g	Cortex Dictamni
急性子	jí xìng zǐ	15g	Semen Impatientis
透骨草	tòu gǔ cǎo	15g	Caulis Impatientis
蒲公英	pú gōng yīng	15g	Herba Taraxaci
侧柏叶	cè bǎi yè	15g	Cacumen Platycladi

Ma Ya-juan and Mei Qun-chao used *Zhōng Yào Tōng No. 1* (中药通I号) [ingredients listed below] to treat 60 patients with gouty arthritis. Total efficacy rate was 96.6%. [68]

大黄	dà huáng	500g	Radix et Rhizoma Rhei
路路通	lù lù tōng	500g	Fructus Liquidambaris
蜂蜜	fēng mì	500g	Mel

He Huan-ping used a self-drafted formula, *Tòng Fēng Sǎn* (痛风散) [ingredients listed below], to treat gouty arthritis. The powdered formula was mixed with Vaseline and applied to the affected area before bedtime. [69]

山慈菇	shān cí gū	Pseudobulbus Cremastrae seu Pleiones
甘草	gān cǎo	Radix et Rhizoma Glycyrrhizae
血竭	xuè jié	Sanguis Draconis
白花蛇舌草	bái huā shé shé cǎo	Herba Hedyotis Diffusae
三棱	sān léng	Rhizoma Sparganii
莪术	é zhú	Rhizoma Curcumae
蒲公英	pú gōng yīng	Herba Taraxaci
地丁	dì dīng	Herba Violae
大钻	dà zuàn	Radix Kadsurae Coccineae
小钻	xiǎo zuàn	Radix Kadsurae Longipedunculatae

Wang Long-chuan uses *Tòng Fēng Zhǐ Tòng Gāo* (痛风止痛膏) [ingredients listed below] to treat gouty arthritis. [70]

川乌	chuān wū	Radix Aconiti
黄柏	huáng bǎi	Cortex Phellodendri Chinensis
青黛	qīng dài	Indigo Naturalis

白芷	bái zhǐ	Radix Angelicae Dahuricae
川芎	chuān xiōng	Rhizoma Chuanxiong
冰片	bīng piàn	Borneolum Syntheticum

Yan Shi uses *Fù Fāng Mǎ Yǐ Gāo* (复方蚂蚁膏) [ingredients listed below] to treat gouty arthritis. Total effective rate is 91.11%.[71]

蚂蚁	mǎ yǐ	ant
秦皮	qín pí	Cortex Fraxini
萆薢	bì xiè	Rhizoma Dioscoreae Hypoglaucae
虎杖	hǔ zhàng	Rhizoma Polygoni Cuspidati
六轴子	liù zhóu zǐ	Rhododendri Mollis Fructus
川芎	chuān xiōng	Rhizoma Chuanxiong
赤芍	chì sháo	Radix Paeoniae Rubra
桂枝	guì zhī	Ramulus Cinnamomi
甘草	gān cǎo	Radix et Rhizoma Glycyrrhizae

Cheng Chun-kui recommends the following formula as a warm medicinal bath to treat acute gouty arthritis. Twice a day; 5 days equal a course of treatment.[72]

蒲公英	pú gōng yīng	30g	Herba Taraxaci
野菊花	yě jú huā	30g	Flos Chrysanthemi Indici
海桐皮	hǎi tóng pí	15g	Cortex Erythrinae
川椒目	chuān jiāo mù	15g	Semen Zanthoxyli
牛膝	niú xī	15g	Radix Achyranthis Bidentatae
川芎	chuān xiōng	20g	Rhizoma Chuanxiong
赤芍	chì sháo	20g	Radix Paeoniae Rubra
艾叶	aì yè	20g	Folium Artemisiae Argyi

Xia Jin-hua reports that *Tòng Fēng Líng Hé Jì* (痛风灵合剂) administered orally, *Zhèn Jiāng Gāo Yào* (镇江膏药) applied as a paste, and *Sì Hǔ Sǎn* (四虎散) plus *xuán míng fěn* (Exsiccated Sodium Sulfate), *zhāng nǎo* (Camphor), and *bái hú jiāo* (white pepper) applied as a powder produce satisfactory therapeutic effects.[73]

B. Tui Na

Zhou Cui-ying selects the acupoints that correspond to the location of joint pain and inflammation, and applies pushing, grasping, pressing, rotation, foulage, and shaking, starting with gentle force and gradually adding pressure. Treatment is administered once or twice a day for 15-30 minutes per session. [74]

For all types of gout, Wu Xu-ping suggests pressing DU 14 (*dà zhuī*), GB 20 (*fēng chí*), and BL 23 (*shèn shù*); kneading and grasping along the three yin channels of hand and the three yin meridians of foot; and pressing LI 10 (*shǒu sān lǐ*), SI 9 (*jiān zhēn*), and LI 4 (*hé gǔ*) for 20 minutes, once a day. 7 sessions equal one course of treatment. Alternatively, one may opt to press and knead *zú zhǐ píng* (足 趾 平), GB 42 (*dì wǔ huì*), and the affected areas of the foot from the small joints of the feet to the ankles; apply heavy pressing and pushing on the soles of the feet and the intermetatarsal spaces of the dorsum; or apply rotation, plucking, and shaking on the toes and ankles for 20 minutes, once a day, for patients with lower extremity pain.[75]

Experimental Studies

The effect of *Fáng Jǐ Huáng Qí Wū Yī Tāng* (防己黄芪乌苡汤) on the peripheral neurotransmitters and on the protective structure and function of the connective tissues surrounding the joints in acute gout:

Chen Wen-zhao, et al. believes that pain factors such as K^+, NE, DA, and 5-HT play an important role in the pain of acute gout. *Fáng Jǐ Huáng Qí Wū Yī Tāng* inhibits the synthesis and delivery of 5-HT while promoting the excretion of 5-HT, thereby decreasing the concentration of 5-HT in both the inflammatory tissue and the blood. The effect of this formula on NE and DA may involve promotion of their excretion and thereby decreasing their concentration; however, it has no effect on their synthesis and delivery, hence their decrease in concentration in inflammatory tissue is insignificant. The effect of *Fáng Jĭ Huáng Qí Wū Yĭ Tāng* on K^+ in inflammatory tissue may be inhibition of its production and delivery while promoting its excretion. The formula significantly lowers the concentration of peripheral pain factors, thereby weakening the stimulatory function of the peripheral pain receptors at the inflammation site, which results in peripheral analgesia. Furthermore, this formula may raise the excitatory transmitters of the hypothalamus, which can induce central analgesia. [76]

The onset of gout is associated with deposition of urate, inflammatory cell infiltrate, tissue necrosis and collagen fibroid degeneration. Experimental results observed by Chen Wen-zhao demonstrate that activity of collagenase was heightened in rat mortise sodium urate acute gout model. *Fáng Jĭ Huáng Qí Wū Yĭ Tāng* (防己黄芪乌苡汤) and colchicin both suppress the activity of collagenase, reduce collagen fiber breakage, that is both can sustain structure and function of connective tissue. *Fáng Jĭ Huáng Qí Wū Yĭ Tāng* is better than colchicin at lowering the activity of acute gout collagenase. [77]

The anti-inflammatory and analgesic effects of *Tòng Fēng Níng Kŏu Fú Yè* (痛风宁口服液) [ingredients listed below]: Li Juan, et al. found that *Tòng Fēng Níng Kŏu Fú Yè*, can inhibit sodium urate (MSU) induced swelling of the metatarsus in rats and lower white blood cells in the synovial fluid of rabbits with MSU-induced acute gouty arthritis. It can suppress swelling of the foot caused by carrageenan and dimethyl benzene, and restrain granulomatous formation. In short, *Tòng Fēng Níng Kŏu Fú Yè* (痛风宁口服液) has anti-inflammatory and analgesic effects. [78]

淫羊藿	yín yáng huò	Herba Epimedii
桔梗	jié gĕng	Radix Platycodi

陈皮	chén pí	Pericarpium Citri Reticulatae
生姜	shēng jiāng	Rhizoma Zingiberis Recens

The treatment of gout with *Hŭ Shēn Tòng Fēng Jiāo Náng* (虎参痛风胶囊): The main ingredient of this formula is *hŭ zhàng* (Rhizoma Polygoni Cuspidati) and *dān shēn* (Radix et Rhizoma Salviae Miltiorrhizae). The main chemical components of *hŭ zhàng* (Rhizoma Polygoni Cuspidati) are polygonin and polydatin, and its functions include dispelling wind, draining dampness, removing phlegm, suppressing cough, clearing heat, resolving toxins, invigorating blood, and transforming stasis. *Dān shēn* (Radix et Rhizoma Salviae Miltiorrhizae) also invigorates blood and transforms stasis. Modern pharmacological research reveals that *hŭ zhàng* (Rhizoma Polygoni Cuspidati) and *dān shēn* (Radix et Rhizoma Salviae Miltiorrhizae) both improve local blood circulation, counter free radicals, relieve inflammation, promote the absorption of exudation from local inflammation, relieve adhesions caused by local inflammation, suppress the formation of scar tissue, and promote the reparation of damaged tissue. Furthermore, *hŭ zhàng* (Rhizoma Polygoni Cuspidati) and *dān shēn* (Radix et Rhizoma Salviae Miltiorrhizae) can effectively relieve pain. [79][80]

Song Wen-chong, Wang Yan-yan, et al. studied the anti-inflammatory effect of *Hŭ Shēn Tòng Fēng Jiāo Náng* on prostaglandin E_2 (PGE_2) of swollen foot tissue in rats. The results indicated that this formula can inhibit swelling and reduce PGE_2 in the albumen-induced swelling of foot tissue in rats. [81][82]

Song Wen-chong, et al. observed the effect of *Hŭ Shēn Tòng Fēng Jiāo Náng* on the blood uric acid levels and renal function of rats with hyperuricemia and uric acid nephropathy. The results revealed that the formula's blood uric acid lowering effect is similar to that of aurigen and that it can decrease the production of uric acid; however, it does not promote the excretion of uric acid. Various dosages of both Hus and allopurinol effectively lower blood uric acid in hyperuricemia. The effect of 500 mg/kg Hus is better than that of allopurinol. Specific stain light microscope and electron microscope ultramicro pathology revealed that Hus can reduce the deposition of uric acid crystals in the kidney, thereby relieving the structural damage and inhibiting renal interstitial fibrosis caused by hyperuricemia. It can also slow the progression of the disease and protect the kidney, as well as lower blood cholesterin and raise immunity and tolerance. [83][84]

Ji Wei, et al. holds that the first treatment principle of gouty arthritis is to discharge turbidity, transform dampness, clear heat, and unblock the collaterals. The classical formula, *Bì Xiè Fēn Qīng Yǐn* (萆薢分清饮), which was modified and renamed *Rè Bì Xiāo Kē Lì Chōng Jì* (热痹消颗粒冲剂), is highly effective with few adverse effects. This patent formula can also lower blood uric acid. [85]

Rè Bì Xiāo Kē Lì Jì (热痹消颗粒剂) [basic ingredients listed below] can significantly reduce MSU-induced swelling of the metatarsus of rats within 4 hours, with lasting effect. It can reduce the content of PGEz and UA in inflammed metatarsus, thereby relieving pain. This result show that the granule has anti-inflammatory and analgesic effects.[86]

萆薢	bì xiè	Rhizoma Dioscoreae Hypoglaucae
虎杖	hǔ zhàng	Rhizoma Polygoni Cuspidati
三七	sān qī	Radix et Rhizoma Notoginseng
黄柏	huáng bǎi	Cortex Phellodendri Chinensis
秦皮	qín pí	Cortex Fraxini

Wang Xiu-hua holds that the pathogenesis of gouty arthritis is damp-heat and blood stasis causing obstruction in the channels and collaterals, while cell factor IL-1β and NO also play an important role. The formula below has been shown to lower IL-1β and NO in the synovial fluid of the knee joint, which indicate that this method has an excellent curative effect on acute gout. [87]

黄柏	huáng bǎi	Cortex Phellodendri Chinensis
丹参	dān shēn	Radix et Rhizoma Salviae Miltiorrhizae
秦艽	qín jiāo	Radix Gentianae Macrophyllae
怀牛膝	huái niú xī	Radix Achyranthis Bidentatae
苍术	cāng zhú	Rhizoma Atractylodis
薏苡仁	yì yǐ rén	Semen Coicis

REFERENCES

[1] Liu Ming-hui. Clinical Observation of 78 Cases of Gout Treated with *Tong Feng Tang* (痛风汤治疗痛风78例临床观察). *New Chinese Medicine* (新中医), 2000, 32 (2): 19-20.

[2] Gao Guo-yu. Professor Liu Zai-peng's Experience in Treating Gouty Arthritis (刘再朋教授治疗痛风性关节炎理念). *China Journal of Chinese Medicine* (中国中医药). 2004, 9 (2): 22-23.

[3] Huang Xiu-zhen, Tao Yu-yao. Clinical Research on the Pattern Differentiation and Treatment of 56 Cases of Gouty Arthritis (辨证治疗痛风性关节炎56例临床观察). *Hubei Journal of Chinese Medicine* (湖北中医杂志). 2003, 19 (2): 23-24.

[4] Fang Ce, Yu Zhi-qiang. The Treatment of 112 Cases of Gouty Arthritis on the Basis of Pattern Differentiation (分型辨治痛风性关节炎112例). *Liaoning Journal of Chinese Medicine* (辽宁中医杂志). 2002,7 (2): 66.

[5] Zhang Chun-hua. Superficial Recognize about Gouty Treatment Based in Pathogenesis Obtained Through Differentiation of Symptoms and Signs (浅识痛风的辨证治疗). *Xinjiang Journal of Chinese Medicine* (新疆中医药). 2005, 23 (6): 5-6.

[6] Yu Li. Understanding the Chinese Medical Treatment of Gouty Arthritis (痛风性关节炎中医治疗体会). *Jilin Journal of Chinese Medicine* (吉林中医药). 2004, 24 (8): 14.

[7] Cao Xiang-yong, Zhang Sheng-hua and Chen Xiao-hong. Understanding the Chinese Medical Treatment of Gout (痛风病中医证治体会). *Practical Chinese Medicine Journal* (实用中医药杂志). 2003, 19 (4): 210-211.

[8] Wu Qi-fu, Yao Zhong-qiang, Li Juan, et al. Clinical Research on the Use of *Tong Feng Qing Chong Ji No. 2* in the Treatment of Acute Gouty Arthritis (痛风清2号冲剂治疗急性痛风性关节炎临床研究). *China Journal of TCM Emergency Medicine* (中国中医急症). 2000, 9 (2): 56-57.

[9] Chen Jin-yi. The Treatment of 55 Cases of Gouty Arthritis with *Yun Pi Li Niao Liang Xue Fang* (运脾利尿凉血方治疗痛风性关节炎55例). *Zhejiang Journal of Chinese Medicine* (浙江中医杂志). 2001, 36 (6): 251.

[10] Wang Zheng. Clinical Observation of the Treatment of 25 Cases of Gouty Arthritis by Draining Turbidity and Unblocking the Collaterals (泻浊通络法为主治疗痛风性关节炎25例临床观察).

Shanghai Journal of Chinese Medicine (上海中医药杂志). 2000, (10): 32-33.

[11] Xu Xiao-fang , Zhu Rong. Understanding the Treatment of Gouty Arthritis from the Perspective of Deficiency Patterns (从虚论治痛风性关节炎体会). *Gansu Journal of Chinese Medicine* (甘肃中医). 2005, 18 (12): 20-22.

[12] Wu Zong-hai. Clinical Observation of the Treatment of Gouty Arthritis with Chinese Medicine (中药治疗痛风性关节炎临床观察). *Chinese Practical Journal of Chinese and Western Medicine* (中华实用中西医杂志). 2003, 16 (11): 1578-1579.

[13] Chen Zu-hong. The Treatment of 55 Cases of Gouty Arthritis with *Dan Xi Tong Feng Jia Jian Fang* (丹溪痛风加减方治疗痛风性关节炎55例). *Shanxi Journal of Chinese Medicine* (陕西中医). 2004, 25 (12): 1093-1095.

[14] He Gang , Li Xue-mei. The Treatment of 24 Cases of Acute Gouty Arthritis with *Si Miao Wan Jia Wei* (四妙丸加味治疗急性痛风关节炎24例). *China Journal of TCM Emergency Medicine* (中国中医急症). 2006, 15 (1): 4.

[15] Yin Lian. Survey of the Use of *Si Miao Wan Jia Wei* in the Treatment of Acute Gouty Arthritis (四妙丸加味治疗急性痛风性关节炎概述). *China Journal of Chinese Medical Science and Technology* (中国中医药科技). 2004, 11 (1): 63-64.

[16] Zhi Liang, Liu Hong-jun, Li Hui-qi, et al. The Treatment of 42 Cases of Gouty Arthritis with *Dang Gui Nian Tong Tang* and *Wen He Gao* (当归拈痛汤合蚊合膏治疗痛风性关节炎42例). *New Chinese Medicine* (新中医). 2005, 37 (1): 78.

[17] Luo Ya-ming. The Treatment of Acute Gouty Arthritis with *Fu Fang Chen Tong San* (复方趁痛散治疗急性痛风性关节炎). *Chinese Journal of the Integration of Chinese Medicine and Western Medicine in the Treatment of Rheumatic Disease* (中国中西医结合风湿病杂志). 1994, (3): 112.

[18] Gao Cheng-fen, Liu Yong-mei. The Treatment of 55 Cases of Acute Gouty Arthritis with Modified *Mu Fang Ji Tang* (加减木防己汤治疗急性痛风性关节炎55例). *Sichuan Journal of Chinese Medicine* (四川中医). 2003, 21 (2): 42-43.

[19] Xu Tian-jing, Chen Zhi-wei. Observation of the Curative Effect of Treating 45 Cases of Acute Gout with Modified *Gui Zhi Shao Yao Zhi Mu Tang* (桂枝芍药知母汤加减治疗急性痛风45例疗效观察). *Journal of Zhejiang College of Chinese Medicine* (浙江中医学院学报). 1998, 22 (4): 19.

[20] Zhao Dong-ying. The Clinical Application of Modified *Xue Fu Zhu Yu Tang* (血府逐瘀汤加减临床运用举隅). *Anhui Journal of Clinical Chinese Medicine* (安徽中医临床杂志). 2000, 12 (5): 438.

[21] Yao Gui-rong, Wang Chang-chun. The Treatment of 46 Cases of Gout with Modified *Xuan Bi Tang* (加味宣痹汤治疗痛风46例). *Hubei Journal of Chinese Medicine* (湖北中医杂志). 2000, 22 (4): 35.

[22] Zhang Jun. The Treatment of 42 Cases of Gouty Arthritis with *Bu Shen Qing Re Zhi Wang Tang* (补肾清热治尪汤治疗痛风性关节炎42例). *Chinese Practical Journal of the Integration of Chinese and Western Medicine* (中华实用中西医结合杂志). 2004, 4 (17): 2593.

[23] Wang Jin-jun. Zhang Huang-sheng's Experience in Treating Gout (张荒生治疗痛风经验). *Practical Journal of TCM Internal Medicine* (实用中医内科杂志). 2006, 20 (1): 23.

[24] Huang Li-ping. The Treatment of 32 Cases of Gout Caused by Damp-heat and Blood Stasis with Dr. Zhu's Empirical Formula with Modifications (朱氏经验方化裁治疗湿热夹瘀痹阻型痛风32例).

Anhui Journal of Clinical Chinese Medicine (安徽中医临床杂志). 2003, 15 (2): 114-115.

[25] He Wei-yan. Professor Gai Guo-zhong's Experience in Treating Acute Gouty Arthritis (盖国忠教授论治急性痛风关节炎经验). *China Journal of TCM Emergency Medicine* (中国中医急症). 2004,9(13):606.

[26] He Ze-min. The Clinical Observation of the Treatment of 40 Cases of Acute Gouty Arthritis with *Zhen Tong Xi Feng Tang* (镇痛息风汤治疗急性痛风性关节炎40例临床观察). *Chinese Practical Journal of Chinese and Western Medicine* (中华实用中西医杂志). 2004, 4(17):3284-3285.

[27] Fu Dong-fang. The Treatment of 50 Cases of Gout with *Yan Hu Ding Tong Tang* (延胡定痛汤治疗痛风50例). *Chinese Practical Journal of Chinese and Western Medicine* (中华实用中西医杂志). 2003, 3 (16): 2115.

[28] Ji Wei, Tan Wen-feng, Lu Yan, et al. The Clinical Observation of the Treatment of Recurrent Attacks of Acute Gouty Arthritis by Expelling Turbidity and Clearing Heat (泄浊清热法治疗反复发作的急性痛风性关节炎的临床研究). *Chinese Practical Journal of Chinese and Western Medicine* (中华实用中西医杂志). 2005, 18 (23): 1733-1735.

[29] Song Ping. Observation of the Curative Effect of the Treatment of 40 Cases of Acute Gouty Arthritis with *Tong Feng Capsule* (痛风胶囊治疗急性痛风性关节炎40例疗效观察). *New Chinese Medicine* (新中医). 2006, 38 (2): 46-47.

[30] Cao Xiao-tian, Chen Ji-bang, Chen Ying-jun, et al. The Preparation of *Xi Tong Ning Capsule* and its Curative Effect in the Treatment of Gout (息痛宁胶囊的制备及对痛风症状的疗效观察). *Chinese Hospital Journal of Pharmacology* (中国医院药学杂志). 2003, 23 (6): 370-372.

[31] Yan Qun-chao, Mo Mu-shun. The Treatment of 100 Cases of Gouty Arthritis with *Tong Feng Ning Pill* (痛风宁片治疗痛风性关节炎100例). *Shanxi Journal of Chinese Medicine* (陕西中医). 2004, 25 (10): 891-892.

[32] Wen Shao-dun. Using *Suan Zhi Qing Capsule* to Treat 107 Cases of Gout-induced Hyperuricemia and Hyperlipidemia (酸脂清胶囊治疗痛风高尿酸伴高脂血症107例). *Shaanxi Journal of Chinese Medicine* (陕西中医). 2006, 27 (2): 180-191.

[33] Zhao Wei and Zhang Long-ji. The Clinical Observation of the Treatment of Gouty Arthritis with *Xin Huang Pill* (新癀片治疗痛风性关节炎临床观察). *Modern Chinese Journal of the Integration of Chinese and Western Medicine* (中华现代中西医杂志). 2005, 3 (7): 634-635.

[34] Zhang Hai-jiang and Xiang Nian-hu. Treat Acute Goutyarthritis 197 Cases with Point Bleedletting (刺络放血疗法治疗急性痛风性关节炎197例). *The People Military Surgeon* (人民军医). 2004, 47 (3): 157.

[35] Li Zhao-wen, Lin Shi-ming, Lin Jun-shan, et al. Controlled Study of the Treatment of 90 Cases of Acute Gouty Arthritis with Point Pricking (刺血疗法治疗急性痛风性关节炎90例对照研究). *Chinese Acupuncture and Moxibustion* (中国针灸). 2004, 24 (5): 311-313.

[36] Wen Shao-dun. The Clinical Observation of the Treatment of Acute Gouty Arthritis of the Foot with the Use of Fire Needling with Varying Intensities of Bloodletting (火针不同刺血量治疗足部急性痛风性关节炎观察). *Chinese Acupuncture and Moxibustion* (中国针灸). 2005, 25 (11): 779-780.

[37] Liu Xin. The Treatment of 61 Cases of Gouty Arthritis with Warming Acupuncture (温针灸

治疗痛风性关节炎61例). *Chinese Acupuncture and Moxibustion* (中国针灸). 2000, (9): 537-538.

[38] Zhang Shu-ying. The Treatment of 32 Cases of Gouty Arthritis with Acupuncture (针刺治疗痛风性关节炎32例). *Clinical Journal of Acupuncture* (针灸临床杂志). 2001, 17 (8): 9-10.

[39] Rao Guang-tao, Chen De-jun and Chen Hong-bin. The Clinical Observation of the Treatment of 109 Cases of Primary Gouty Arthritis with Acupuncture and Medicinals (针刺与药物对照治疗原发性痛风性关节炎109例疗效观察). *Chinese Acupuncture and Moxibustion* (中国针灸). 1993, (1): 8.

[40] Cheng Chun-kui. *Treating Rheumatism with Chinese Medicine and Western Medicine* (风湿病的中西医治疗). Chongqing: Chongqing University Press. 1997.81.

[41] Wu Zi-li. Observation of the Analgesic Effects of Needling UB 27 in the Treatment of Gout (针刺小肠俞对痛风镇痛效果的观察). *Sichuan Journal of Chinese Medicine* (四川中医). 1994, (10): 54.

[42] Duan Wei-ping. The Clinical Observation of the Treatment of 48 Cases of Gouty Arthritis with the Combination of Acupuncture and Medicinal Therapy (针药结合治疗痛风性关节炎48例临床观察). *Zhejiang Journal of Chinese Medicine* (浙江中医杂志). 2003, (4): 159.

[43] Yang Jin-hong, Luo Yong-li. The Treatment of 48 Cases of Acute Gouty Arthritis with Acupuncture and External Application of Medicinals (针刺配合药物外敷治疗急性痛风性关节炎48例). *Chinese Acupuncture and Moxibustion* (中国针灸). 2000, (7): 395-396.

[44] Jiang Xing-peng, Li Fu, Chen Wei. The Treatment of Gouty Arthritis with Acupuncture and External Application of Chinese Medicinals (针刺加中药薰洗治疗痛风性关节炎). *China Journal of Clinical Rehabilitation* (中国临床康复). 2005, 9 (18): 61.

[45] Li Yang-zhen. The Treatment of 32 Cases of Gouty Arthritis with Collateral Bloodletting (刺络治疗痛风性关节炎32例). *Chinese Acupuncture and Moxibustion* (中国针灸). 2006, 26 (2): 150.

[46] Xu Hao, Mao Hong-rong. The Treatment of 38 Cases of Gouty Arthritis with Acupuncture and Laser Therapy (针刺配合激光治疗痛风性关节炎38例). *Hubei Journal of Chinese Medicine* (湖北中医杂志). 2003, 25 (2): 43-44.

[47] Zhao Fen. Damp-heat Type Bi Syndrome [Gout] (湿热痹证[痛风]). *New Chinese Medicine* (新中医). 1985, (4): 10.

[48] Jiang Xi, Zhu Wan-hua. Understanding the Treatment of Gout by Draining Turbidity and Transforming Stasis (泄浊化瘀治疗痛风的经验体会). *Jiangsu Journal of Chinese Medicine* (江苏中医). 1990, (3): 7.

[49] Wang Jing-chun, Wang Zhi-ping, Cui Guo-wei. Understanding Pattern Differentiation and Treatment of Gouty Arthritis: A Study of 23 Cases (痛风性关节炎23例分型辨治体会). *New Chinese Medicine* (新中医). 1995, (6): 21.

[50] Liu Meng-zhou. Understanding the Treatment of Gouty Arthritis (痛风性关节炎的证治体会). *Journal of Liaoning University of Chinese Medicine* (辽宁中医学院学报). 2004, 6 (4): 284-285.

[51] Zheng Ping-dong. Treat Gout with Promoting Blood Circulation to Remove Meridian Obstruction, Dissipating Phlegm and Expelling Turbid (活血通络、化痰泄浊法治疗痛风之探讨). *Shanghai Journal of Chinese Medicine* (上海中医药杂志). 2004, 38 (12).

[52] Wang Fan-hong, Shi Zheng-fang. The Treatment of 28 Cases of Primary Gout with Chinese

Medicine (中医药治疗原发性痛风28例). *Zhejiang Journal of Chinese Medicine* (浙江中医杂志). 1994, (5): 208.

[53] Xia Han. The Treatment of 40 Cases of Gout with Modified *Dang Gui Nian Tong Tang* (当归拈痛汤加减治疗痛风40例疗效分析). *Journal of Chinese Medicine* (中医杂志). 1987, (2): 31.

[54] Zhang Bo. Discussion of Guo Zhong-yuan's Experience in Treating Gouty Arthritis (郭中元治疗痛风性关节炎经验论谈). *Hebei Journal of Chinese Medicine* (河北中医). 1993, 15 (6): 5.

[55] Jiang Xi, Zhu Wan-hua. Understanding the Treatment of Gout by Draining Turbidity and Transforming Stasis (泄浊化瘀治疗痛风的经验体会). *Jiangsu Journal of Chinese Medicine* (江苏中医). 1990, (3): 7.

[56] Yang Jia-ren. Case Histories of Gout (痛风验案). *Sichuan Journal of Chinese Medicine* (四川中医). 1989, (11): 35.

[57] Zhang Rui-yi. An Introduction to Luo Yu-tian's Experience in the Treatment of Gout (罗禹田老中医治疗痛风经验介绍). *Chinese Medicine Traumatology Journal* (中医骨伤科杂志). 1987, 3 (4): 47.

[58] Yan Dong-mei, Yan Xiao-ping. The Treatment of Gouty Arthritis (痛风性关节炎的中医辨治). *China Clinician* (中国临床医师). 2003, 31 (5): 52-53.

[59] Chen Li-ming. Discussion on the Significance of Binding Constraint of Phlegm-Stasis in the Onset and Treatment of Gout (略论痰瘀互结在痛风发病与治疗中的意义). *China Journal of Chinese Medicine News* (中国中医药信息杂志). 2004, 11 (5): 458-459.

[60] Wang Xiao-fang, Zhang En-shu. Ren Da-ran's Experience in the Treatment of Gout with *Hua Zhuo Qu Yu Tong Feng Fang* (任达然用"化浊祛瘀痛风方"治疗痛风的经验). *Jiangsu Journal of Chinese Medicine* (江苏中医药). 2005, 26 (6): 9-10.

[61] Zhang Rui-bin. Understanding the Treatment of Gouty Arthritis with Chinese Medicine (痛风性关节炎中医治疗体会). *Shandong Journal of Chinese Medicine* (山东中医杂志). 2003, 22 (7): 413-414.

[62] Chen Jin-yi, Yu Guo-hua. Observation of the Curative Effect of Decreasing Gouty Hyperuricemia by Invigorating the Spleen and Leaching Out Dampness (运脾渗湿法降低痛风症血尿酸浓度疗效观察). *Zhejiang Journal of Chinese Medicine* (浙江中医杂志). 1992, (1):12.

[63] Yao Jie-ming. *Report of Medical Data* (医学情报资料通讯). Shu Guang Hospital of the Shanghai University of Traditional Chinese Medicine (上海中医学院附属曙光医院编). 1989, (2): 39.

[64] Fan Yi-shan. The Treatment of 14 Cases of Gout with *Tong Feng Yin* (痛风饮治疗痛风14例). *Journal of Yunan University of Chinese Medicine* (云南中医学院学报). 1991, 14 (3): 45.

[65] Duan Hua-duan, Zhao Dian-fa, Zhao Ji-wei. The Clinical Observation of the Treatment of Gout by Promoting Urination, Expelling Stones, Clearing Heat and Resolving Toxicity (利尿排石清热解毒法治疗痛风疗效观察). *Liaoning Journal of Chinese Medicine* (辽宁中医杂志). 2005, 32 (7): 678-679.

[66] Huang Xuan-zhu, Zeng Suan-xiang, Liu Dong-zhou, et al. Observation of the Curative Effect of the External Application of *Shuang Bai Gao* on Acute Gouty Arthritis (双柏膏外敷辅助治疗急性痛风性关节炎的疗效观察). *Nursing Journal* (护理学杂志). 2006, 21 (3): 38-39.

[67] Liu Guang-zhen. The Clinical Observation of the Treatment of Acute Gouty Arthritis with *Juan Bi Xi Ji* (蠲痹洗剂治疗急性痛风性关节炎的临床观察). *Journal of External Treatment in Chinese Medicine* (中医外治杂志). 2004, 13 (6): 4-5.

[68] Ma Ya-juan, Mei Qun-chao. The Clinical Observation of the Treatment of Acute Gouty Arthritis with *Chinese Medicine No. I* (中药通I号治疗急性痛风性关节炎临床观察). *Hubei Journal of Chinese Medicine* (湖北中医杂志). 2006, 28 (2): 44.

[69] He Huan-ping. Clinical Analysis of the External Application of *Tong Feng San* in the Treatment of Gouty Arthritis: A Study of 43 Cases (外用痛风散治疗痛风性关节炎43例临床分析). *China Journal of Chinese Medicine News* (中国中医药信息杂志). 2000, 7 (1): 48.

[70] Wang Long-chuan. *Tong Feng Zhi Tong Gao* in the Treatment of 233 Cases of Gouty Arthritis (痛风止痛膏治疗痛风性关节炎233例). *Journal of External Treatment in Chinese Medicine* (中医外治杂志). 2001, 10 (6): 10-11.

[71] Yan Shi. External Application of *Fu Fang Ma Yi Gao* in the Treatment of 45 Cases Gouty Arthritis (复方蚂蚁膏外敷治疗痛风性关节炎45例). *Journal of External Treatment in Chinese Medicine* (中医外治杂志). 2001, 10 (1): 11.

[72] Cheng Chun-kui. Chinese Medicine and Western Medicine in the Treatment of Rheumatism (风湿病的中西医治疗). *Chongqing: Chongqing University Press*(重庆:重庆大学出版社). 1997. 81.

[73] Xia Jin-hua. The Treatment of 100 Cases of Gout with Internal and External Treatment (内外并治痛风100例). *Jiangsu Journal of Chinese Medicine* (江苏中医). 1994, (12): 13.

[74] Zhou Cui-ying, Sun Su-ping, Fu Xin-li. Chinese and Western Medical Diagnosis of Rheumatism (风湿病中西医诊疗学). *Beijing: China Chinese Medicine Publishing House*(北京:中国中医药出版社). 1998: 425.

[75] Xu Ke-zhi and Li Li. External Treatment of Internal Disease (内科疾病外治法). *Beijing: Chinese Medical Science and Technology Publishing House*(北京:中国中医药出版社). 1998:295.

[76] Chen Wen-zhao, Wu Shi-liang, Gu Duan-sheng, et al. The Effect of *Fang Ji Huang Qi Wu Yi Tang* on the Peripheral Neurotransmitters in Acute Gout (防己黄芪乌苡汤对急性痛风外周神经递质的影响). *China Journal of Medicine* (中国医药学报). 1997, 12 (4): 25.

[77] Chen Wen-zhao, Liu Yan-ling, Wu Shi-liang, et al. The Effect of *Fang Ji Huang Qi Wu Yi Tang* on Collagenase and Collagen Fibers of Rats with Gout (防己黄芪乌苡汤对痛风大鼠胶原酶及胶原纤维的影响). *Chinese Medicine Bonesetting* (中医正骨). 1999, 11 (2): 7.

[78] Li Juan, Yi Ming-juan, Guo Rong-xiao, et al. The Empirical Study of the Oral Administration of *Tong Feng Ning* in the Treatment of Acute Gouty Arthritis (痛风宁口服液治疗急性痛风性关节炎实验研究). *Huaxi Journal of Medicine* (华西医学杂志). 1998, 13 (3): 159.

[79] Zhang Bai-jia and Liu Liu. Advancement in the Pharmacological Research of *Dan Shen* Water Bath (丹参水溶部分药理研究进展). *Chinese Herbal Medicine* (中草药). 1996, 27 (10): 634-636.

[80] Zhang Xi-yun. The Chemical Composition, Pharmacological Action and Extraction of *Hu Zhang* (虎杖的化学成分、药理作用及提取分离). *Tianjin Medicine* (天津药学). 1999, 11(3):13-14.

[81] Song Wen-chong, Chen Chao. *Hu Shen Tong Feng Capsule*'s Anti-inflammatory Effect and its Effect on Tissue PGE2 (虎参痛风胶囊的抗炎作用及对组织PGE2含量的影响). *Chinese Practical Journal of Chinese and Western Medicine* (中华实用中西医杂志). 2003, 3 (16): 1416-1418.

[82] Wang Yan-yan, Chen Chao, Yang Hong-fa. *Hu Shen Tong Feng Capsule*'s Anti-Inflammatory Effect to Foot Swelling of Rat (虎参痛风胶囊对大鼠足肿的抗炎作用). *Chinese Hospital Journal of*

Pharmacology (中国医院药学杂志). 2005, 25 (3):206-208.

[83] Song Wen-chong, Wang Ya-qin and Chen Chao. *Hu Shen Tong Feng Capsule*'s Effect on Hyperuricemia and Uric acid Nephropathy in Rats (虎参痛风胶囊对高尿酸血症及尿酸性肾病大鼠的影响). *China Journal of Pharmacology* (中国药理学通报). 2004, 20 (3): 342-346.

[84] Qian Jing-ping and Chen Chao. The Effect of *Hu Shen Tong Feng Capsule* on Blood Uric Acid and its Analgesic Effect on Mice (虎参痛风胶囊对小鼠血尿酸的影响及其镇痛作用). *China Journal of New Medicinals and the Clinic* (中国新药与临床杂志). 2004, 23 (12): 878-890.

[85] Ji Wei, Zhu Xuan-xuan, Tan Wen-feng, et al. The Effect of *Re Bi Xiao Ke Li* on Recurrent Attacks of Hyperuricemia in Acute Gouty Arthritis (热痹消颗粒冲剂对反复发作的急性痛风性关节炎血尿酸的影响). *Chinese Practical Journal of Chinese and Western Medicine* (中华实用中西医杂志). 2004, 4 (17): 1761-1764.

[86] Zhu Xuan-xuan, Chen Zhen, Ji Wei, et al. The Empirical Study of *Re Bi Xiao* in the Treatment of Acute Gouty Arthritis (热痹消治疗急性痛风性关节炎的实验研究). *China Medicine Standard* (中国药品标准). 2002, 3 (1): 57-60.

[87] Wang Xiu-hua. The Effect of Treating Acute Gouty Arthritis by Clearing Heat and Dispelling Dampness on Cell Factor IL-1β and NO in the Knee Joints of Rabbits (清热祛湿法对兔膝关节急性痛风性关节炎细胞因子IL-1β和NO的影响). *Chinese Medicine Bonesetting* (中医正骨). 2001, 13 (4): 5.

Rheumatoid Arthritis

by **Deng Zhao-zhi,**
Professor & Chief Physician
of Chinese Internal Medicine,
the Second Teaching Hospital
of Guangzhou University of CM,
Guangzhou, China

Chen Wei,
Professor & Chief Physician
of Chinese Internal Medicine,
the Second Teaching Hospital
of Guangzhou University of CM,
Guangzhou, China

He Yi-ting,
Professor & Chief Physician
of Chinese Internal Medicine,
the Second Teaching Hospital
of Guangzhou University of CM,
Guangzhou, China

Zhu Li-qun,
Chief Physician,
the Second Teaching Hospital
of Guangzhou University of CM,
Guangzhou, China

OVERVIEW

Rheumatoid arthritis (RA) is a chronic systemic disease of unknown etiology that gradually affects the joints as well as their surrounding tissues by means of non-infective inflammation. It is characterized by the formation of continuous, recurrent, and progressive arthrosynovitis, effusions, cell proliferation, and pannus. It commonly affects the small joints of the hands, wrists, and feet symmetrically. RA may lead to the destruction of articular cartilage and bones, and eventually cause arthrocleisis, deformity, and functional impairment. The clinical manifestations of RA are varied and multiple, alternating between episodes of attack and relief with a high mutilation rate. The disease is given its name and categorized as a diffuse connective tissue disease because of the fact that it leads to multisystemic damage (e.g., hydrohymenitis, arteritis, scleritis, iritis, interstitial pneumonia, renal amyloidosis, neuropathy, lymphadenectasis, splenomegaly, and rheumatoid nodules) and the fact that it is an inflammatory reaction as a result of a disordered immune system. Both genetic and environmental factors control the course, scope, and type of the inflammatory reaction. RA occurs worldwide in all races and ethnic groups. Recent researches regarding HLA genes indicate that RA has a genetic basis. The reported incidence rate of RA in China and other countries vary (0.3%-1.5%) due to the difference in the level of understanding of the diagnostic criteria.

Biomedicine considers genetic factors to be the cause of RA. Infectious agents may induce the onset of RA but they are not the direct cause. Many factors play a role in the complicated process of immunological derangement in the joints and throughout the entire body. Single or multiple external antigens may trigger the onset, while other factors (e.g., environmental, psychological, postpartum, or post-menopausal) may also give rise to RA. Common complications include chronic gastritis or gastrointestinal bleeding, bone marrow depression, renal functional impairment, pulmonary interstitial fibrosis, bone fractures, ulceration or necrosis of the extremities, and infections (lung infection is most common, while the incidence of cryptococcus infection of CNS and specific infections (e.g., TB) has increased over the past few years). Currently, most of these complications are serious enough to be major causes of death in RA patients, some of which may be related to the long-term use of glucocorticoids and immunodepressants. It is not difficult to arrive at a diagnosis based on characteristic clinical symptoms, X-ray findings of specific changes in the joints, presence of the three characteristics of rheumatism, an elevated ESR, and changes in peripheral seroimmunity. The diagnosis of RA is mainly based on the standard diagnostic criteria proposed by ARA in 1987. If more than 4 of the total 7 conditions are present, a diagnosis of RA is confirmed.

Since the root of RA cannot be treated, the greatest objective of biomedical treatment is to prevent joint destruction, protect joint function, and help improve the patients' quality of life. Modern medicine holds that early diagnosis followed by proper use of disease-modifying antirheumatic drugs (DMARDs) is the key to the preventing mutilation. Once the diagnosis of RA is confirmed, combination therapy should be started immediately. During the window phase of the first three months, NSAIDs and DMARDs should be administered. One class of appropriate NSAIDs will do, while the best choice of DMARDs is a combination of methotrexate, sulfasalazine, and hydroxychloroquine (MTX+SSZ+HCQ). Although the therapeutic regimen depends on the patient's condition, the MTX+SSZ+HCQ combination is recommended as the first-line therapy. When choosing drugs of the same therapeutic effect, especially second-line drugs, doctors should select those of different classes and mechanisms of action, and at the same time, avoid prescribing those with identical side effects. In spite of these efforts, the therapeutic efficacy is still not satisfactory, as the treatment can only relieve some of the symptoms or stop the progression of the disease, but it cannot cure the disease. Furthermore, most of the drugs produce adverse effects; for instance, NSAIDs may give rise to poor appetite, nausea, vomiting, skin rashes, hematocytopenia, or nervous system impairment. Drugs that improve the condition, such as gold preparations and cytotoxic drugs may cause bone marrow depression, hepatotoxicity, reproductive system toxicity, or other adverse effects. The use of biological agents to treat RA has been gaining popularity in the past few years, and is still under study. There are many methods to treat RA using biological agents, e.g., IFN-ee resistant T lymphocyte, anti-cytokine therapy (mainly directed at TNF, interleukin-1, and granulocyte macrophage colony stimulating factor), and gene therapy. Since biological agents have the advantage of highly selective pharmacological action with minor side effects, they are expected to have a larger application market.

RA is categorized as a *bi* syndrome in Chinese medicine.

CHINESE MEDICAL ETIOLOGY AND PATHOMECHANISM

Even as early as *Yellow Emperor's Inner Classic* (黄帝内经, *Huáng Dì Nèi Jīng*), the notion that wind, cold, and dampness invade the human body and cause *bi* has been proposed, as it was said: "The three evils, wind, cold, and dampness, mix and combine to form *bi*." (风寒湿三气杂至合而为痹也。) *Bi* syndromes were divided into 3 categories of moving *bi* (行痹, *xíng bì*), painful *bi* (痛痹, *tòng bì*), and fixed *bi* (着痹, *zhuó bì*), according to their etiology. There were also mentions of visceral *bi* (五脏痹, *wŭ zàng bì*) and *bi* of the five body constituents (五体痹, *wŭ tĭ bì*). Ever since, increasing numbers of Chinese medicine doctors have contributed to this theory, eventually completing the etiology and pathomechanism of *bi* syndromes. A contemporary expert of Chinese medicine, Jiao Shu-de, studied and absorbed the experiences of his predecessors and referred to modern research. Integrating this gathered knowledge with his own comprehension, he created the term "lame *bi*" (尪痹 , *wāng bì*), and proposed a general summary on its etiology, pattern, pulse manifestation, and treatment, all of which are widely acknowledged by practitioners of Chinese medicine.

1. Chinese Medical Perspective of RA Etiology

(1) Constitutional Insufficiency and Liver and Kidney Depletion

Constitutional insufficiency gives rise to liver and kidney depletion. The liver governs the sinews and the kidney governs the bones. Sinews and bones are supported by blood, essence, and the fluid of the liver and kidney, and are also dependant upon the warmth of the liver and kidney yang qi. Kidney yang is also called "true yang", "original yang", or "life gate (*mìng mén*) fire." It warms and nourishes the *zang-fu*, and is the foundation of body's yang qi. The kidney stores essence, engenders marrow, and governs the bones; it is the office of labor. The liver and kidney are of the same source; together, they nourish the sinews and bones. Kidney deficiency results in insufficiency of the marrow and debilitation of true qi. When wind, cold, and dampness combine together, if cold and dampness are predominant, they will invade the deficient kidney. As a result, there is obstruction in the channels and collaterals, qi and blood cannot flow properly, and the joints are blocked. The deficient kidney (water) is unable to nourish the liver (wood), and thus the sinews and bones lose their source of nourishment, eventually leading to looseness of the bones and hypertonicity of the sinews, deformity of the joints, and inability to bend and stretch. In severe cases, the muscles and tendons shorten, and the elbow is unable to bend.

(2) The Six External Evils Exploit and Invade the Deficient Body

Insufficiency of right qi renders the body susceptible to the invasion of evils. For instance, living in a damp environment, wading in cold water, and exposure to cold and rainy weather allow the body to be invaded by external evils, which impair the circulation of qi and blood and give rise to *bi* syndromes. *Yellow Emperor's Inner Classic - Basic Questions, Treatise on Bi Syndromes* (黄帝内经素问 · 痹论, *Huáng Dì Nèi Jīng Sù Wèn - Bì Lùn*) states: "What is known as *bi*, is the contraction of wind, cold, and dampness." (所谓痹者，各以其时，重感于风寒湿之气也。) Wind evil is swift and changeable; it invades the many joints and causes wandering pain. Cold evil is congealing and stagnating, and causes contracture and tautness; it invades the sinews and bones, inhibits bending and stretching, and causes qi and blood stagnation, which leads to pain. Damp evil is sticky, stagnant, and heavy; it invades the body and causes continuous and unremitting swelling and distention. If one contracts yang heat evil or if the constitution is one of yang exuberance, and one also contracts wind cold damp evil, the long-term constraint will transform into heat and invade the channels, collaterals, and blood vessels, and spread over the entire body. The blood and the heat will then bind together. Since heat is a yang evil, it can easily damage the body fluids and consume qi; it decocts the body fluid to form phlegm; the resulting phlegm-heat stasis obstructs the joints and causes swelling, distention, and deformity.

(3) Imbalance of the Seven Emotions

Anger causes qi counterflow and excessive thinking causes qi to knot. Both lead to the disharmonious movement of the qi dynamic, resulting in constraint and stagnation. Qi is the commander of blood, and blood is the mother of qi; they are intimately related. Long-term emotional imbalance disrupts the circulation of blood. Qi governs warming, and blood governs moistening. All the functions of the *zang-fu* rely on the moisture and nourishment of qi and blood, and thus long-term impairment of qi and blood flow will eventually affect the *zang-fu*. Furthermore, it causes obstruction in the channels and vessels, giving rise to *bi*. Emotional imbalance during the remission stage of disease can induce a relapse or worsen the condition.

(4) Imbalance between Work and Rest, and Sexual Intemperance

Excessive physical labor damages nutritive and defensive qi and blood, and leads to yang qi insufficiency. The interstices (腠 理 , *còu lǐ*) become empty, the exterior defense becomes insecure, and the evil qi pour into the channels, collaterals, joints, and flesh. Excessive sexual activity gradually depletes the essential qi and makes the body prone to the invasion of evils. On the other hand, too much rest weakens the transportative and transformative functions of the spleen and stomach, thereby leading to a decrease in the production of qi and blood. Furthermore, too much leisure and rest hinder the circulation of qi and blood. People whose lifestyles involve very little physical activity develop brittle bones and weak sinews, which eventually lead to liver and kidney deficiency detriment. Even slight carelessness can easily make them susceptible to evils that exploit this deficiency and invade the body. The evils will then struggle with the blood, block the flow of yang qi, impair the circulation of qi, blood, and fluids, and induce the generation of phlegm-stasis, which infiltrate into the joints.

2. Chinese Medical Perspective of RA Pathomechanism

"The three evils, i.e., wind, cold, and dampness, mix and combine to form *bi*." (风寒湿三气杂至合而为痹也。) This is considered not only the etiology and pathomechanism of *bi* syndromes, but also those of RA. Among the pathomechanisms of *bi* syndromes, the internal factor of right qi deficiency plays the most crucial role, while the invasion of external evils is the important cause of disease onset. *Yellow Emperor's Inner*

Classic: Basic Questions - Treatise on Needling Methods (黄帝内经素问 · 刺法论, *Huáng Dì Nèi Jīng Sù Wèn - Cì Fǎ Lùn*) states: "As long as there is right qi in the interior, the evils cannot invade." (正气存内，邪不可干。) *Yellow Emperor's Inner Classic: Divine Pivot, The Beginnings of the Hundred Diseases* (黄帝内经灵枢 · 百病始生, *Huáng Dì Nèi Jīng Líng Shū - Bǎi Bìng Shǐ Shēng*) mentions: "Wind, cold, and heat cannot harm the body if there is no right qi deficiency…the combination of right qi deficiency and exogenous pathogens is what causes the formation of disease." (风雨寒热不得虚，邪不能独伤人……此必因虚邪之风，与其身形，两虚相得，乃客其形。) Right qi deficiency is basically liver and kidney depletion; it is the most important internal factor of the disease onset, and plays an important role in the entire course of the disease. It determines the body's ability to fight against the pathogens; regulates qi, blood, yin, and yang; influences the waxing and waning of evil qi and right qi; and determines the prognosis of the illness. According to the disease condition and the struggle between evil qi and right qi, RA can be divided into 3 stages: early, middle, and late.

(1) Early Stage: Evil Excess and Right Qi Deficiency

In the early stage, the chief pathomechanism is liver and kidney depletion with concurrent external evil obstruction. The former is the root and the latter is the branch. The primary clinical manifestations are that of evil excess. The nature of cold evil is to congeal and stagnate, while damp evil tends to impede the normal flow of qi and blood. Invasion of the body by cold-damp evil causes obstruction and stagnation of the qi and blood of the channels and vessels. When movement is inhibited, symptoms such as pain, swelling, and distention of the joints and flesh arise. Invasion of the skin and flesh by cold-damp evil causes disharmony of qi and blood and inhibited flow of qi in the channels and vessels; hence, there is numbness. Cold-damp damages the yang qi of the body, stripping yang of its warming function, and thus giving rise to cold limbs that are worse upon exposure to cold; it also obstructs the collaterals, impeding the flow of channel qi and giving rise to cold pain in the joints of the limbs that is temporarily relieved by warmth and movement. Yang qi depletion leads to malnourishment of the sinews, which causes inability of the joints to bend and stretch. Wind-cold-damp evil obstructs the flow of yang qi and damages the yang qi, leading to local aversion to wind and cold. The clinical manifestations of this stage include symmetrical redness, swelling, and hot pain of multiple joints. The pain is either wandering or fixed, and often occurs in the small joints of the extremities. Fusiform swelling can be seen in the proximal interphalangeal joints. Swelling and pain often occur in the metacarpal (or metatarsal) joint, wrist joint, knee joint, elbow joint, ankle joint, and sometimes in the temporal mandibular joint as well. The cricoarytenoid joint (the joint between the cricoid and arytenoids; located in the larynx) may also be involved.

(2) Middle Stage: A Prolonged Disease Course of Deficiency-Excess Complex

Whether a condition is one of deficiency or excess is decided by exuberance and debilitation of right and evil. The progression of disease to this stage may be a result of difficulty in arriving at a diagnosis during the early stage, failure of the patient to promptly seek medical attention, lack of treatment, or erroneous treatment. Since the patient has root deficiency, i.e., liver and kidney depletion, in addition to a prolonged disease course, the evil qi lingering in the body gradually consumes and damages the right qi, and hence, there are signs of a deficiency-excess complex. The disease condition fluctuates unsteadily and unceasingly, alternating between remission and relapse for many years. The prolonged disease course greatly debilitates the health and further depletes the right qi. The overall health is poor, and the body is emaciated. The evil qi obstructs the channels and vessels, and over a long period of time, affects the movement and distribution of qi, blood, and body fluids. Blood stagnates and forms stasis, while the body fluids stop flowing and transform into phlegm. The phlegm-turbidity and static blood will further obstruct the channels and collaterals, and give rise to signs and symptoms such as stasis macules of the skin, nodules surrounding the joints, and inhibited bending and stretching. Clinical manifestations may also include limited range of articular motion or joint swelling, distention, and deformity. Severe struggle between right and evil may manifest as fever and red, swollen, hot, and painful joints (or a subjective sensation of hot joints but the joints are not hot to the touch). Cold evil congealing and stagnating leads to the inhibited flow of yang qi, which is then unable to reach the limbs, and thus commonly manifests as pain, swelling, and distention of the small joints, and in chronic cases, there may even be morning stiffness. Liver and kidney depletion gives rise to spasms and contracture of the sinews and numbness of the skin. In chronic cases, there may also be soreness and weakness of the lumbus and knees, dizziness, and unclear vision.

(3) Late Stage: Liver and Kidney Insufficiency, Qi and Blood Depletion, and Phlegm-Stasis Bind

If treatment is not administered promptly to prevent articular deformity, protect articular function, and improve the patient's quality of life, the disease will get progressively worse. The main focus of the disease shifts from evil excess to liver and kidney deficiency. Because of the resulting lingering evils and insufficient right qi, a prolonged disease course allows the evils to infiltrate into the bones, consuming blood and essence, damaging sinews and bones, and causing shifting or dislocation of the joints. It also causes inability of the PIPs to extend and hyperextension of the distal interphalangeal joints (goose-neck deformity). Chronic *bi* injures kidney yang and obstructs the waterways, and over time, this excessive accumulation of water-damp transforms into phlegm. Chronic rheumatism leads to disorder of the visceral qi dynamic. As a result, qi, blood, and phlegm-turbidity obstruct one another and form phlegm-stasis. Phlegm-stasis and water-damp interact, giving way to further transformation, e.g., dampness gathers and becomes phlegm, blood gathers and forms stasis, and phlegm obstructs the flow of blood. Phlegm-stasis and water-damp bind together and prolong the course of the disease, leading to stubborn *bi*. Phlegm-stasis obstructing the skin and flesh gives rise to round or oval-shaped nodules, which can be fixed or mobile, with or without tenderness. Chronic *bi* can affect not only the channels and collaterals, but also the *zang-fu* organs as well, manifesting as pathological changes of the corresponding *zang-fu*, of which the most common is heart *bi*. The clinical signs and symptoms of heart *bi* include flusteredness, vexation, hasty panting upon exertion, and, in severe cases, puffy swelling of the limbs and body.

To summarize, the pathogenesis of RA is different from that of other general *bi* syndromes. The disease is mainly a result of constitutional weakness and postnatal taxation detriment, which allows the external pathogens, i.e., wind, cold, and dampness, to invade the body and obstruct the channels and collaterals. Cold congealing in the collaterals or heat amassment in the channels and collaterals cause the liver and kidney to become deficient and phlegm and stasis to intermix. The location of the disease is in the sinews and bones, and the basic pathomechanism is the combination of constitutional (root) deficiency; qi and blood insufficiency; liver and kidney depletion; and wind, cold, and dampness obstructing the channels and infiltrating into the joints. The disease affects the bones, joints, sinews, and muscles. The root of the disease is deficiency, while the branch is excess (deficiency-excess complex).

CHINESE MEDICAL TREATMENT

Pattern Differentiation and Treatment

RA is a chronic and recurrent disease whose root lies in right qi depletion and liver and kidney insufficiency, and whose branch involves wind, cold, and dampness invading the body and causing obstruction in the joints, channels, and collaterals, and eventually giving rise to phlegm and stasis. The key point in pattern differentiation is to determine the extent of right qi deficiency and evil excess; the extent of the depletion of the qi, blood, yin, and yang of the *zang-fu*; and the extent of predominance of wind, cold, dampness (heat), phlegm, and stasis. The following treatment principles can be employed: dispel wind and disperse cold; transform dampness and clear heat; expel phlegm and disperse stasis; unblock the collaterals and relieve pain; tonify and boost qi and blood; and enrich and tonify the liver and kidney.

(1) Wind-cold-damp *Bi*

【Syndrome Characteristics】

Pain in the joints and muscles with inhibited bending and stretching. If wind evil is predominant, the pain is wandering and can involve many joints; if cold evil is predominant, the pain is severe, and is aggravated by cold and relieved by warmth; if dampness is predominant, the pain is fixed and heavy, and there is diffuse joint swelling with numbness of the skin, accompanied by exterior symptoms such as aversion to cold and fever. The tongue is pale with white coating that is either thin or greasy. The pulse is floating or wiry, tight, soft, and moderate.

【Treatment Principle】

Dispel wind, disperse cold, transform dampness, unblock the collaterals, and relieve pain.

【Commonly Used Medicinals】

Fáng fēng (Radix Saposhnikoviae), *fáng jǐ* (Radix Stephaniae Tetrandrae), and *fú líng* (Poria) are used to expel wind, disperse cold, and transform dampness; *qiāng huó* (Rhizoma et Radix Notopterygii), *dú huó* (Radix Angelicae Pubescentis), and *zhì chuān wū* (Radix Aconiti Praeparata) are used to disperse cold and transform dampness; *guì zhī* (Ramulus Cinnamomi) and *gān cǎo* (Radix et Rhizoma Glycyrrhizae) can be used to harmonize nutritive qi and unblock the collaterals.

【Representative Formula】

Modified *Juān Bì Tāng* (蠲痹汤)

【Ingredients】

羌活	qiāng huó	10g	Rhizoma et Radix Notopterygii
姜黄	jiāng huáng	15g	Rhizoma Curcumae Longae
当归	dāng guī	15g	Radix Angelicae Sinensis
赤芍	chì sháo	10g	Radix Paeoniae Rubra
黄芪	huáng qí	10g	Radix Astragali
防风	fáng fēng	6g	Radix Saposhnikoviae
炙甘草	zhì gān cǎo	5g	Radix et Rhizoma Glycyrrhizae Praeparata cum Melle
独活	dú huó	10g	Radix Angelicae Pubescentis
乌头	wū tóu	10g	Radix Aconiti Kusnezoffii (decocted first)
炙麻黄	zhì má huáng	10g	Herba Ephedrae (honey-fried)
白芍	bái sháo	10g	Radix Paeoniae Alba
薏苡仁	yì yǐ rén	15g	Semen Coicis
桂枝	guì zhī	10g	Ramulus Cinnamomi
川芎	chuān xiōng	10g	Rhizoma Chuanxiong
生姜	shēng jiāng	5g	Rhizoma Zingiberis Recens

【Formula Analysis】

Qiāng huó (Rhizoma et Radix Notopterygii) and *dú huó* (Radix Angelicae Pubescentis) are important herbs for treating *bi* syndromes. *Herbal Foundation for Decoctions* (汤液本草, *Tāng Yè Běn Cǎo*) states: "*Qiāng huó* (Rhizoma et Radix Notopterygii) strongly moves qi. It is good for dispelling wind and transforming dampness in the foot taiyang channel to relieve pain of the entire body." (羌活气雄，治足太阳风湿相搏，一身尽痛者，非此不能除。) *Qiāng huó* (Rhizoma et Radix Notopterygii) is good for treating water-damp and wandering wind. It is specific for treating wind cold damp *bi* above the waist, especially the shoulder and back. *Dú huó* (Radix Angelicae Pubescentis) treats water dampness and hidden wind. It is specific for treating cold-damp in the lower body. *Huáng qí* (Radix Astragali) boosts defensive qi. *Yì yǐ rén* (Semen Coicis) eliminates dampness and unblocks obstruction. *Bái sháo* (Radix Paeoniae Alba) regulates blood. *Gān cǎo* (Radix et Rhizoma Glycyrrhizae) harmonizes all the herbs. *Bái sháo* (Radix Paeoniae Alba) and *gān cǎo* (Radix et Rhizoma Glycyrrhizae) moderate spasms and relieve pain. *Wū tóu* (Radix Aconiti Kusnezoffii) seeks out wind, disperses cold, warms the channels, and relieves pain. *Wū tóu* (Radix Aconiti Kusnezoffii) is a toxic herb that is extremely acrid and hot. In The dosage of *wū tóu* (Radix Aconiti Kusnezoffii) should be small in the beginning, and gradually increased if necessary. *Wū tóu* (Radix Aconiti Kusnezoffii) should be decocted for a long time to minimize its toxic nature. Honey can be added to the formula if necessary, to boost blood, nourish the sinews, relax tension, and relieve pain; it can also control the dry heat toxins of *wū tóu* (Radix Aconiti Kusnezoffii).

【Modifications】

- For predominance of wind evil, emphasis should be placed on prescribing medicinals that dispel wind. Medicinals that nourish and invigorate blood can also be added. "To treat wind, first treat the blood; when the blood moves, the wind will naturally be extinguished." (治风先治血，血行风自灭。) Appropriate medicinals include *fáng fēng* (Radix Saposhnikoviae) 15g, *jī xuè téng* (Caulis Spatholobi) 15g, and *gǎo běn* (Rhizoma et Radix Ligustici) 10g.

➢ For yang qi deficiency and cold exuberance, add *shú fù zǐ* (Radix Aconiti Lateralis Preparata) 10g (decocted first), *zhì chuān wū* (Radix Aconiti Praeparata) 10g (decocted first), and *zhì cǎo wū* (Radix Aconiti Kusnezoffii Praeparata) 10g (decocted first) to warm yang, disperse cold, and relieve pain.

➢ For exuberant dampness, add *zhū líng* (Polyporus) 10g, *zé xiè* (Rhizoma Alismatis) 15g, *cāng zhú* (Rhizoma Atractylodis) 10g, and *hòu pò* (Cortex Magnoliae Officinalis) 10g to fortify the spleen and dry dampness. In addition, using *guì zhī* (Ramulus Cinnamomi) and *zé xiè* (Rhizoma Alismatis) together can help eliminate joint swelling and distention by relieving fluid accumulation in the joint cavity.

➢ For severe pain, add *yán hú suǒ* (Rhizoma Corydalis) 10g and *piàn jiāng huáng* (Rhizoma Wenyujin Concisum) 10g to move qi, invigorate blood, and relieve pain.

(2) Wind-damp-heat *Bi*

【Syndrome Characteristics】

Joint pain involving one or more joints. The affected joints are hot, red, swollen, and tender with limited range of motion. The symptoms are relieved by cold and aggravated by heat. Other signs and symptoms include morning stiffness, thirst, reddish urine, dry stool, a red tongue with yellow coating, and a rapid pulse.

【Treatment Principle】

Clear heat, transform dampness, relieve spasms, and unblock the collaterals.

【Commonly Used Medicinals】

Huáng lián (Rhizoma Coptidis), *huáng bǎi* (Cortex Phellodendri Chinensis), *tǔ fú líng* (Rhizoma Smilacis Glabrae), and *bì xiè* (Rhizoma Dioscoreae Hypoglaucae) are used to clear heat and dry dampness. *Qín jiāo* (Radix Gentianae Macrophyllae), *sāng zhī* (Ramulus Mori), and *luò shí téng* (Caulis Trachelospermi) are used to clear heat and dispel wind. *Chuān shān lóng* (Rhizoma Dioscoreae Nipponicae), *sī guā luò* (Retinervus Luffae Fructus) are used to dispel wind and unblock the collaterals.

【Representative Formula】

A modified combination of *Xuān Bì Tāng* (宣痹汤) plus *Sān Miào Săn* (三妙散).

【Ingredients】

防己	fáng jĭ	10g	Radix Stephaniae Tetrandrae
生薏苡仁	shēng yì yĭ rén	30g	Semen Coicis (raw)
苍术	cāng zhú	10g	Rhizoma Atractylodis
防风	fáng fēng	10g	Radix Saposhnikoviae
黄柏	huáng băi	10g	Cortex Phellodendri Chinensis
土茯苓	tŭ fú líng	30g	Rhizoma Smilacis Glabrae
川萆薢	chuān bì xiè	30g	Rhizoma Dioscoreae Hypoglaucae
蚕沙	cán shā	20-30g	Faeces Bombycis
怀牛膝	huái niú xī	10g	Radix Achyranthis Bidentatae

Boil the above ingredients in 500 ml water until reduced to a 200 ml decoction. Take warm, 1 batch a day.

【Formula Analysis】

Fáng jĭ (Radix Stephaniae Tetrandrae), *fáng fēng* (Radix Saposhnikoviae), and *yì yĭ rén* (Semen Coicis) course wind, dispel dampness, and remove obstruction in the joints. *Cāng zhú* (Rhizoma Atractylodis) dries dampness and fortifies the spleen. *Huáng băi* (Cortex Phellodendri Chinensis), *tŭ fú líng* (Rhizoma Smilacis Glabrae), and *bì xiè* (Rhizoma Dioscoreae Hypoglaucae) clear heat and drain dampness. *Cán shā* (Faeces Bombycis) is used to diffuse *bi* and transform dampness. *Huái niú xī* (Radix Achyranthis Bidentatae) dispels wind-damp, invigorates blood, and strengthens the sinews and bones.

【Modifications】

- For severe joint pain, add *rĕn dōng téng* (Caulis Lonicerae Japonicae)

15g, *luò shí téng* (Caulis Trachelospermi) 15g, *sāng zhī* (Ramulus Mori) 30g, *mù guā* (Fructus Chaenomelis) 15g, and *yán hú suǒ* (Rhizoma Corydalis) 10g to strengthen the effects of clearing heat and relieving pain.

➢ For exuberant heat, add *shuǐ niú jiǎo* (Cornu Bubali) 10g, *bái huā shé shé cǎo* (Herba Hedyotis Diffusae) 15g, and *lián qiào* (Fructus Forsythiae) 10g to clear heat and resolve toxins.

➢ For exuberant damp-turbidity, add *huá shí* (Talcum) 15g and *chì xiǎo dòu* (Semen Phaseoli) 15g to separate the clear from the water-damp.

(3) Kidney Deficiency and Congealing Cold

【Syndrome Characteristics】

Soreness and weakness of the lumbus and knees; fatigue and lack of strength; preference for warmth and aversion to cold; pain, swelling, and deformity of joints of the fingers, wrists, knees, ankles, and toes; morning stiffness; a pale red tongue with white coating; and thready and weak pulse.

【Treatment Principle】

Tonify the kidney and disperse cold; transform dampness and scatter wind; strengthen the sinews and bones; and unblock the channels and collaterals.

【Commonly Used Medicinals】

Xù duàn (Radix Dipsaci), *bǔ gǔ zhī* (Fructus Psoraleae), *shú dì huáng* (Radix Rehmanniae Praeparata), *yín yáng huò* (Herba Epimedii), and *niú xī* (Radix Achyranthis Bidentatae) are used to tonify the liver and kidney and strengthen the sinews and bones. *Zhì fù piàn* (Radix Aconiti Lateralis Preparata), *má huáng* (Herba Ephedrae), and *guì zhī* (Ramulus Cinnamomi) are used to disperse cold and unblock the collaterals.

【Representative Formula】

Modified *Bǔ Shèn Qū Hán Zhì Wāng Tāng* (补肾祛寒治尪汤)

【Ingredients】

续断	xù duàn	12g	Radix Dipsaci
补骨脂	bǔ gǔ zhī	12g	Fructus Psoraleae
熟地	shú dì	12g	Radix Rehmanniae Praeparata
淫羊藿	yín yáng huò	20g	Herba Epimedii
制附片	zhì fù piàn	6-12g	Radix Aconiti Lateralis Praeparata
骨碎补	gǔ suì bǔ	20g	Rhizoma Drynariae
桂枝	guì zhī	9g	Ramulus Cinnamomi
赤芍	chì sháo	12g	Radix Paeoniae Rubra
白芍	bái sháo	12g	Radix Paeoniae Alba
知母	zhī mǔ	12g	Rhizoma Anemarrhenae
独活	dú huó	12g	Radix Angelicae Pubescentis
麻黄	má huáng	3-6g	Herba Ephedrae
苍术	cāng zhú	10g	Rhizoma Atractylodis
威灵仙	wēi líng xiān	12g	Radix et Rhizoma Clematidis
伸筋草	shēn jīn cǎo	30g	Herba Lycopodii
牛膝	niú xī	9g	Radix Achyranthis Bidentatae
松节	sōng jié	15g	Lignum Pini Nodi
炙山甲	zhì shān jiǎ	9g	Squama Manis (liquid-fried)
地鳖虫	dì biē chóng	10g	Eupolyphaga seu Steleophaga
寻骨风	xún gǔ fēng	12g	Herba Aristolochiae Mollissimae
自然铜	zì rán tóng	6-9g	Pyritum (soaked in vinegar and decocted first)
透骨草	tòu gǔ cǎo	20g	Caulis Impatientis

Boil the above ingredients in 500ml water until reduced to a 200ml decoction. Take warm, 1 batch a day.

【Formula Analysis】

This formula is a modified version of the combination of *Guì Zhī Sháo Yào Zhī Mǔ Tāng* (桂枝芍药知母汤) and *Hǔ Gǔ Sǎn* (虎骨散). *Chuān duàn* (Radix Dipsaci), *bǔ gǔ zhī* (Fructus Psoraleae), *shú dì* (Radix Rehmanniae Praeparata), *yín yáng huò* (Herba Epimedii), and *niú xī* (Radix Achyranthis Bidentatae) tonify the liver and kidney. *Zhì fù piàn* (Radix Aconiti Lateralis Preparata) and *guì zhī* (Ramulus Cinnamomi) warm the channels, disperse cold, and *fáng fēng* (Radix Saposhnikoviae) dispel and guard against wind. *Má huáng* (Herba Herba Ephedrae) disperses cold. *Cāng zhú* (Rhizoma Atractylodis) dispels dampness and prevents the repeated contraction of the three evils. *Dú huó* (Radix Angelicae Pubescentis), *wēi líng xiān* (Radix et Rhizoma Clematidis), *shēn jīn cǎo* (Herba Lycopodii), *xún gǔ fēng* (Herba Aristolochiae Mollissimae), *zì rán tóng* (Pyritum), and *tòu gǔ cǎo* (Caulis Impatientis) dispel wind, transform dampness, unblock the collaterals, and relieve pain. *Sōng jié* (Lignum Pini Nodi) frees the joints from obstruction. *Zhì shān jiǎ* (liquid-fried Squama Manis) and *dì biē chóng* (Eupolyphaga seu Steleophaga) invigorate blood, break stasis, and strengthen the effect of relieving pain. *Bái sháo* (Radix Paeoniae Rubra) softens the sinews. *Chì sháo* (Radix Paeoniae Rubra) clears heat and transforms stasis. *Zhī mǔ* (Rhizoma Anemarrhenae) enriches the kidney, clears heat, and balances out the excessively drying nature of the formula.

【Modifications】

➢ If the joints of the upper extremities are severely affected, remove *niú xī* (Radix Achyranthis Bidentatae), and add envoys to the upper limbs, i.e., *piàn jiāng huáng* (Rhizoma Wenyujin Concisum) 10-12g and *qiāng huó* (Rhizoma et Radix Notopterygii) 12g to invigorate blood, transform stasis, dispel wind, and eliminate dampness.

➢ For pronounced blood stasis symptoms, add *hóng huā* (Flos Carthami) 10g, *zào jiǎo cì* (Spina Gleditsiae) 10g, *rǔ xiāng* (Olibanum) 6g, *mò yào* (Myrrha) 6g, or *sū mù* (Lignum Sappan) 15g to invigorate blood and transform stasis.

➢ For fatigue, hypertonicity, and stiffness of the joints, remove *fáng fēng* (Radix Saposhnikoviae), *cāng zhú* (Rhizoma Atractylodis), and *sōng jié* (Lignum Pini Nodi), and add *shēng yì yǐ rén* (raw Semen Coicis) 30g, *mù guā* (Fructus Chaenomelis) 12g, and *bái jiāng cán* (Bombyx Batryticatus) 10g to relax the sinews and free joint obstruction.

➢ For severe joint pain, increase the dosage of *zhì fù piàn* (Radix Aconiti Lateralis Praeparata), and add *cǎo wū* (Radix Aconiti Kusnezoffii) 6-9g to strengthen the effects of dispersing cold and relieving pain.

➢ For thick, greasy tongue coating with poor appetite and distention of the stomach duct, remove *shú dì* (Radix Rehmanniae Praeparata), and add *chén pí* (Pericarpium Citri Reticulatae) 10g, *shā rén* (Fructus Amomi, added later) 6g (decocted last), and *jiāo sān xiān* (scorch-fried Fructus Crataegi, Fructus Hordei Germinatus, and Massa Medicata Fermentata) 10g each to move qi, fortify the spleen, promote digestion, and harmonize the stomach.

(4) Liver and Kidney Deficiency with Phlegm-stasis Bind

【Syndrome Characteristics】

A prolonged disease course with the following manifestations: swelling, pain, and deformity of the joints, limited range of motion, pronounced morning stiffness, a purple and darkish color of the skin, and possible subcutaneous nodules or stubborn numbness of the limbs. Common accompanying symptoms include: soreness and weakness of the lumbus and knees, shortness of breath and lack of strength, dizziness and tinnitus, palpitation and chest oppression, a lusterless facial complexion, pale nails, a dusky tongue with stasis macules, and a tight, thready and rough pulse.

【Treatment Principle】

Tonify and boost the liver and kidney, while simultaneously invigorating blood, transforming stasis, dispelling phlegm, and unblocking the collaterals.

【Commonly Used Medicinals】

Táo rén (Semen Persicae), *hóng huā* (Flos Carthami), *dāng guī* (Radix Angelicae Sinensis), *dì lóng* (Pheretima), *niú xī* (Radix Achyranthis Bidentatae), *jiāng huáng* (Rhizoma Curcumae Longae), and *jī xuè téng*

(Caulis Spatholobi) are used to invigorate blood and transform stasis. *Bàn xià* (Rhizoma Pinelliae), *dǎn nán xīng* (Arisaema cum Bile), *zhǐ qiào* (Fructus Aurantii), and *jié gěng* (Radix Platycodonis) are used to eliminate dampness and transform phlegm. *Yuán hú* (Rhizoma Corydalis) and *chuān xiōng* (Rhizoma Chuanxiong) are used to unblock the collaterals and relieve pain. *Bā jǐ tiān* (Radix Morindae Officinalis), *yín yáng huò* (Herba Epimedii), *bǔ gǔ zhī* (Fructus Psoraleae), *dù zhòng* (Cortex Eucommiae), *xù duàn* (Radix Dipsaci), and *gǒu jǐ* (Rhizoma Cibotii) are used to tonify the liver and kidney and strengthen the sinews and bones. *Dāng guī* (Radix Angelicae Sinensis), *shú dì* (Radix Rehmanniae Praeparata), *bái sháo* (Radix Paeoniae Alba), *hé shǒu wū* (Radix Polygoni Multiflori), and *jī xuè téng* (Caulis Spatholobi) are used to nourish and tonify the blood.

【Representative Formula】

A modified combination of *Dú Huó Jì Shēng Tāng* (独活寄生汤) plus *Shēn Tòng Zhú Yū Tāng* (身痛逐瘀汤)

【Ingredients】

独活	dú huó	10g	Radix Angelicae Pubescentis
桑寄生	sāng jì shēng	30g	Herba Taxilli
杜仲	dù zhòng	12g	Cortex Eucommiae
牛膝	niú xī	10g	Radix Cyathulae
当归	dāng guī	10g	Radix Angelicae Sinensis
川芎	chuān xiōng	12g	Rhizoma Chuanxiong
地黄	dì huáng	10g	Radix Rehmanniae
芍药	sháo yào	12g	Radix Paeoniae Alba
党参	dǎng shēn	15g	Radix Codonopsis
山萸肉	shān yú ròu	9-12g	Fructus Corni
淫羊藿	yín yáng huò	10-30g	Herba Epimedii
骨碎补	gǔ suì bǔ	10g	Rhizoma Drynariae
桂枝	guì zhī	6g	Ramulus Cinnamomi
甘草	gān cǎo	6g	Radix et Rhizoma Glycyrrhizae
黄芪	huáng qí	15g	Radix Astragali

桃仁	táo rén	10g	Semen Persicae
红花	hóng huā	10g	Flos Carthami
秦艽	qín jiāo	10g	Radix Gentianae Macrophyllae
地龙	dì lóng	30g	Pheretima
茯苓	fú líng	10g	Poria
白芥子	bái jiè zǐ	10g	Semen Sinapis
胆南星	dǎn nán xīng	10g	Arisaema cum Bile

Boil the above ingredients in 500ml water until reduced to a 200ml decoction. Take warm, 1 batch a day.

【Formula Analysis】

Dú huó (Radix Angelicae Pubescentis) is acrid, bitter, and slightly warm. It can dispel wind cold damp evil from the lower body, alleviate *bi*, and relieve pain. *Fáng fēng* (Radix Saposhnikoviae) dispels wind and overcomes dampness. *Sāng jì shēng* (Herba Taxilli), *niú xī* (Radix Achyranthis Bidentatae), *dù zhòng* (Cortex Eucommiae), and *gǔ suì bǔ* (Rhizoma Drynariae) tonify the liver and kidney and strengthen the sinews and bones. *Sì Wù Tāng* (四物汤) nourishes and invigorates blood. *Dǎng shēn* (Radix Codonopsis) and *huáng qí* (Radix Astragali) are used to tonify qi. *Shān yú ròu* (Fructus Corni) and *yín yáng huò* (Herba Epimedii) warm and tonify kidney yang. *Guì zhī* (Ramulus Cinnamomi) warms yang, transforms qi, and unblocks the collaterals. *Táo rén* (Semen Persicae), *hóng huā* (Flos Carthami), *dāng guī* (Radix Angelicae Sinensis), *qín jiāo* (Radix Gentianae Macrophyllae), *dì lóng* (Pheretima), and *niú xī* (Radix Achyranthis Bidentatae) invigorate blood, transform stasis, unblock the collaterals, and relieve pain. *Qín jiāo* (Radix Gentianae Macrophyllae) dispels wind and unblocks the collaterals. *Bái jiè zǐ* (Semen Sinapis) and *dǎn nán xīng* (Arisaema cum Bile) transform phlegm and unblock the collaterals.

【Modifications】

- For marked swelling, add *zé lán* (Herba Lycopi) 15g, *zé xiè*

(Rhizoma Alismatis) 10g, *shuǐ zhì* (Hirudo) 10g, and *zhū líng* (Polyporus) 10g to drain dampness, invigorate blood, and disperse swelling.

➢ For severe pain, add *quán xiē* (Scorpio) 10g and *dì biē chóng* (Eupolyphaga seu Steleophaga) 10g to track down and dispel wind, expel rheum, and disperse stasis; or, add *é zhú* (Rhizoma Curcumae) 10g and *mǎ qián zǐ* (Semen Strychni preparata) 0.3-0.6g to invigorate blood and relieve pain; or, add *bái jiè zǐ* (Semen Sinapis) 10g to dispel and eliminate the phlegm between the skin and membrane.

➢ For an emaciated body, add *zǐ hé chē* (Placenta Hominis) 15g, *zhū jǐ suǐ* (Suis Spinae Medulla) 20g, *guī jiǎ jiāo* (Colla Carapax et Plastrum Testudinis) 10g, *lù jiǎo jiāo* (Colla Cornus Cervi) 10g, and *ē jiāo* (Colla Corii Asini) 15g to tonify deficiency and support right qi.

➢ For aching or stabbing pain in the joints, add *wū shāo shé* (Zaocys) 10g and *qí shé* (Agkistrodon) 10g to track down wind, unblock the collaterals, and relieve pain.

➢ For a tendency towards yin deficiency, add *Zuǒ Guī Wán* (左归丸) to enrich yin, tonify the kidney, replenish essence, and boost marrow.

➢ For a tendency towards yang deficiency, add *Yòu Guī Wán* (右归丸) to warm and tonify kidney yang, replenish essence, and boost marrow.

Additional Treatment Modalities

1. Chinese Patent Medicine

(1) ***Wāng Bì Chōng Jì*** (尪痹冲剂): Tonifies and boosts the liver and kidney, dispels wind, invigorates blood, unblocks the collaterals, and relieves pain. For stubborn *bi* type RA that manifests as mild swelling, pain, heaviness, and numbness of the skin and flesh, the channels and vessels, and the joints; soreness and weakness of the lumbus and knees; fear of cold and preference for warmth; and cold limbs. In severe cases, there may be joint swelling and deformity with inability to bend and

stretch, stiffness, contraction of the sinews, emaciation, crippling of the feet, or inability to walk. The tongue is pale with white glossy coating. The pulse is slippery and thready. Take one packet, 2-3 times a day.

(2) ***Hán Shī Bì Chōng Jì*** (寒湿痹冲剂): Warms yang, dispels cold, and expels dampness. Used to treat cold pain, swelling, and heaviness of the joints of the limbs, local aversion to cold, and skin that is neither red nor hot to the touch, accompanied by a pale, dusky tongue with white greasy or white glossy coating, and a wiry and tight, wiry and moderate, or deep and slow pulse. Take one packet, 3 times a day.

(3) ***Shī Rè Bì Chōng Jì*** (湿热痹冲剂): Clears heat, eliminates dampness, invigorates blood, and unblocks the collaterals. For pain, redness, burning, and swelling of the joints that are relieved by exposure to cold; pain which is exacerbated by the slightest pressure; inability of the joints to bend and stretch; and, in severe cases, difficulty in walking or inability to move, which may involve one or more joints. Usually accompanied by fever, thirst, chest oppression, restlessness, a tongue that is covered with yellow and greasy, or yellow and dry coating, and a slippery and rapid pulse. For oral administration. Take 1-2 packets, 3 times a day. Reduce the dosage for children.

(4) ***Yū Xuè Bì Chōng Jì*** (瘀血痹冲剂): Invigorates blood, transforms stasis, unblocks the collaterals, and relieves pain. For excruciating pain of the flesh and joints (most of which are stabbing, unremitting, fixed, or one that refuses pressure) and local swelling (sometimes accompanied by hard nodules or stasis maculae). Other possible accompanying symptoms include a somber facial complexion, dry skin, a purple and dusky tongue with stasis macules, and a thready and rough pulse. Take 1 packet, 3 times a day.

(5) ***Yì Shèn Juān Bì Wán*** (益肾蠲痹丸): Warms and tonifies kidney yang, alleviates *bi*, and unblocks the collaterals. Suitable for stubborn *bi* of the kidney deficiency and evil obstruction type, the signs and

symptoms of which include red, swollen, painful, and inflexible joints with morning stiffness, emaciation, or stiffness and deformity. For oral administration; take 1 packet 3 times a day with warm water. To be taken after meals. Cautions: 1) Those that are already on many other types of medicinal therapy should gradually reduce the dosage of those medicinals after the symptoms are relieved; they must not stop the treatment abruptly. 2) Occasionally, there may be allergic reactions to the medicinals, such as itchy skin, thirst, constipation, or discomfort of the stomach duct. If an itchy skin or papular eruption occurs, then it is an allergic reaction to insect medicinals. An oral decoction made from *dì fū zǐ* (Fructus Kochiae) 30g, *xú cháng qīng* (Radix et Rhizoma Cynanchi Paniculati) 15g, *bái xiān pí* (Cortex Dictamni) 30g can relieve these adverse reactions.

(6) ***Fēng Shī Mǎ Qián Piàn*** (风湿马钱片): Dispels wind, eliminates dampness, invigorates blood, and relieves pain. For pain in the joints and flesh with an inability to bend and stretch. The pain can be fixed, numb and heavy, wandering, accompanied by convulsions, or recurrent, accompanied by joint deformity. For oral administration; take 4 tablets, 3 times a day. Children over 7 years of age can be given half the dosage of adults.

(7) ***Mù Guā Wán*** (木瓜丸): Dispels wind, disperses cold, warms the channels, unblocks the collaterals, relieves pain, and strengthens the sinews and bones. For shoulder, arm, lumbar, leg, and heel pain in the elderly due to chronic unremitting *bi* syndrome that is recurrent and causes damage to the right qi. Also for numbness of the limbs, pain of the whole body, soreness and heaviness of the lumbus and legs, lack of strength in the feet and knees, and a weak body due to wind damp cold evil. Take 9g, 2 times a day.

(8) ***Dú Huó Jì Shēng Wán*** (独活寄生丸): Dispels wind-damp, disperses cold, nourishes the liver and kidney, tonifies qi and blood, and relieves

pain. For cold pain of the lumbus and knees, inflexible or numb joints, and fear of cold and preference for warmth; accompanied by a pale tongue with white coating, and a thready and weak pulse. Take 1 pill, 2 times a day.

(9) ***Kūn Míng Shān Hǎi Táng Piàn*** (昆明山海棠片): Dispels wind, eliminates dampness, relaxes the sinews, quickens the collaterals, clears heat, and resolves toxins. For oral administration; take 2 tablets, 3 times a day. Warning: Those with impaired kidney function should use with caution.

(10) ***Zhèng Qīng Fēng Tòng Níng*** (正清风痛宁): Has anti-inflammatory, analgesic, and immunoregulatory effects. Treats obstruction of the collaterals by *bi* pathogens. Take 1 tablet, twice a day.

(11) ***Huǒ Bǎ Huā Gēn Piàn*** (火把花根片): Dispels wind, eliminates dampness, relaxes the sinews, quickens the collaterals, clears heat, and resolves toxins. Treats obstruction of the collaterals by *bi* pathogens. Take 4-6 tablets, 3 times a day.

2. Acupuncture and Moxibustion

Acupuncture can course and unblock the channels and collaterals, regulate and harmonize qi and blood, dispel wind, eliminate dampness, invigorate blood, transform stasis, disperse swelling, and relieve pain. Modern medical research shows that acupuncture can regulate the immune system and improve hemorrheology in RA patients. Local acupoints or points on the corresponding channel pathways are often selected. *Ashi* points can also be chosen. If wind or heat evil is predominant, apply superficial needling with filiform needle or tap the affected areas with a plum-blossom needle. If cold is predominant, perform moxibustion or deep insertion with needle retention. If there is severe pain, ginger moxibustion can be performed. For damp evil obstruction, apply acupuncture in conjunction with moxibustion, or apply warming needle with plum-blossom needling and cupping therapy.

(1) Body Acupuncture

【Treatment Principle】

Tonify the liver and kidney, strengthen the sinews and bones, unblock the collaterals, and relieve pain.

【Point Combination】

BL 11	dà zhù	大杼
BL 23	shèn shù	肾俞
ST 36	zú sān lǐ	足三里
SP 6	sān yīn jiāo	三阴交

【Point Modification】

➢ For the MCPJ and wrist joint, add SJ 4 (*yáng chí*), LI 4 (*hé gǔ*), and SI 3 (*hòu xī*).

➢ For the knee joint, add ST 35 (*dú bí*), BL 60 (*kūn lún*), KI 3 (*tài xī*), and GB 40 (*qiū xū*).

➢ For the shoulder, elbow, and vertebral joints, add LI 15 (*jiān yú*), SI 9 (*jiān zhēn*), SJ 14 (*jiān liáo*), LI 11 (*qū chí*), *Hua Tuo jia ji* points, and *ashi* points.

【Manipulation】

Deep insertion. Apply supplementation to deficiency patterns and drainage to excess patterns. Retain the needles for 10-20 minutes. Warming-needle or moxibustion can also be applied.

【Analysis of Acupoints】

BL 11 (*dà zhù*) is the influential point of the bones; it unblocks the collaterals and relieves pain. BL 23 (*shèn shù*) tonifies the liver and kidney and strengthens the sinews and bones; it is good for relieving soreness of the lumbus and back. ST 36 (*zú sān lǐ*) is the *he*-sea point of the foot yangming stomach channel. It can fortify the spleen and strengthen the stomach to nourish the source of qi and blood. SP 6 (*sān yīn jiāo*) can fortify the spleen and resolve liver qi constraint. The combination of all of these points achieves the effect of boosting qi, nourishing blood, unblocking the collaterals, and relieving pain.

1) Wind-cold-damp *Bi*

【Treatment Principle】

Disperse cold, eliminate dampness, dispel wind, and unblock the collaterals.

【Point Combination】

DU 14	dà zhuī	大椎
RN 6	qì hǎi	气海
RN 4	guān yuán	关元
RN 8	shén quē	神阙

【Point Modification】

➢ For the shoulder joint, add SJ 14 (*jiān liáo*), LI 16 (*jù gǔ*), and LI 11 (*qū chí*).

➢ For the elbow joint, add LI 11(*qū chí*), LU 5 (*chǐ zé*), HT 3 (*shào hǎi*), and LI 10 (*shǒu sān lǐ*).

➢ For the wrist joint, add SJ 4 (*yáng chí*), LI 5 (*yáng xī*), PC 7 (*dà líng*), LI 4 (*hé gǔ*), and SJ 5 (*wài guān*).

➢ For the metacarpophalangeal joint, add EX-UE9 (*bā xié*), LI 4 (*hé gǔ*), and LI 3 (*sān jiān*).

➢ For the finger joints, add *sì fèng* (EX-UE10).

➢ For the hip joint, add GB 30 (*huán tiào*), GB 29 (*jū liáo*), and GB 34 (*yáng líng quán*).

➢ For the knee joint, add *nèi xī yǎn* (EX-LE4), *xī yǎn* (EX-LE5), ST 34 (*liáng qiū*), BL 40 (*wěi zhōng*), GB 33 (*xī yáng guān*), LV 8 (*qū quán*), and GB 34 (*yáng líng quán*).

➢ For the ankle joint, add BL 60 (*kūn lún*), KI 3 (*tài xī*), ST 41 (*jiě xī*),

GB 40 (*qiū xū*), and KI 2 (*rán gŭ*).

➢ For the metatarsal joint, add *bā fēng* (EX-LE10), ST 44 (*nèi tíng*), and LV 3 (*tài chōng*).

➢ For the vertebral joints, alternate between DU14 (*dà zhuī*), DU12 (*shēn zhù*), DU3 (*yāo yáng guān*), and corresponding *Hua Tuo jia ji* points. For each session, 6-10 points can be chosen according to the number of involved joints and the patient's tolerance to acupuncture.

【Manipulation】

Mild supplementation and drainage with needle retention for 20-30 minutes, plus warming-needle method or pole moxa. RN 4 (*guān yuán*), RN 6 (*qì hăi*), and RN 8 (*shén quē*) can be selected for moxibustion. Apply pole moxibustion for 20-30 minutes, or 7-9 cones of ginger moxibustion.

2) Wind-damp-heat *Bi*

【Treatment Principle】

Clear heat, dispel wind, eliminate dampness, and unblock the collaterals.

【Point Combination】

DU 14	dà zhuī	大椎
DU 12	shēn zhù	身柱
LI 11	qū chí	曲池

Local points are the same as those selected for wind-cold-damp *bi* (see the section on "wind-cold-damp *bi*"). For affected joints, needle along the corresponding channels. Select 6-10 points per treatment session.

【Point Modification】

➢ For profuse sweating, add LI 4 (*hé gŭ*) and KI 7 (*fù liū*).

➢ For vexation, add HT 7 (*shén mén*).

【Manipulation】

First, needle DU 14 (*dà zhuī*), DU 12 (*shēn zhù*), and LI 11 (*qū chí*) with medium stimulation; do not retain the needles. Next, needle the acupoints surrounding the red swollen joints with medium stimulation, and retain the needles for 10-15 minutes. When withdrawing the needles, try to enlarge the pinhole to induce bleeding (drainage technique). Then, select distal points along the corresponding channels, and apply drainage with medium stimulation, retaining the needles for 10-15 minutes; treat once a day. If exterior evils have not been released, the resulting disharmony of nutritive and defensive qi will cause profuse sweating. Treat this by supplementing LI 4 (*hé gǔ*) and draining KI 7 (*fù liū*). For heat evil harassing the heart and causing vexation and agitation, drain HT 7 (*shén mén*) with medium stimulation.

3) Liver and Kidney Deficiency with Retention of Evils

【Treatment Principle】

Support right qi, dispel evil, invigorate blood, and unblock the collaterals.

【Point Combination】

BL 18	gān shù	肝俞
BL 23	shèn shù	肾俞
ST 36	zú sān lǐ	足三里

Local points are the same as those selected for wind-cold-damp *bi* (see the section on "wind-cold-damp *bi*"). Select 6-10 points per treatment session.

【Point Modification】

Bleed the swollen joints with a three-edged needle. For night sweating and tidal fever, add HT 6 (*yīn xì*) and DU 14 (*dà zhuī*).

【Manipulation】

Supplement BL 18 (*gān shù*), BL 23 (*shèn shù*), and ST 36(*zú sān lǐ*), without needle retention. Apply drainage followed by supplementation to local points. If the skin of the affected area is not hot and has aversion to cold, apply warming-needle method or pole moxa once a day or once every other day. If there is fusiform swelling and distention with deformity in the finger joints, bleed *sì fèng* (EX-UE10) with a three-edged needle. Other swollen and deformed joints can be treated with diffuse bleeding using a three-edged needle. For tidal fever and night sweating, drain HT 6 (*yīn xì*) and DU 14 (*dà zhuī*).

(2) Auricular Acupuncture

【Point Combination】

corresponding auricular points			耳区相应部位
adrenal gland	TG 2p	shèn shàng xiàn	肾上腺
shen men	TF 4	shén mén	神门

【Manipulation】

Administer treatment once a day, with filiform needles. Retain needles for 20-30 minutes per session, or, apply needle implantation or ear seeding to auricular acupoints. Press and knead the seeded points until there is a sensation of burning pain, 1-2 minutes per point. The seeds can be left on the ear for 3-5 days.

【Cautions】

A. Proper disinfection should be applied to prevent infection. If there is any skin breakage or lesion, avoid using any kind of stimulation (e.g., acupuncture or ear seeding) on that area.

B. It is best not to administer acupuncture to women during the 2nd to 5th months of pregnancy, especially those with a history of habitual miscarriage. During the 5th to 9th months of pregnancy, it is best to avoid points such as uterus, ovary, endocrine, lumbosacral vertebrae, and abdomen; this prevents the induction of a miscarriage or abortion.

C. Elderly patients with high blood pressure or arteriosclerosis should rest well before and after each acupuncture session.

(3) Direct Current Medicinal Iontonphoresis

Iontonphoresis is a process that involves the use of electrical currents to drive ions of medicinals into the body tissues. The medium used in this case is the liquid obtained from soaking Chinese medicinals in 50% alcohol made from distilled water or 50-proof Chinese white liquor (spirits distilled from sorghum).

(4) Moxibustion

Moxibustion is an appropriate treatment for most RA patients. Through the warm stimulation, it achieves the effects of moving qi, unblocking the collaterals, invigorating blood, and expelling stasis. The various types of moxibustion include scarring moxibustion, also called suppurative moxibustion. It is performed by spreading garlic juice on the skin, placing a moxa cone directly on the skin, and then burning the moxa until the skin blisters and suppurates. This moxibustion method is good for stubborn cases of RA. The size of the moxa cone used for scarring moxibustion is that of a soybean or a grain of wheat. 10-20 cones can be used on each point. Treatment is performed once a day; three days equal a course. Extreme caution must be exercised when administering scarring moxibustion so as to avoid causing severe burns.

Other common types of moxibustion include:

A. Mild moxibustion or sparrow-pecking moxibustion: 15-20 minutes each point, once a day or once every other day. 10 sessions equal a course.

B. Ginger (garlic) moxibustion: Use soybean-sized moxa cones; 3-6 cones each point, once a day or once every other day. 10 sessions equal a course.

C. Non-scarring moxibustion: Use moxa cones that are the size of wheat grains; 3-6 cones each point, once a day or once every other day. 10 sessions equal a course.

One can also perform moxibustion on BL 11 (*dà zhù*), *ashi* points,

points along the governing vessel [from DU14 (*dà zhuī*) to DU 2 (*yāo shù*)], LI 11 (*qū chí*), and SP 10 (*xuè hǎi*). Select 4-6 points per session.

As RA has a long disease course, moxibustion provides the patient with a convenient supplementary treatment modality that family members can perform on them at home in their spare time.

(5) Plum-Blossom Needle

The usage of the plum-blossom needle is similar to that of the above-mentioned treatment modalities. It can be divided into 2 techniques: stimulation along the channels and stimulation on the focal points. The former technique involves tapping along the corresponding channel pathways, from the distal end to the proximal end, or vice versa. Afterwards, a red line along with the channel pathway can be seen on the skin (small petechia). The latter technique involves tapping on the relevant acupoints surrounding the involved joints, including *ashi* points (usually denotes spots that are most tender or most sensitive). After tapping on the *ashi* points, move on to ST 34 (*liáng qiū*), ST 35 (*dú bí*), GB 34 (*yáng líng quán*), and GB 33 (*xī yáng guān*). For joint pain of the upper limbs, tap along the hand taiyin lung channel, the hand jueyin pericardium channel, the hand shaoyin heart channel, the hand yangming large intestine channel, the hand shaoyang *san jiao* channel, and the hand taiyang small intestine channel. Finally, tap on LI 15 (*jiān yú*), SJ 14 (*jiān liáo*), LI 11 (*qū chí*), LI 4 (*hé gǔ*), SJ 5 (*wài guān*), LU 5 (*chǐ zé*), and GB 33 (*xī yáng guān*).

【Manipulation】

After local disinfection, hold the needle handle and use the strength of the wrist to tap perpendicularly on the skin. The percussion should be accurate, and the strength should be well-distributed. The intensity of percussion can be either light or heavy. Light percussion refers to the minute amount of tapping strength required just to make the skin rosy-colored and induce local hyperemia. Heavy percussion refers to the greater strength required to cause slight bleeding. Plum-blossom needling can be administered once a day or once every other day. 15 sessions equal a course.

Plum-blossom needling has certain analgesic effects, but it is only suitable for treating chronic or mild RA. During the acute inflammation stage, plum-blossom needling is ineffective.

3. Cupping

Materials that can be used to perform cupping include bamboo cups, porcelain cups, glass cups, and metal cups.

(1) Simple Cupping

This method involves the use of cups alone (without medicinals or tools). It includes retained cupping, moving cupping, and flash cupping. Retained cupping involves creating suction by using fire or boiling to exhaust the air inside the cup, and then quickly placing the cup on the skin. The cup is retained for a while and then removed. Based on the different techniques applied after retention of the cups, retained cupping can be divided into the following sub-categories: rotation cupping, press cupping, and shake cupping. Moving cupping is also called push cupping or slide cupping. After the cups are placed on the skin, push the cup around to enlarge the treatment area. Flash cupping involves removing the cup immediately after it is placed on the skin, repeating this over and over until the skin becomes red. There is another technique called sound cupping which involves strongly pushing or rotating the cup after it is placed on the skin, a procedure that produces an audible noise.

(2) Combined Cupping

This method refers to the use of medicinals or medical tools during or after the cupping. Depending on the different equipment used, combined cupping can be divided into the following sub-categories: cupping with needle retention, medicinal cupping, infrared cupping, ultra-violet cupping, and laser cupping. To remove the cups, with one hand, tilt the cup, and with the other hand, press the skin by the edge of the cup to release the suction. During cupping with needle retention, if there is any bleeding or exudation after the cup and needle are removed, it can be cleaned with a sterilized, dry cotton ball.

【Cautions】

- Make sure the treatment room is warm before performing cupping, so as to prevent the patient from catching a cold.
- For weak patients, elderly, children, nervous patients, or those new to cupping, use smaller cups. The patient should be lying down during the treatment. The practitioner should observe the patient's complexion and expression closely, and ask the patient how she/he is feeling; to rule out or promptly deal with any abnormal conditions should they arise.
- Select the right spot or points for cupping. It is best to choose the parts of the body that has sufficient muscles and substantial subcutaneous tissue but with little hair.
- When removing the cups, the movement should be steady, accurate, gentle, and quick.
- Tell the patients not to move during the cupping procedure, to prevent accidents such as dropping the cup. If there are many cups, do not place them too close to one other on the skin, to prevent the cups from pulling excessively on the skin and causing pain, and to prevent the cups from pressing on one other and falling.
- If there is local redness or itching after removal of a cup, do not scratch the area. The redness and itching will dissipate on its own within a few hours or days.

➢ Do not repeatedly cup the same location until the mark from the last cup has dissipated.

➢ On patients with serious, deep, or painful conditions, the cups can be retained for a longer duration of time. On patients with less serious, superficial, or paralytic conditions, the cups should be retained for only a short while. If the musculature of the cupped area is thick, the cups can be retained for a longer while; if the musculature is thin, the cups should only be retained for a short while. The cups can be retained for a longer amount of time during cold days but shorter amount of time during hot days.

➢ The technique to remove the cups should be gentle and steady. Hard pushing or rotation can hurt the skin and are thus not recommended. Cupping is contraindicated in the following conditions: extreme hunger, extreme fullness, extreme fatigue, extreme thirst, high fever, severe edema, extreme nervousness, extreme hypersensitivity of the skin, skin breakage, poor skin elasticity, severe skin disorders, tumor, hemophilia, and active tuberculosis. Cupping is also contraindicated during menstruation and pregnancy.

4. Medicinal Steams and Washes

This method has advantages of being convenient and easy to learn, and having remarkable effects without pain. It is the preferred treatment for patients who are unable to take medication. (Note: It is not enough for RA patients to be treated with steams and washes alone. The combination of both internal and external treatment can ensure satisfactory results.)

【Manipulation】

Steaming and washing the fingers, elbows, and knees: Pour the medicinal decoction in a basin. Place the affected area of the body over the basin and cover (body part and basin) with a cloth sheet to let the steam fumigate the body part. After steaming, use the medicinal dregs as a hot compress (by placing the dregs in a cloth sack) to wash the affected area. Finally, rub the body part gently with a towel and keep it away from drafts.

【Cautions】

The medicinals used for steaming and washing cannot be taken internally. During the process of steaming and washing, move the affected joint to circulate qi and blood, thereby gradually improving joint mobility. Treatment is administered 1-2 times a day, for 30 or more minutes per session. Each batch of medicinals can be used for 2-3 days, and 20 days equal a course of treatment. When the decoction cools down, it should be re-heated before re-using. During the treatment period, the patient should rest well and avoid overstrain. The amount of water used to decoct the medicinals is important. It can be neither too much nor too little. Too much water can dilute the concentration of the medicinals, and too little can weaken the potency of the medicinals. Medicinal steams and washes may be combined with other treatments to increase the therapeutic effect.

5. External Application

1) *Bì Tòng Dìng* (痹痛定): Consists of *shēng chuān wū* (raw Radix Aconiti) 20g, *yáng jīn huā* (Flos Daturae) 2g, *nào yáng huā* (Flos Rhododendri Mollis) 16g, *lù yīng* (Sambucus chinensis Lindl.) 20g, *zǐ ròu guì* (Cortex Cinnamomi) 20g, *huā jiāo* (Pericarpium Zanthoxyli) 6g, and *zhāng nǎo* (Camphora) 3g. The medicinals are ground into a coarse powder, and then soaked in 300ml of 75% alcohol for 5-7 days. After filtering out the decoction and discarding the dregs, apply the liquid on the affected area with a cotton swab, twice a day.

2) Decoct *fù zǐ* (Radix Aconiti Lateralis Praeparata) 50-100g, *cǎo wū* (Radix Aconiti Kusnezoffii) 50-100g, *chuān wū* (Radix Aconiti) 50-100g, *yǔ bái fù* (Rhizoma Typhonii) 50-100g, *qiāng huó* (Rhizoma et Radix

Notopterygii) 40-80g, *dú huó* (Radix Angelicae Pubescentis) 40-80g, *tòu gǔ cǎo* (Caulis Impatientis) 40-80g, *guì zhī* (Ramulus Cinnamomi) 30-50g, *gān jiāng* (Rhizoma Zingiberis) 30-50g, *gān sōng* (Radix et Rhizoma Nardostachyos) 30-50g, *dāng guī* (Radix Angelicae Sinensis) 10-30g, *xì xīn* (Radix et Rhizoma Asari) 10-30g, and *dì biē chóng* (Eupolyphaga seu Steleophaga) 10-30g with water for about 1 hour. When the liquid decoction cools down to around 40℃, soak the affected body part in it, 1-2 times a day. The decoction from each batch of medicinals can be used 2-3 times. The nature of the medicinals in this formula is harsh and therefore cannot be ingested. After each treatment session, any part of the body that has touched the decoction should be washed thoroughly with warm water.

3) Medicinals Used for Steams, Washes, or External Application:

A. Decoct *shēng chuān wū* (raw Radix Aconiti) 15g, *shēng cǎo wū* (raw Radix Aconiti Kusnezoffii) 15g, *shēng fù zǐ* (raw Radix Aconiti Lateralis) 15g, *shēng bàn xià* (raw Rhizoma Pinelliae) 15g, *yáng jīn huā* (Flos Daturae) 3-6g, and *bīng piàn* (Borneolum Syntheticum) 6g and use the liquid to steam the affected area for 30-40 minutes each time, twice a day. Or, grind the herbs and blend the powder with water, yellow rice wine, or vinegar to make a paste. Apply the paste on the swollen joints, once a day. Good for RA of the cold-damp prevalence type.

B. Decoct *shēng chuān wū* (raw Radix Aconiti) 20g, *shēng cǎo wū* (raw Radix Aconiti Kusnezoffii) 20g, *shēng nán xīng* (raw Rhizoma Arisaematis) 20g, *shēng bàn xià* (raw Rhizoma Pinelliae) 20g, *guì zhī* (Ramulus Cinnamomi) 30g, *sāng zhī* (Ramulus Mori) 30g, *ròu guì* (Cortex Cinnamomi) 30g, *gān jiāng* (Rhizoma Zingiberis) 20g, *má huáng* (Herba Ephedrae) 25g, *xì xīn* (Radix et Rhizoma Asari) 15g, *mù fáng jǐ* (Radix Stephaniae Tetrandrae) 30g, *qín jiāo* (Radix Gentianae Macrophyllae) 30g, *táo rén* (Semen Persicae) 20g, *hóng huā* (Flos Carthami) 20g, *fáng fēng* (Radix Saposhnikoviae) 30g, *cāng zhú* (Rhizoma Atractylodis) 30g, *sī guā luò* (Retinervus Luffae Fructus) 20g, and *zǐ huā dì dīng* (Herba Violae) 30g in 3000ml water until reduced to 1500ml of liquid. Wash the affected area with the decoction, twice a day, for 30-60 minutes each time.

C. Medicated Baths: Decoct medicinals that dispel wind, eliminate dampness, relax the sinews, quicken the collaterals, invigorate blood, and transform stasis, and use the liquid to wash the affected joints. Add warm water (45-50°C) to the decoction according to the ratio of 1:2, decoction to water. Pour the medicated bath decoction in a bathtub and let the patient lie down or place the affected limb in the tub for 30 minutes each time, 2 times a day. 15 days equal a course of treatment.

6. Simple Prescriptions And Empirical Formulas

(1) *Fù Fāng Mǎ Qián Zǐ Sǎn* (复方马钱子散) [by Ji Fu-le]

制马钱子	zhì mǎ qián zǐ	250g	Semen Strychni (prepared)
制川乌	zhì chuān wū	30g	Radix Aconiti (prepared)
制草乌	zhì cǎo wū	30g	Radix Aconiti Kusnezoffii Praeparata
乳香	rǔ xiāng	30g	Olibanum
没药	mò yào	30g	Myrrha
木瓜	mù guā	50g	Fructus Chaenomelis
麻黄	má huáng	30g	Herba Ephedrae
苍术	cāng zhú	30g	Rhizoma Atractylodis
威灵仙	wēi líng xiān	30g	Radix et Rhizoma Clematidis
牛膝	niú xī	80g	Radix Cyathulae
乌蛇	wū shé	30g	Zaocys
全蝎	quán xiē	20g	Scorpio
僵蚕	jiāng cán	30g	Bombyx Batryticatus
防己	fáng jǐ	30g	Radix Stephaniae Tetrandrae
蜂房	fēng fáng	30g	Nidus Vespae
醋制自然铜	zì rán tóng	50g	Pyritum (processed with vinegar)
甘草	gān cǎo	30g	Radix et Rhizoma Glycyrrhizae

Take warm, one batch a day, in several portions. This formula is good for treating cold-damp *bi* presenting with severe, wandering joint pain.

Comments

Mǎ qián zǐ (Semen Strychni), *chuān wū* (Radix Aconiti), and *cǎo wū* (Radix Aconiti Kusnezoffii) must be processed according to the guidelines set forth in the pharmacopeia, otherwise they should not be included in any formula.

(2) *Wǔ Téng Tāng* (五藤汤) [by Zhou Lin-kuan & Zhang Jian-hua]

青风藤	qīng fēng téng	15g	Caulis Sinomenii
雷公藤	léi gōng téng	6-9g	Tripterygium Wilfordii
忍冬藤	rěn dōng téng	15g	Caulis Lonicerae Japonicae
海风藤	hǎi fēng téng	15g	Caulis Piperis Kadsurae
络石藤	luò shí téng	15g	Caulis Trachelospermi
蕲蛇	qí shé	10g	Agkistrodon
蜈蚣	wú gōng	3 pieces	Scolopendra
仙灵脾	xiān líng pí	12g	Herba Epimedii
当归	dāng guī	30g	Radix Angelicae Sinensis
白芥子	bái jiè zǐ	10g	Semen Sinapis
鸡血藤	jī xuè téng	30g	Caulis Spatholobi
生黄芪	shēng huáng qí	30g	Radix Astragali (raw)

Take warm, one batch a day, divided into several portions. Actions: tonifies qi, nourishes blood, clears heat, relaxes the sinews, and quickens the collaterals. Good for treating damp-heat *bi*.

(3) *Wài Yòng Shè Xiāng Jiǔ Lóng Gāo* (外用麝香九龙膏) [by Wang Ling-xi, Wang Dong-gang, and Wang Dong-qiang]

麝香	shè xiāng	0. 2g	Moschus
樟脑	zhāng nǎo	3g	Camphora
天龙	tiān lóng	7g	Scolopendra
地龙	dì lóng	7g	Pheretima
海龙	hǎi lóng	7g	Syngnathus

穿山龙	chuān shān lóng	7g	Rhizoma Dioscoreae Nipponicae
穿山甲	chuān shān jiǎ	7g	Squama Manis
守宫	shǒu gōng	7g	Gekko Swinhoana
乌蛇	wū shé	7g	Zaocys
白花蛇	bái huā shé	7g	Agkistrodon
水蛇	shuǐ shé	7g	Enhydris Caro
川乌	chuān wū	7g	Radix Aconiti
草乌	cǎo wū	7g	Radix Aconiti Kusnezoffii
马钱子	mǎ qián zǐ	7g	Semen Strychni
黄芪	huáng qí	20g	Radix Astragali
当归	dāng guī	20g	Radix Angelicae Sinensis
鹿角胶	lù jiǎo jiāo	20g	Colla Cornus Cervi
黄酒	huáng jiǔ	500g	yellow (rice or millet) wine

Grind all the herbs except for *shè xiāng* (Moschus) and *zhāng nǎo* (Camphora) into a fine powder, and decoct the powder in yellow wine to make a paste. Spread the paste on a piece of cloth (32cm by 22cm) and sprinkle the separately powdered *shè xiāng* (Moschus) and *zhāng nǎo* (Camphora) on the paste. Apply directly on the affected area. Change the dressing once every three days. Ten times equal a course. 2-3 courses are generally required to produce a noticeable effect. Actions of the formula: warms the channels, disperses cold, quickens the collaterals, and relieves pain. Suitable for a weak constitution with joint pain that is aggravated by cold and relieved by warmth.

(4) *Qīng Rè Juān Bì Tāng* (清热蠲痹汤)

生石膏	shēng shí gāo	60g	Gypsum Fibrosum (raw)
知母	zhī mǔ	20g	Rhizoma Anemarrhenae
黄柏	huáng bǎi	10g	Cortex Phellodendri Chinensis
丹皮	dān pí	15g	Cortex Moutan
赤芍	chì sháo	20g	Radix Paeoniae Rubra
紫草	zǐ cǎo	15g	Radix Arnebiae
蒲公英	pú gōng yīng	30g	Herba Taraxaci

丹参	dān shēn	30g	Radix et Rhizoma Salviae Miltiorrhizae
地龙	dì lóng	12g	Pheretima
炮山甲	páo shān jiă	10g	Squama Manis (blast-fried)
地鳖虫	dì biē chóng	6g	Eupolyphaga seu Steleophaga
桃仁	táo rén	10g	Semen Persicae
红花	hóng huā	10g	Flos Carthami
苡仁	yĭ rén	12g	Semen Coicis

Decoct the medicinals and take one batch a day, divided into 2 portions. Actions: clears heat, invigorates blood, alleviates *bi*, and unblocks the collaterals. Suitable for RA of the heat stasis type.

(5) *Mă Yĭ Wán* (蚂蚁丸)

蚂蚁	mă yĭ	30g	Formica Fusca
首乌	shŏu wū	30g	Radix Polygoni Multiflori
熟地黄	shú dì huáng	30g	Radix Rehmanniae Praeparata
人参	rén shēn	30g	Radix Ginseng
五味子	wŭ wèi zĭ	30g	Fructus Schisandrae Chinensis

Crush and sift the medicinals, then add water to make pills of 2.5g each. Take 1 pill every three days. 10 pills equal a course of treatment, and 2 courses are required. Actions: tonifies the kidney, fortifies the spleen, strengthens the sinews and bones, and boosts qi and blood. Suitable for chronic RA.

(6) *Huó Luò Xĭ Fāng* (活络洗方)

生川乌	shēng chuān wū	30g	Radix Aconiti (raw)
木瓜	mù guā	30g	Fructus Chaenomelis
炒艾	chăo ài	30g	Folium Artemisiae Argyi (dry-fried)
防风	fáng fēng	30g	Radix Saposhnikoviae
五加皮	wŭ jiā pí	30g	Cortex Acanthopanacis
地龙	dì lóng	30g	Pheretima
当归	dāng guī	30g	Radix Angelicae Sinensis

羌活	qiāng huó	30g	Rhizoma et Radix Notopterygii
土鳖虫	tǔ biē chóng	30g	Eupolyphaga seu Steleophaga
伸筋草	shēn jīn cǎo	30g	Herba Lycopodii

Wrap all the medicinals in gauze and place the gauze in a basin. Add cold water and decoct over a fire. After boiling for 5 minutes, remove the basin from the fire and immediately use the decoction to steam the affected areas of the body. Once the decoction cools down to a tolerable temperature (not hot), use it to wash the affected areas for 1 hour, 1-2 times a day. The decoction from each batch of medicinals can be used for 5-7 days continuously. Contraindicated in cases of skin breakage or suppurative skin disorders.

(7) *Yín Ěr Jī Dàn Tāng* (银耳鸡蛋汤)

银耳	yín ěr	50g	Tremella (white wood-ear mushroom)
鸡蛋	jī dàn	one	egg

Soak the white wood-ear mushrooms in water for 2 hours. Cut off the stems and remove any sediment. Tear the mushrooms into pieces. Boil them in water over a low flame until they are thoroughly cooked. Then, add an egg into the soup and stir. Add some rock sugar as desired. Take the soup two hours after meals as a dessert. Actions: boosts yin and engenders fluids. For RA of the qi and yin deficiency type.

(8) *Chuān Wū Zhōu* (川乌粥)

生川乌	shēng chuān wū	3-5g	Radix Aconiti (raw)
粳米	jīng mǐ	30g	Oryza sativa L. (polished round-grained non-glutinous rice)
姜汁	jiāng zhī	10 drops	ginger juice
蜂蜜	fēng mì	as desired	Mel (honey)

Cook the rice into porridge. Add *chuān wū* (raw Radix Aconiti) when the water boils, and continue to cook over a low flame. When the porridge is done, add the desired amount of ginger juice and honey. Cook again for another 1-2 minutes. Serve warm. Actions: disperses cold, eliminates dampness, warms the channels, and relieves pain. For RA of the cold-damp *bi* type. Contraindicated in cases of pregnancy, hot pain, and fever. Cannot be taken together with *bàn xià* (Rhizoma Pinelliae), *guā lóu* (Fructus Trichosanthis), *bèi mŭ* (Bulbus Fritillaria) and *bái jí* (Rhizoma Bletillae).

PROGNOSIS

As a chronic, recurrent inflammatory disease, the prognosis of RA is connected to the following four factors:

1. The Nature of the Evil, the Location of Invasion, the Degree of Recurrence, and the Length of the Disease Course

Of all the *bi* evils, cold-damp and toxic heat are more difficult to eliminate, while wind evil is relatively easier to expel. *Prescriptions of Universal Benefit - The Gateway to All Bi* (普济方·诸痹门, *Pŭ Jì Fāng - Zhū Bì Mén*) states: "Among all the *bi* syndromes, those caused by prevalence of wind tend to be easy to recover from." (诸痹风胜者则易愈……。) Regarding the location of invasion, *Yellow Emperor's Inner Classic - Basic Questions: Treatise on Bi Syndromes* (黄帝内经素问·痹论, *Huáng Dì Nèi Jīng Sù Wèn: Bì Lùn*) elaborates: "When *bi* evils enter the *zang* organs, the condition is fatal; when *bi* evils linger in the sinews and bones, the disease is chronic; when *bi* evils linger in the skin, the disease is easy to recover from." (痹其入脏者死，其留连筋骨间者久，其留皮肤间者易已。) If the *bi* evils are exuberant, it is difficult to eliminate them, and the lingering evils often cause recurrent attacks and a poor prognosis. Modern medicine holds that a high RF titre in the early stage of RA indicates a poor prognosis. Other conditions that point to a poor prognosis include an accelerated disease progression, manifestations other than joint symptoms (e.g., lesions organ damage, vasculitis, neuropathy, iritis, or scleritis), recurrence of rheumatoid nodules, and accumulation of fluid in the joint cavity.

2. Age, Gender, and Constitution

Disturbance of articular function in the early stage indicates a poor prognosis. High RF titre, elevation of ESR/CRP, eminent changes in radiology, and rheumatoid nodules are connected to the progression of the disease. The prognosis for middle-aged and elderly patients is worse than that for young patients. The prognosis for female patients over 50 years of age tend to be poor. Disturbance of articular function occur earlier in males than in females. Patients with weak constitutions respond less sensitively to treatment, and hence the evils can easily penetrate deeper into their bodies, resulting in a poor prognosis.

3. Early Recognition and Prompt Treatment

Early diagnosis, early testing of RA-related antibodies (e.g., AKA, CCP, RA-33, and the three examinations for the diagnosis of autoimmune disorders), radiological examinations, and early treatment can improve the prognosis. Statistics show that 15%-20% of RA patients, after recovering from one attack episode, do not suffer from subsequent attacks for at least one year. In addition, the disease condition of 10%-15% patients progress rapidly, and these patients develop joint destruction or deformity within a period of 2 years. The remaining 70% of patients present with recurrent, periodical attacks of multiple-joint inflammation, which is gradually relieved by prompt and appropriate treatment.

4. Improve Living Conditions, Regulate the Diet, Seek Spiritual Counseling, and Perform Functional Exercises

Living in a damp and cold environment, lack of regularity in one's daily life, excessive work or rest, improper diet, depression, and lack of exercise can all lead to a poor prognosis. Refer to the chapter on "preventive healthcare" for more details.

PREVENTIVE HEALTHCARE

(1) First-Degree Prevention

Avoid exposure to wind, cold and dampness. Physical exercise, increased intake of nutritious food, leading a balanced lifestyle, and maintaining a positive outlook and cheerful state of mind can all increase immunity and are essential for the healing process. As many cases of RA are related to bacterial or viral infection, prompt and effective management of the infection is an important measure for the prevention of RA.

(2) Second-Degree Prevention

Since there are no radical cures, patients can do functional exercises (to prevent articular deformity and muscular atrophy) while they are under medication for pain management. Immunosuppressants and surgery may be a viable option for some patients. Commonly used treatment modalities include medicinal therapy, exercise therapy, physical therapy, relaxation therapy, psychotherapy, and surgery.

(3) Third-Degree Prevention

For RA patients with 3rd to 4th degree functional impairment of the joints, the use of orthopedic instruments and other assistant devices are required as an auxiliary treatment. For severely damaged joints or articular dysfunction, prosthetic joint replacement can be selectively applied to facilitate the recovery of articular function.

Lifestyle Modification

- Live in a dry, warm environment with good ventilation.

- Avoid exposure to wind and cold.
- Maintain a healthy balance between work and rest.
- Take preventive measures against infection, and seek early treatment.

Dietary Recommendation

Most scholars presume that there are no special dietary guidelines for RA patients. RA is a chronic consumptive disease, and biomedical treatment involves the use of anti-rheumatic drugs whose side effects often include poor appetite and disorders of the digestive tract. These side effects eventually give way to insufficient absorption of nutrition and protein, leading to malnutrition and anemia. Therefore, the diet of an RA patient must consist of sufficient protein and a variety of vitamins and minerals. In Chinese medicine, it is believed that "medicinals and foods are equally effective." Foods high in protein and calories, rich in cellulose, and easily absorbed are preferred. In addition, patients should eat foods that are beneficial to them according to their body constitution and the type of *bi* syndrome that they are being treated for.

Generally speaking, for a thin body with effulgent ministerial fire, cooling foods such as lotus seed piths and lily bulbs can be eaten to drain heat and boost yin. For a fat body with qi deficiency and excessive phlegm, eat *yì yǐ rén* (Semen Coicis), *shān yào* (Rhizoma Dioscoreae) and *bái biǎn dòu* (Semen Lablab Album), to fortify the spleen and transform dampness. For exuberant wind evil, eat fermented soybeans and shepherd's purse; for prevalence of cold evil, use fennel, cinnamon twig, and wild pepper [*huā jiāo* (Pericarpium Zanthoxyli)] as seasonings; for prevalence of dampness, eat *yì yǐ rén* (Semen Coicis), *chì xiǎo dòu* (Semen Phaseoli), and *chǎo bái biǎn dòu* (dry-fried Semen Lablab Album); for prevalence of heat, eat duck roasted with *tōng xīn cǎo* (Crotalaria assamica Benth.), green vegetables, and fruits; for lumbar soreness caused by kidney deficiency, eat walnuts and pig kidneys; for qi insufficiency, eat *huáng qí* (Radix Astragali), hen stewed with *dà zăo* (Fructus Jujubae), soft-shelled turtle, and snakeheaded fish (a.k.a. snakehead mullet).

In addition to the above guidelines, the following recipes are recommended:

(1) *Gŏu Qĭ Yáng Shèn Tāng* (枸杞羊肾汤)

枸杞叶	gŏu qĭ yè	30g	Folium Lycii
羊肾	yáng shèn	2 pairs	goat kidney
羊肉	yáng ròu	250g	mutton
葱	cōng	1 stalk	scallion
五味佐料	wŭ wèi zuŏ liào	as desired	"five flavors" seasoning (powdered star anise, clove, cinnamon, fennel, and brown pepper)
粳米	jīng mĭ	50g	Oryza sativa L. polished round-grained non-glutinous rice

Boil the *gŏu qĭ yè*, goat kidney, and mutton, and then add the scallion and seasoning. Once the soup is done, add the rice and cook into a porridge. Take every morning and evening. Replenishes essence, boosts marrow, and warms the spleen and kidney. Good for dual deficiency of yin and yang, and for patients with fear of the cold in the winter and aversion to heat in the summer.

(2) *Mù Guā Tāng* (木瓜汤)

木瓜	mù guā	4	Fructus Chaenomelis (Chinese quince fruit)
白蜜	bái mì	1000g	(fine-quality) honey

Steam the quince fruits. When they are well cooked, peel off the skin, and blend the fruit to a paste. Add honey and stir the two ingredients together in a clean porcelain container. Take 1-2 spoonfuls of the juice with warm, boiled water every morning. Unblocks *bi* and relieves pain; good for pain of the sinews and bones due to damp-heat obstruction in the channels and collaterals.

(3) *Shēng Jiāng Zhōu* (生姜粥)

生姜	5 slices	ginger
粳米	50g	polished round-grained (non-glutinous) rice
连须葱	several stalks	scallion with rootlets
米醋	as desired	vinegar

Cook the rice into porridge. Grind the ginger and boil it with the rice. When done, add the scallions and vinegar. After taking the porridge, cover the body with blankets to induce sweating. Resolves the exterior and disperses cold. For RA of the wind-cold obstruction type.

(4) *Bái Mù Ěr Guì Yuán Tāng* (白木耳桂圆汤)

白木耳	200g	tremella (white wood-ear mushroom)
桂圆	100g	flesh of the longan fruit

Wash the mushrooms and remove the stems. Place them in a pot with water, bring to a boil, and cook over a low flame. When the mushrooms are half softened, add the longan and continue to cook until the mushrooms are thoroughly cooked and the flavor of the longan has been released into the soup. Take two spoonfuls of the warm soup every morning. For RA of the cold-heat complex type. Indications: swollen and painful joints and muscles, local heat, fear and aversion of cold but aversion to heat when bundled up, feverish sensation in the palms and soles with less noticeable sensation of heat in the body, aversion to cold upon exposure of the skin, a red or pale tongue with white or yellow coating, and a pulse that is wiry, slippery, and slightly rapid, or deep, thready, slippery, and slightly rapid.

(5) *Táo Rén Tāng* (桃仁汤)

桃仁	táo rén	15g	Semen Persicae (peach kernel)
粳米	jīng mǐ	160g	polished round-grained (non-glutinous) rice

Grind the peach kernels into a paste and mix it with water. After filtering the liquid and discarding the dregs, use the liquid to cook the rice into porridge. Take once a day. The quantity of the ingredients shown above is for one serving. For RA of the blood stasis type. Indications: fixed, stabbing joint pain that is worse at night and relieved by movement, a dark purple tongue, and a rough or intermittent pulse.

(6) *Fú Líng Fěn Zhōu* (茯苓粉粥)

茯苓粉	fú líng	30g	Poria (powdered)
白米	bái mǐ	30g	polished white rice
大枣	dà zǎo	7 pc	Fructus Jujubae

After boiling the rice in a pot, add *dà zǎo* (Fructus Jujubae) and continue to cook. When the porridge is done, add the *fú líng* powder and stir with a chopstick. Add some sugar to taste. This porridge can be taken as breakfast or at any time. Good for RA of the phlegm obstruction type. Indications: local swelling, no redness of the skin, shortness of breath, a weak body, dizziness, poor appetite, abdominal distention, an enlarged and tender tongue with white glossy coating, and a wiry and slippery, or deep and slow pulse.

(7) *Yuán Shēn Dùn Zhū Gān* (元参炖猪肝)

猪肝	zhū gān	500g	pork liver
元参	yuán shēn	15g	Radix Scrophulariae
菜油	cài yóu	as desired	vegetable oil
葱	cōng	2 stalks	scallion
生姜	shēng jiāng	9 slices	ginger
酱油	jiàng yóu	as desired	soy sauce
白糖	bái táng	30g	white sugar
黄酒	huáng jiǔ	as desired	yellow (rice or millet) wine
豆粉	dòu fěn	as desired	soybean flour

Wash the pork liver and put it in a pot with *yuán shēn* (Radix

Scrophulariae). Add water and boil for 1 hour, then take out the liver and cut it into slices. Pour vegetable oil into a saucepan and briefly stir-fry the scallion and ginger. Put the liver slices in the saucepan, and add a small amount of soy sauce, sugar, wine, and soup (made from boiling the liver and *yuán shēn*). After cooking for a little while longer to reduce the volume of the soup, add the soybean flour to make the soup thick and transparent. To be consumed in one sitting or divided into portions to be eaten with meals. Good for liver and kidney yin deficiency. Indications: a somber and lusterless facial complexion accompanied by dizziness, vexing heat of the five centers, soreness and weakness of the lumbus and knees, fatigue, a red tongue with scanty coating, and a thready or rapid pulse.

(8) *Shēn Qí Jú Xìng Yǐn* (参芪桔杏饮)

人参	rén shen	5g	Radix Ginseng
黄芪	huáng qí	30g	Radix Astragali
杏仁	xìng rén	10g	Armeniacae Semen Amarum
丝瓜	sī guā	60g	Fructus Retinervus (silk melon)

Boil the above ingredients in water for 20 minutes. After filtering out the dregs, the liquid decoction can be taken as a beverage (in place of tea) with no limitation of timing or quantity. Tonifies qi, transforms phlegm, relaxes the sinews, unblocks the collaterals, and relieves pain. Good for all types of *bi* syndromes caused by qi deficiency and phlegm-turbidity obstruction.

Regulation of Emotional and Mental Health

RA is a life-long disease. Its tendency for recurrence and poor diagnosis leads to depression, which can eventually give rise to anxiety, hopelessness, anger, despair, and in some cases, thoughts of suicide. Clinicians must not overlook the importance of these emotions. In addition to showing patience and providing emotional counseling (or refer the patient to a psychotherapist if necessary), obtaining the cooperation of the patient's family and friends is also a crucial part of the treatment process. Chinese medicine advocates using life cultivation as the primary focus of treatment. This means that in order to prevent illness, one must adapt to climate changes, regulate the emotions, and lead a balanced life. In addition, RA patients can rejuvenate their spirit by strengthening their body constitution and facilitating recovery with exercises such as *tài jí quán* (太极拳; also written as "tai chi chuan" in the older romanization systems for Mandarin Chinese), traditional Chinese sword-play, deep breathing exercises, and gymnastics.

CLINICAL EXPERIENCE OF RENOWNED PHYSICIANS

Empirical Formulas

1. Jiao Shu-de Uses *Bǔ Shèn Qū Hán Zhì Wāng Tāng* (补肾祛寒治尪汤) to Treat Lame *Bi* due to Kidney Deficiency with Exuberant Cold

【Ingredients】

川续断	chuān xù duàn	12-20g	Radix Dipsaci
补骨脂	bǔ gǔ zhī	9-12g	Fructus Psoraleae
熟地黄	shú dì huáng	12-24g	Radix Rehmanniae Praeparata
淫羊藿	yín yáng huò	9-12g	Herba Epimedii
制附片	zhì fù piàn	6-12g	Radix Aconiti Lateralis Praeparata
骨碎补	gŭ suì bŭ	10-20g	Rhizoma Drynariae
桂枝	guì zhī	9-15g	Ramulus Cinnamomi
赤芍	chì sháo	9-12g	Radix Paeoniae Rubra
白芍	bái sháo	9-12g	Radix Paeoniae Alba
知母	zhī mŭ	9-12g	Rhizoma Anemarrhenae
独活	dú huó	10-12g	Radix Angelicae Pubescentis
防风	fáng fēng	10g	Radix Saposhnikoviae

麻黄	má huáng	3-6g	Herba Ephedrae
苍术	cāng zhú	6-10g	Rhizoma Atractylodis
威灵仙	wēi líng xiān	12-15g	Radix et Rhizoma Clematidis
伸筋草	shēn jīn cǎo	30g	Herba Lycopodii
牛膝	niú xī	9-15g	Radix Achyranthis Bidentatae
松节	sōng jié	15g	Lignum Pini Nodi
炙山甲	zhì shān jiǎ	6-9g	Squama Manis (liquid-fried)
地鳖虫	dì biē chóng	6-10g	Eupolyphaga seu Steleophaga
炙虎骨	zhì hǔ gǔ	9-12g	Os Tigris (liquid-fried)

Note: Since the tiger is an endangered animal currently under the protection of the national wilderness preservation program, *hǔ gǔ* (Os Tigris) can be replaced by *tòu gǔ cǎo* (Caulis Impatientis), *xún gǔ fēng* (Herba Aristolochiae Mollissimae), or *zì rán tóng* (Pyritum, soaked in vinegar and decocted first).

【Indications】

Lame *bi* of the Kidney deficiency and exuberant cold type.

【Formula Analysis】

The primary medicinals, *xù duàn* (Radix Dipsaci), *bǔ gǔ zhī* (Fructus Psoraleae), *shú dì huáng* (Radix Rehmanniae Praeparata), and *zhì fù piàn* (Radix Aconiti Lateralis Preparata), tonify the kidney, disperse cold, replenish essence, tonify blood, and enrich and nourish the liver and kidney to strengthen the sinews and bones. The adjuvant medicinals, *gǔ suì bǔ* (Rhizoma Drynariae), *yín yáng huò* (Herba Epimedii), *zhì hǔ gǔ* (prepared Os Tigris), *bái sháo* (Radix Paeoniae Alba), *guì zhī* (Ramulus Cinnamomi), *dú huó* (Radix Angelicae Pubescentis), and *wēi líng xiān* (Radix et Rhizoma Clematidis), tonify kidney yang, strengthen the sinews and bones, disperse wind and cold, unblock the channels and collaterals, relieve spasms, and relax the sinews. Other adjuvant medicinals, *fáng fēng* (Radix Saposhnikoviae), *má huáng* (Herba Ephedrae), *cāng zhú* (Rhizoma Atractylodis), *zhī mǔ* (Rhizoma Anemarrhenae), *zhì shān jiǎ* (liquid-fried

Squama Manis), *shēn jīn cǎo* (Herba Lycopodii), *chì sháo* (Radix Paeoniae Rubra), *sōng jié* (Lignum Pini Nodi), and *dì biē chóng* (Eupolyphaga seu Steleophaga), disperse wind-cold, dispel wind-damp, invigorate blood, transform stasis, unblock the channels, dissipate binds, relax the sinews, quicken the collaterals, enrich the kidney, and clear heat. *Huái niú xī* (Radix Achyranthis Bidentatae) is used as an envoy to strengthen the sinews and bones, dissipate static blood, and guide the effects of the medicinals to the kidney.

【Modifications】

This formula can be used alone or combined with other formulas or medicinals according to pattern differentiation.

➢ For severe involvement of the upper limbs, remove *huái niú xī* (Radix Achyranthis Bidentatae) and add *piàn jiāng huáng* (Rhizoma Wenyujin Concisum) 10g and *qiāng huó* (Rhizoma et Radix Notopterygii) 10g to dispel wind, eliminate dampness, and invigorate blood.

➢ For pronounced blood stasis, add *hóng huā* (Flos Carthami) 10g, *zào jiǎo cì* (Spina Gleditsiae) 5-6g, *rǔ xiāng* (Olibanum) 6g, *mò yào* (Myrrha) 6g, or *sū mù* (Lignum Sappan) 15-20g to strengthen the effects of invigorating blood and transforming stasis.

➢ For marked pain of the lumbus and legs, remove *sōng jié* (Lignum Pini Nodi) and *cāng zhú* (Rhizoma Atractylodis), add *sāng jì shēng* (Herba Taxilli) 30g, and increase the dosages of *xù duàn* (Radix Dipsaci) and *bǔ gǔ zhī* (Fructus Psoraleae). Chew 1-2 pieces of *zhì hú táo ròu* (honey-fried walnut flesh) with the decoction to tonify the kidney and strengthen the lumbus.

➢ For joint stiffness and spasm, remove *cāng zhú* (Rhizoma Atractylodis), *fáng fēng* (Radix Saposhnikoviae), and *sōng jié* (Lignum Pini Nodi), and add *shēng yì yǐ rén* (Semen Coicis) 30-40g, *mù guā* (Fructus Chaenomelis) 9-12g, and *bái jiāng cán* (Bombyx Batryticatus) 10g to relax the sinews and quicken the collaterals.

➢ For severe joint pain, increase the dosage of *zhì fù piàn* (Radix Aconiti Lateralis Preparata) and add *zhì căo wū* (Radix Aconiti Kusnezoffii Praeparata) 6-9g and one third of a vial of *Qī Lí Săn* (七厘散) [taken with the decoction] to disperse cold and relieve pain.

[Jiao Shu-de. *Essentials of Jiao Shu-de's Clinical Experience* (焦树德临床经验辑要). Beijing: China Medical Science and Technology Publishing House.2001.6]

2. Jiao Shu-de Uses *Jiā Jiăn Bŭ Shèn Zhì Wāng Tāng* (加减补肾治尪汤) to Treat Lame *Bi* due to Kidney Deficiency with Branch Heat (Mild Pattern)

【Ingredients】

生地	shēng dì	15-20g	Radix Rehmanniae Recens
川续断	chuān xù duàn	15-18g	Radix Dipsaci
骨碎补	gŭ suì bŭ	15g	Rhizoma Drynariae
桑寄生	sāng jì shēng	30g	Herba Taxilli
补骨脂	bŭ gŭ zhī	6g	Fructus Psoraleae
桂枝	guì zhī	6-9g	Ramulus Cinnamomi
白芍	bái sháo	15g	Radix Paeoniae Alba
知母	zhī mŭ	12g	Rhizoma Anemarrhenae
威灵仙	wēi líng xiān	12-15g	Radix et Rhizoma Clematidis
酒炒黄柏	huáng băi	12g	Cortex Phellodendri Chinensis (wine-fried)
炙山甲	zhì shān jiă	9g	Squama Manis (liquid-fried)
羌活	qiāng huó	9g	Rhizoma et Radix Notopterygii
独活	dú huó	9g	Radix Angelicae Pubescentis
红花	hóng huā	9g	Flos Carthami
制附片	zhì fù piàn	3-5g	Radix Aconiti Lateralis Praeparata
忍冬藤	rĕn dōng téng	30g	Caulis Lonicerae Japonicae
络石藤	luò shí téng	20-30g	Caulis Trachelospermi
地鳖虫	dì biē chóng	9g	Eupolyphaga seu Steleophaga
伸筋草	shēn jīn căo	30g	Herba Lycopodii
生薏苡仁	shēng yì yĭ rén	30g	Semen Coicis (raw)

One batch a day, decocted twice until it becomes a thick decoction (300 ml). Divide into two equal portions of 150 ml each and take one portion, twice a day.

【Indications】

Kidney deficiency with branch heat (mild).

【Formula Analysis】

After of the patient is treated for kidney deficiency with cold exuberance, the yang is gradually revitalized and some of the evils dissipate. At this time, one should reduce the dosages of warm and drying herbs such as *zhì fù piàn* (Radix Aconiti Lateralis Preparata), *guì zhī* (Ramulus Cinnamomi), and *má huáng* (Herba Ephedrae). Remove *shú dì huáng* (Radix Rehmanniae Praeparata), *yín yáng huò* (Herba Epimedii), *cāng zhú* (Rhizoma Atractylodis), *fáng fēng* (Radix Saposhnikoviae), and *sōng jié* (Lignum Pini Nodi), and add the herbs that tonify the kidney, quicken the collaterals, course stagnation, and clear heat, i.e., *shēng dì huáng* (Radix Rehmanniae), *huáng bǎi* (Cortex Phellodendri Chinensis), *rěn dōng téng* (Caulis Lonicerae Japonicae), *luò shí téng* (Caulis Trachelospermi), *hóng huā* (Flos Carthami), *sāng jì shēng* (Herba Taxilli), and *yì yǐ rén* (Semen Coicis). Keep the following medicinals in the formula to further tonify the kidney, dispel wind, disperse cold, and transform dampness: *xù duàn* (Radix Dipsaci), *bǔ gǔ zhī* (Fructus Psoraleae), *gǔ suì bǔ* (Rhizoma Drynariae), *zhī mǔ* (Rhizoma Anemarrhenae), *chì bái sháo* (Radix Paeoniae Alba), *dú huó* (Radix Angelicae Pubescentis), *wēi líng xiān* (Radix et Rhizoma Clematidis), *zhì shān jiǎ* (liquid-fried Squama Manis), *dì biē chóng* (Eupolyphaga seu Steleophaga), and *shēn jīn cǎo* (Herba Lycopodii).

[Jiao Shu-de. *Essentials of Jiao Shu-de's Clinical Experience* (焦树德临床经验辑要). Beijing: China Medical Science and Technology Publishing House. 2001.6]

3. Jiao Shu-de Uses *Bŭ Shèn Qīng Rè Zhì Wāng Tāng* (补肾清热治尫汤) to Treat Lame *Bi* due to Kidney Deficiency with Branch Heat (Severe Pattern)

【Ingredients】

生地	shēng dì	15-20g	Radix Rehmanniae Recens
川续断	chuān xù duàn	15g	Radix Dipsaci
地骨皮	dì gŭ pí	10g	Cortex Lycii
骨碎补	gŭ suì bŭ	15g	Rhizoma Drynariae
桑枝	sāng zhī	30g	Ramulus Mori
赤芍	chì sháo	12g	Radix Paeoniae Rubra
秦艽	qín jiāo	20-30g	Radix Gentianae Macrophyllae
知母	zhī mŭ	12g	Rhizoma Anemarrhenae
炒黄柏	chăo huáng băi	12g	Cortex Phellodendri Chinensis (dry-fried)
威灵仙	wēi líng xiān	15g	Radix et Rhizoma Clematidis
羌活	qiāng huó	6-9g	Rhizoma et Radix Notopterygii
独活	dú huó	9g	Radix Angeliae Pubescentis
制乳香	zhì rŭ xiāng	6g	Olibanum (prepared)
制没药	zhì mò yào	6g	Myrrha (prepared)
地鳖虫	dì biē chóng	9g	Eupolyphaga seu Steleophaga
白僵蚕	bái jiāng cán	9g	Bombyx Batryticatus
蚕沙	cán shā	10g	Faeces Bombycis
红花	hóng huā	10g	Flos Carthami
忍冬藤	rĕn dōng téng	30g	Caulis Lonicerae Japonicae
透骨草	tòu gŭ căo	20g	Caulis Impatientis
络石藤	luò shí téng	30g	Caulis Trachelospermi

Decoct and take twice a day. After the heat evil has been eliminated, gradually add medicinals that tonify the kidney and disperse cold.

【Indications】

Kidney deficiency with branch heat (severe).

【Formula Analysis】

This formula is derived from *Qián Xíng Săn* (潜行散), a formula created by Zhu Dan-xi, and *Qīng Rè Sàn Bì Tāng* (清热散痹汤), a formula created by Jiao Shu-de himself. The primary medicinals, *xù duàn* (Radix Dipsaci), *gŭ suì bŭ* (Rhizoma Drynariae), *shēng dì huáng* (Radix Rehmanniae), *zhī mŭ* (Rhizoma Anemarrhenae), *huáng băi* (Cortex Phellodendri Chinensis), *dì gŭ pí* (Cortex Lycii), and *chì sháo* (Radix Paeoniae Rubra), tonify the kidney and clear heat. The adjuvant medicinals, *sāng zhī* (Ramulus Mori), *qín jiāo* (Radix Gentianae Macrophyllae), *rĕn dōng téng* (Caulis Lonicerae Japonicae), *luò shí téng* (Caulis Trachelospermi), *cán shā* (Faeces Bombycis), and *wēi líng xiān* (Radix et Rhizoma Clematidis), clear heat, dispel wind, eliminate dampness, and free obstruction. *Qiāng huó* (Rhizoma et Radix Notopterygii), *dú huó* (Radix Angelicae Pubescentis), *bái jiāng cán* (Bombyx Batryticatus), *rŭ xiāng* (Olibanum), *mò yào* (Myrrha), *dì biē chóng* (Eupolyphaga seu Steleophaga), and *hóng huā* (Flos Carthami) dispel wind and overcome dampness; they guide the effects of all the medicinals deep into the bones to track down and remove the evils that have entered the bones.

【Modifications】

- For constipation, add *táo rén* (Semen Persicae) 10g and *zhì dà huáng* (Radix et Rhizoma Rhei Praeparata) 3g-6g to unblock the bowels and free the stool.
- For thirst with a preference for cold drinks, add *shēng shí gāo* (raw Gypsum Fibrosum) 30g (decocted first) to clear the heat.

[Jiao Shu-de. *Essentials of Jiao Shu-de's Clinical Experience* (焦树德临床经验辑要). Beijing: China Medical Science and Technology Publishing House.2001.6]

4. Zheng Hui-bo Uses *Zhèng Shì Hŭ Zhèng Săn* (郑氏虎挣散) to Treat Yang Deficiency with Obstruction of the Collaterals by Cold-damp *Bi*

【Ingredients】

制马钱子	zhì mă qián zĭ	30g	Semen Strychni (prepared)
制附片(浸泡)	zhì fù piàn	30g	Radix Aconiti Lateralis Praeparata (steeped)
山甲珠	shān jiă zhū	30g	Squama Manis

蜈蚣	wú gōng	15 pieces	Scolopendra
蕲蛇	qí shé	10g	Agkistrodon
虎骨(用透骨草等代)	hǔ gǔ	20g	Os Tigris (can be replaced by *tòu gǔ cǎo* [Caulis Impatientis])

Preparation method for *mǎ qián zǐ* (Semen Strychni): First, remove the hair and soak the herb in healthy boy's urine for 7 days, changing the urine daily. Next, dry the herb in the sun. Meanwhile, decoct *má huáng* (Herba Ephedrae) 20g and *gān cǎo* (Radix et Rhizoma Glycyrrhizae) 20g in a pot, filter and discard the dregs, and throw the *mǎ qián zǐ* into the decoction. Cook over a low flame until the essence of the decoction has seeped into the *mǎ qián zǐ*. Remove the herb from the pot and dry it in the sun. Grind the herb into a powder and add honey to make pills of 3g each. Take one pill, 3 times a day (this is a safe and effective dose).

【Indications】

Cold-damp *bi*

【Formula Analysis】

The primary medicinal, *zhì mǎ qián zǐ* (prepared Semen Strychni), resolves toxins and dissipates binds. *Zhì fù piàn* (Radix Aconiti Lateralis Preparata) warms yang and dissipates binds. *Shān jiǎ zhū* (Squama Manis), *wú gōng* (Scolopendra), *qí shé* (Agkistrodon), and *hǔ gǔ* (Os Tigris) quicken the collaterals and relieve pain.

[Shan Shu-jian, Chen Zi-hua. *The Golden Mirror of the Clinical Experience of Famous Ancient and Modern Physicians* (古今名医临证金鉴). Beijing: China Publishing House of Chinese Medicine.1999]

5. Ren Ji-xue Uses an Empirical Formula to Treat Chronic *Bi* Syndromes with Qi Stagnation and Blood Stasis

【Ingredients】

酒炒当归	jiǔ chǎo dāng guī	20g	Radix Angelicae Sinensis (wine-fried)

肉桂炒熟地	ròu guì chǎo shú dì huáng	10g	Radix Rehmanniae Praeparata (dry-fried with Cortex Cinnamomi)
姜汁炒白芍	jiāng zhī chǎo bái sháo	30g	Radix Paeoniae Alba (fried with ginger juice)
蜈蚣	wú gōng	one piece	Scolopendra
全蝎	quán xiē	3g	Scorpio
土鳖虫	tǔ biē chóng	10g	Eupolyphaga seu Steleophaga
蜂房	fēng fáng	15g	Nidus Vespae
乌梢蛇	wū shāo shé	15g	Zaocys
山甲珠	shān jiǎ zhū	10g	Squama Manis
苍耳子	cāng ěr zǐ	10g	Fructus Xanthii
仙灵脾	xiān líng pí	10g	Herba Epimedii
仙茅	xiān máo	10g	Rhizoma Curculiginis

【Indications】

Chronic *bi* with qi stagnation and blood stasis

【Formula Analysis】

The chief medicinals, *dāng guī* (Radix Angelicae Sinensis), *ròu guì chǎo shú dì huáng* [Radix Rehmanniae Praeparata (dry-fried with Cortex Cinnamomi)], and *jiāng zhī chǎo bái sháo* [Radix Paeoniae Alba (fried with ginger juice)], regulate, harmonize, and nourish blood to remove obstruction in the collaterals. As the deputies, *wú gōng* (Scolopendra), *quán xiē* (Scorpio), *tǔ biē chóng* (Eupolyphaga seu Steleophaga), and *fēng fáng* (Nidus Vespae) chase wind, alleviate spasms, relieve pain, and track down stasis in the channels and collaterals. The assistant medicinals, *wū shé* (Zaocys), *jiǎ zhū* (Squama Manis), *cāng ěr zǐ* (Fructus Xanthii) strengthen nutritive and defensive qi, regulate qi and blood, and eliminate *bi* evils from the interior and exterior aspects of the body. The envoys, *xiān líng pí* (Herba Epimedii) and *xiān máo* (Rhizoma Curculiginis), boost kidney yang, tonify the *mìng mén* (命门; life gate) fire, and warm the qi of the interior and exterior aspects of the body. Once the right qi is restored and evil qi is eliminated, the disease condition will improve on its own.

【Modifications】

➢ For generalized heaviness and puffy swelling (a.k.a. superficial edema), add *bái jiè zǐ* (Semen Sinapis) 10g and *xī xiān cǎo* (Herba Siegesbeckiae) 50g to dispel dampness and disperse cold.

➢ For slight fever, remove *xiān líng pí* (Herba Epimedii) and *xiān máo* (Rhizoma Curculiginis), and add *cǎo guǒ* (Fructus Tsaoko) 10g, *zhī mǔ* (Rhizoma Anemarrhenae) 10g, and *shí gāo* (Gypsum Fibrosum) 15g to outthrust evils and clear heat.

[Shan Shu-jian, Chen Zi-hua. *The Golden Mirror of the Clinical Experience of Famous Ancient and Modern Physicians* (古今名医临证金鉴). Beijing: China Publishing House of Chinese Medicine.1999]

6. Xie Hai-zhou Uses *Bì Tòng Níng* (痹痛宁) to Treat Bi Syndromes due to Kidney Deficiency with Cold Exuberance and Obstruction in the Channels and Collaterals

【Ingredients】

鹿角霜	lù jiǎo shuāng	12g	Cornu Cervi Degelatinatum
当归	dāng guī	15g	Radix Angelicae Sinensis
肉桂	ròu guì	10g	Cortex Cinnamomi
制附子	zhì fù zǐ	10g	Radix Aconiti Lateralis Praeparata
细辛	xì xīn	5g	Radix et Rhizoma Asari
羌活	qiāng huó	10g	Rhizoma et Radix Notopterygii
独活	dú huó	10g	Radix Angelicae Pubescentis
防己	fáng jǐ	15g	Radix Stephaniae Tetrandrae
白芍	bái sháo	10g	Radix Paeoniae Alba
蜈蚣	wú gōng	3g	Scolopendra
地龙	dì lóng	10g	Pheretima
生地	shēng dì	30g	Radix Rehmanniae Recens
生薏苡仁	shēng yì yǐ rén	30g	Semen Coicis (raw)
生甘草	shēng gān cǎo	12g	Radix et Rhizoma Glycyrrhizae (raw)
生黄芪	shēng huáng qí	30g	Radix Astragali (raw)
乌梢蛇	wū shāo shé	10g	Zaocys

Decoct with water, divide the decoction into two portions and take one portion, twice a day.

【Indications】

Cold pain, swelling, distention, and deformity in the flesh and joints of the limbs, accompanied by inhibited bending and stretching and aching pain of the lumbus and knees.

【Formula Analysis】

Lù jiăo shuāng (Cornu Cervi Degelatinatum) and *zhì fù zĭ* (Radix Aconiti Lateralis Praeparata) tonify kidney yang and strengthen the sinews and bones. *Guì zhī* (Ramulus Cinnamomi) warms yang, unblocks the channels, and regulate nutritive and defensive qi. *Xì xīn* (Radix et Rhizoma Asari), *qiāng huó* (Rhizoma et Radix Notopterygii), *dú huó* (Radix Angelicae Pubescentis), *fáng jĭ* (Radix Stephaniae Tetrandrae), and *shēng yì yĭ rén* (raw Semen Coicis) dispel wind-damp and disperse cold. *Shēng huáng qí* (raw Radix Astragali), *dāng guī* (Radix Angelicae Sinensis), *chì sháo* (Radix Paeoniae Rubra), and *shēng dì huáng* (Radix Rehmanniae Recens) tonify qi and nourish blood. *Dì lóng* (Pheretima), *wú gōng* (Scolopendra), and *wū shāo shé* (Zaocys) unblock the channels and quicken the collaterals. *Shēng gān căo* (raw Radix et Rhizoma Glycyrrhizae) harmonizes all the medicinals.

[Zhang Jun-ting. *Essential TCM Diagnostic and Treatment Skills* (中医诊疗特技精典). Beijing: Chinese Medicine Classics Publishing House, 1994]

7. Zhu Chen-yu Uses *Sì Téng Yī Xiān Tāng* (四藤一仙汤) to Treat *Bi* Syndromes due to Wind Cold Damp Obstruction with Qi and Blood Stagnation

【Ingredients】

海风藤	hăi fēng téng	20g	Caulis Piperis Kadsurae
络石藤	luò shí téng	15g	Caulis Trachelospermi
鸡血藤	jī xuè téng	30g	Caulis Spatholobi

钩藤	gōu téng	10g	Ramulus Uncariae Cum Uncis
威灵仙	wēi líng xiān	10g	Radix et Rhizoma Clematidis
生黄芪	shēng huáng qí	30g	Radix Astragali (raw)
桂枝	guì zhī	10g	Ramulus Cinnamomi
白芍	bái sháo	10g	Radix Paeoniae Alba
生姜	shēng jiāng	3 pieces	Rhizoma Zingiberis Recens
大枣	dà zǎo	5 pieces	Fructus Jujubae

Decoct the herbs with water. Take one dose a day (after meal).

【Indications】

Wind cold damp obstruction with qi and blood stagnation manifesting as pain and numbness of the joints and flesh, inhibited bending and stretching, impaired mobility, and severe pain upon pressure. Commonly seen in rheumatic or rheumatoid arthritis and gout.

【Formula Analysis】

Hǎi fēng téng (Caulis Piperis Kadsurae), *luò shí téng* (Caulis Trachelospermi), *gōu téng* (Ramulus Uncariae Cum Uncis), and *wēi líng xiān* (Radix et Rhizoma Clematidis) dispel wind, eliminate dampness, unblock the channels, and quicken the collaterals. *Huáng qí* (Radix Astragali) and *jī xuè téng* (Caulis Spatholobi) tonify qi and nourish blood. *Guì zhī* (Ramulus Cinnamomi) regulates and harmonizes nutritive and defensive qi.

【Modifications】

- For moving *bi*, add *fáng fēng* (Radix Saposhnikoviae) 10g and *qín jiāo* (Radix Gentianae Macrophyllae) 10g to dispel wind and unblock the collaterals.
- For cold *bi*, add *páo fù zǐ* (blast-fried Radix Aconiti Lateralis) 10g and *xì xīn* (Radix et Rhizoma Asari) 5g to warm the channels, disperse cold, and eliminate *bi*.
- For damp *bi*, add *fáng jǐ* (Radix Stephaniae Tetrandrae) 10g, *cán shā* (Faeces Bombycis) 15g, and *bái zhú* (Rhizoma Atractylodis

Macrocephalae) 15g to fortify the spleen and dispel dampness.

- For heat *bi*, add *Zǐ Xuě Sǎn* (紫雪散) to clear heat and resolve toxins.
- For joint deformity, add *dà wú gōng* (Scolopendra) 10g and *bái jiāng cán* (Bombyx Batryticatus) 15g to relax the sinews and quicken the collaterals.

[Qiu De-wen and Sha Feng-wu. *A Collection of the Expert Experience of Famous Old TCM Physicians of China* (中国名老中医药专家学术经验集). Guizhou Technology Publishing House. 1995.5]

Selected Case Studies

1. Jiao Shu-de's Case Study: The Treatment of Lame *Bi* by Tonifying the Kidney and Dispersing Cold

Patient: Ren; 48 year-old male.

【Initial Visit】

October 28th, 1971: The patient's chief complaint was pain, swelling, deformity, and stiffness of the joints for over 1 year.

【History of Present Illness】

In September, 1970, the patient had been digging an underground tunnel for extended periods of time. One day, he suddenly came down with a high fever of over 40℃ , followed by redness, swelling, and pain of the left knee and ankle with difficulty in walking. After half a year of treatment, the symptoms seemed to have gotten worse. Both the wrist and index finger joints started to turn red and swollen with pain, stiffness, and deformity. He suffered severe loss of mobility and could not even extend his limbs in the morning. Both knees, particularly the left knee, were swollen and deformed with inhibited bending and stretching. Both ankles were severely swollen. After undergoing relevant examinations at a medical college affiliated hospital, he was diagnosed with RA (the current ESR was 55 mm/h). He was then transferred to the TCM department of the hospital. After taking 80 batches of Chinese medicinals, the symptoms did not show any improvement, and the ESR rose to 118 mm/h. At last, he came to our hospital.

【Present Signs and Symptoms】

Swelling, pain, deformity, and limited range of motion in both knees, wrists and finger joints. In addition, both hip joints were rigid and stuck in a certain position (120° angle between the legs and the trunk, with inability to flex or extend). Both shoulders and elbows were stiff with loss of mobility. He was carried into the hospital by family members. His other signs and symptoms included intermittent fever, fear of cold, vexing heat in the heart, poor appetite, occasional nausea, 1-2 bowel movements a day, reddish-yellow urine, white and glossy tongue coating, and a wiry and rapid pulse. An X-ray examination confirmed the diagnosis of RA.

【Pattern Differentiation】

The underground environment is cold and wet. Long-term exposure to this type of environment makes one susceptible to the invasion of wind cold damp evil, which causes *bi* syndromes. Cold and dampness have a tendency to damage the kidney, and kidney deficiency leads to a decreased resistance to evils, allowing the cold and dampness to penetrate deeper into the body. The kidney governs the bones. Cold evil enters the bones and remains there for a long period of time, causing the bones to lose their nourishment and become distorted or contracted with spasms. The limbs are thus unable to flex or extend normally and the feet are severely swollen and feel as if they are about to fall off, and the patient has a desire to vomit. According to the pulse manifestation, signs, and symptoms, the diagnosis of lame *bi* can be determined. Although there are (branch) heat signs, the condition is essentially a cold pattern.

【Treatment Principle】

Tonify the kidney, disperse cold, dispel wind, and unblock the collaterals.

【Prescription】

Modified *Bŭ Shèn Qū Hán Zhì Wāng Tāng* (补肾祛寒治尪汤)

制附片	zhì fù piàn	10g	Radix Aconiti Lateralis Praeparata
骨碎补	gŭ suì bŭ	12g	Rhizoma Drynariae
桂枝	guì zhī	10g	Ramulus Cinnamomi
赤芍	chì sháo	10g	Radix Paeoniae Rubra
白芍	bái sháo	10g	Radix Paeoniae Alba
麻黄	má huáng	6g	Herba Ephedrae
知母	zhī mŭ	10g	Rhizoma Anemarrhenae
防风	fáng fēng	12g	Radix Saposhnikoviae
威灵仙	wēi líng xiān	12g	Radix et Rhizoma Clematidis
白术	bái zhú	10g	Rhizoma Atractylodis Macrocephalae
炙山甲	zhì shān jiă	10g	Squama Manis (liquid-fried)
生姜	shēng jiāng	10g	Rhizoma Zingiberis Recens
甘草	gān căo	6g	Radix et Rhizoma Glycyrrhizae

6 batches of the above prescription were prescribed.

After the course of treatment, all the symptoms showed improvement. The same formula was prescribed again, with the addition of *shēn jīn căo* (Herba Lycopodii) 30g, and an increase in the dosage *hŭ gŭ* (Os Tigris) to 12g. The patient was instructed to take the formula over a long period of time.

【Second Visit】

March 10th, 1972: The patient could walk by himself again, without a cane. The wrist and finger joints of both hands were able to move freely without tenderness (in spite of deformity). There knees were still slightly swollen. *Huáng qí* (Radix Astragali) 30g was added to the previous prescription. By March 17th, the patient was able to ride a bicycle. The same formula was prescribed again.

【Third Visit】

May 3rd, 1972: The patient's appetite improved, and the deformity of the ankles no longer influenced normal physical activities. He complained only of occasional slight pain and sensation of swelling in the wrists and ankles. After a total of 22 visits and 110 batches of medicinals, the patient's condition was stabilized, and he was instructed to take the formula in powdered form for a long period of time to consolidate the treatment effect.

制附片	zhì fù piàn	45g	Radix Aconiti Lateralis Praeparata
骨碎补	gŭ suì bŭ	54g	Rhizoma Drynariae
川断	chuān duàn	60g	Radix Dipsaci
桂枝	guì zhī	36g	Ramulus Cinnamomi
赤芍	chì sháo	60g	Radix Paeoniae Rubra
白芍	bái sháo	60g	Radix Paeoniae Alba
知母	zhī mŭ	36g	Rhizoma Anemarrhenae
防风	fáng fēng	45g	Radix Saposhnikoviae
苍术	cāng zhú	30g	Rhizoma Atractylodis
白术	bái zhú	30g	Rhizoma Atractylodis Macrocephalae
威灵仙	wēi líng xiān	120g	Radix et Rhizoma Clematidis
麻黄	má huáng	36g	Herba Ephedrae
细辛	xì xīn	12g	Radix et Rhizoma Asari
松节	sōng jié	45g	Lignum Pini Nodi
伸筋草	shēn jīn căo	120g	Herba Lycopodii
炙山甲	zhì shān jiă	36g	Squama Manis (liquid-fried)
地龙	dì lóng	45g	Pheretima
皂角刺	zào jiăo cì	21g	Spina Gleditsiae
泽泻	zé xiè	30g	Rhizoma Alismatis

The medicinals were ground into a fine powder. A dose of 3g was taken each time, 2 times a day, with warm yellow rice wine.

【Fourth Visit】

January 27th, 1973: The swelling in the knees were relieved, and the joints were notably smaller. The same formula was prescribed, with the addition of *dāng guī wěi* (Radix Angelicae Sinensis [tail]) 36g, *jiāo shén qū* (scorch-fried Massa Medicata Fermentata) 30g, *piàn jiāng huáng* (Rhizoma Wenyujin Concisum) 30g, and *hóng huā* (Flos Carthami) 36g, and an increase in the dosage of *chuān duàn* (Radix Dipsaci) to 90g.

制附片	zhì fù piàn	45g	Radix Aconiti Lateralis Praeparata
骨碎补	gŭ suì bŭ	54g	Rhizoma Drynariae
川断	chuān duàn	90g	Radix Dipsaci
桂枝	guì zhī	36g	Ramulus Cinnamomi
赤芍	chì sháo	60g	Radix Paeoniae Rubra
知母	zhī mŭ	36g	Rhizoma Anemarrhenae
防风	fáng fēng	45g	Radix Saposhnikoviae
苍术	cāng zhú	30g	Rhizoma Atractylodis
白术	bái zhú	30g	Rhizoma Atractylodis Macrocephalae
威灵仙	wēi líng xiān	120g	Radix et Rhizoma Clematidis
麻黄	má huáng	36g	Herba Ephedrae
细辛	xì xīn	12g	Radix et Rhizoma Asari
松节	sōng jié	45g	Lignum Pini Nodi
伸筋草	shēn jīn căo	120g	Herba Lycopodii
炙山甲	zhì shān jiă	36g	Squama Manis (liquid-fried)
地龙	dì lóng	45g	Pheretima
皂角刺	zào jiăo cì	21g	Spina Gleditsiae
泽泻	zé xiè	30g	Rhizoma Alismatis
当归尾	dāng guī wěi	36g	Radix Angelicae Sinensis (tail)
焦神曲	jiāo shén qū	30g	Massa Medicata Fermentata (scorch-fried)
片姜黄	piàn jiāng huáng	30g	Rhizoma Wenyujin Concisum
红花	hóng huā	30g	Flos Carthami

The medicinals were ground into powder for oral administration. A dose of 3g was taken each time, 2 times a day, with warm yellow rice wine.

【Fifth Visit】

May 29th, 1973: Articular function improved significantly. The patient could squat down with ease and stand for more than 1 hour without feeling tired, and he could even ride several tens of *lǐ* (里 ; a Chinese mile, equivalent to 1/2 kilometer or about 1/3 mile) on his bicycle. His pulse was more moderate and forceful than before. His tongue coating was normal. There was only slight pain in the left wrist and ankle. The same formula was prescribed to consolidate the treatment effect.

Follow-up visit in the summer of 1975: The patient had returned to his full-time job for the past half year. The shape of the wrists, fingers and left knee did not completely return to normal, but this did not affect his normal daily activities, nor was their any more pain or functional impairment.

In the summer of 1979, the patient came for another follow-up visit: His ESR was 13 mm/h, and RF was still positive. The patient insisted on continuing with his full-time job and was physically capable of performing the taxing labor.

Comments

The patient's illness was caused by long-term exposure to cold and dampness. The main symptoms were joint pain, swelling, deformity, and stiffness; swelling of the feet that feels as if the feet are about to fall off; and a desire to vomit. Careful analysis of the symptoms led to the diagnosis of lame *bi*.

Dr. Jiao believes that lame *bi* is caused by exposure to wind cold damp evil in a cold and wet environment. Cold and dampness have a tendency to damage the kidney, and the resulting kidney deficiency leads to a decreased resistance to evils, which allows the invasion of cold and dampness to penetrate deeper into the body. Wind, cold, and dampness invasion of the liver, kidney, sinews, and bones gives rise to lame *bi*. In addition, the evils in the exterior and interior aspects of the body (i.e., cold-damp, phlegm-turbidity, static blood, and bandit wind) influence one other, congeal and gather together, obstruct the channels and collaterals, and disrupt the flow of qi and blood; this aggravates the progression of the disease, and is the key pathomechanism of this complex disease called lame *bi*. Treatment should be specific to the presenting pattern. The main treatment principles are tonifying the kidney and dispersing cold, assisted by transforming dampness, dispersing wind, nourishing the liver, softening the sinews, dispelling stasis, and unblocking the collaterals; hence Dr. Jiao created *Bŭ Shèn Qū Hán Zhì Wāng Tāng* (补肾祛寒治尪汤). Since the liver and kidney are of the same source, tonification of the kidney also nourishes the liver. Invigorating blood and unblocking the collaterals can dispel stasis and lead to the generation of new blood. When kidney qi flourishes, essence and blood are sufficient and thus marrow is replenished, the bones are strengthened, and the joints, sinews, and vessels are nourished, leading to the gradual restoration of normal joint function. During treatment, attention must be paid to the regulation and protection of the spleen and stomach to consolidate the foundation of acquired constitution.

[Jiao Shu-de. *Essentials of Jiao Shu-de's Clinical Experience* (焦树德临床经验辑要). Beijing: China Medical Science and Technology Publishing House.2001. 6]

2. Lou Duo-feng's Case Study: Blood Stasis and Evil Coagulation

Patient: Ma; 56 year-old housewife.

【Initial Visit】

April 6th, 1992: The patient had been suffering from generalized swelling and pain for the past 36 years, with deformity of the hand for the past 6 years. In June, 1956, she was exposed to wind for several days after childbirth. Ten days later, she had severe pain in the finger joints. A month later, the pain spread to multiple joints all over the body. She was diagnosed with "postnatal pain" at a local county hospital. The symptoms were temporarily relieved by glucocorticoids and gradually got worse. 10 years later, her fingers developed fusiform swelling. 20

years later, both hands developed the typical goose-neck deformity characteristic of RA. The patient had taken glucocorticoids on and off for 30 years and she had started taking diclofenac sodium in the recent 3 months. Present symptoms: multiple joint pain of the entire body with soreness and stiffness, particularly in the four limbs and mandibular joint. She had difficulty in opening the mouth, fear of cold, fatigue, and depression. She had a family history of RA (third sister and nephew also had RA). PE: thin body, pale facial complexion, muscular atrophy and spasms in the four limbs, and typical RA hands. The tongue was pale and dusky with thin white coating. The pulse was wiry, thready, and rough. Lab: Hb 10.5g/L, WBC $7.0*10^9$/L, N 0.76, L 0.23, ESR 60mm/h, ASO (-), RF (+), X-ray: damage in the finger joints with deformity and fusion of carpal bones.

【Pattern Differentiation】

Blood stasis and evil coagulation.

【Treatment Principle】

Nourish and invigorate blood, alleviate *bi*, and unblock the collaterals.

【Prescription】

当归	dāng guī	30g	Radix Angelicae Sinensis
丹参	dān shēn	30g	Radix et Rhizoma Salviae Miltiorrhizae
鸡血藤	jī xuè téng	30g	Caulis Spatholobi
桂枝	guì zhī	12g	Ramulus Cinnamomi
独活	dú huó	20g	Radix Angelicae Pubescentis
千年健	qiān nián jiàn	30g	Rhizoma Homalomenae
木瓜	mù guā	18g	Fructus Chaenomelis
炒山甲	chǎo shān jiǎ	12g	Squama Manis (dry-fried)
香附	xiāng fù	30g	Rhizoma Cyperi
川牛膝	chuān niú xī	30g	Radix Cyathulae
陈皮	chén pí	15g	Pericarpium Citri Reticulatae
甘草	gān cǎo	9g	Radix et Rhizoma Glycyrrhizae

9 batches were prescribed.

【Second Visit】

April 19th: After taking 9 batches of the above formula, the pain and swelling were lessened. She had frequent night urination and experienced puffy swelling (superficial edema) of the lower limbs which would appear in the evening. 6 batches of the same formula were prescribed, with the addition of *zhì fù zǐ* (Radix Aconiti Lateralis Praeparata) 6g and *fú líng* (Poria) 20g.

【Third Visit】

April 26th: Swelling and pain improved, lower limb edema and frequent night urination became less noticeable. *Tián qī* (radix notoginseng) 3g was added to the previous formula. 10 batches of the medicinals were ground into fine powder and made into pills with water. 9g of pills were taken each time, 3 times a day.

【Fourth Visit】

July 6th: The patient continued with the medicinal therapy. Although the deformity of the hands did not improve, the swelling and pain were eliminated. The patient was able to climb the stairs by herself again, and had better muscle tone in the four limbs. The formula was prescribed again to consolidate the treatment effects. 5 batches of the medicinals were ground into fine powder, and made into pills with water.

Follow-up visit on June 18th, 1993: The patient's condition was stabilized. Glucocorticoids and other anti-rheumatoid drugs had been withdrawn.

Comments

The patient was exposed to external evils shortly after childbirth. Since the patient was deficient in qi and blood, the external evils easily invaded the channels and collaterals and induced the disease. She took glucocorticoids on and off for over 30 years, which damaged her body and further consumed yin and blood (glucocorticoid, a hormone, is considered a yang evil, which has the tendency to damage yin and blood). This aggravated the illness and led to deformity of the hand joints. The prolonged course of disease damaged both yin and yang, and gave rise to signs and symptoms of yin and yang deficiency, such as fear of cold, fatigue, thin body, pale facial complexion, atrophied muscles and spasms of the four limbs, puffy swelling (superficial edema) of the lower limbs, and frequent night urination. Dr. Lou selected *dāng guī* (Radix Angelicae Sinensis), *guì zhī* (Ramulus Cinnamomi), and *dú huó* (Radix Angelicae Pubescentis) to nourish and invigorate blood, warm yang, alleviate *bi*, and unblock the collaterals. The addition of *shān yú ròu* (Fructus Corni) to tonify both yin and yang, and *bái sháo* (Radix Paeoniae Alba) to nourish blood and moderate spasms, can enhance the therapeutic effects.

[Qiu De-wen, Sha Feng-tong. *A Collection of the Expert Experience of Famous Old TCM Physicians of China* (中国名老中医药专家学术经验集). Guizhou Technology Publishing House.1995.5]

3. Ding Gan-ren's Case Studies

(1) Wind, Damp and Phlegm Entering the Collaterals and Blocking Nutritive and Defensive Qi

Patient: Chen You; adult female; farmer.

【Initial Visit】

The patient presented with diffuse swelling and pain on the back of the right hand radiating to the arm with loss of mobility, accompanied by fear of cold, generalized fever, a white and glossy tongue coating, and a soft, slippery, and rapid pulse.

【Pattern Differentiation】

Wind damp phlegm entering the collaterals and blocking nutritive and defensive qi.

【Treatment Principle】

Dispel wind, transform phlegm, dispel stasis, and unblock the collaterals.

【Prescription】

清水豆卷	qīng shuǐ dòu juǎn	12g	Semen Sojae Germinatum
青防风	qīng fáng fēng	3g	Radix Saposhnikoviae
秦艽	qín jiāo	6g	Radix Gentianae Macrophyllae
半夏	bàn xià	6g	Rhizoma Pinelliae
枳实炭	zhǐ shí	3g	Fructus Aurantii Immaturus (carbonized)
炒竹茹	zhú rú	6g	Caulis Bambusae in Taenia (dry-fried)
蚕沙	cán shā	9g	Faeces Bombycis
姜黄	jiāng huáng	2.4g	Rhizoma Curcumae Longae
海桐皮	hǎi tóng pí	9g	Cortex Erythrinae
生赤芍	chì sháo	6g	Radix Paeoniae Rubra (raw)
大贝母	bèi mǔ	9g	Bulbus Fritillaria
藏红花	zàng hóng huā	2.4g	Stigma Croci
桑枝	sāng zhī	12g	Ramulus Mori
指迷茯苓丸(包)	Zhǐ Mí Fú Líng Wán	24g	(wrapped)

【Second Visit】

The patient still had diffuse swelling and pain on the back of the right hand radiating to the arm with loss of mobility. The tongue coating was thin and glossy. The previous formula was modified.

清水豆卷	qǐng shuǐ dòu juǎn	24g	Semen Sojae Germinatum
防风	fáng fēng	3g	Radix Saposhnikoviae
秦艽	qín jiāo	6g	Radix Gentianae Macrophyllae
生赤芍	shēng chì sháo	6g	Radix Paeoniae Rubra (raw)
连翘	lián qiào	9g	Fructus Forsythiae
忍冬藤	rěn dōng téng	15g	Caulis Lonicerae Japonicae
蚕沙	cán shā	9g	Faeces Bombycis
姜黄	jiāng huáng	2.4g	Rhizoma Curcumae Longae
海桐皮	hǎi tóng pí	9g	Cortex Erythrinae
桂枝	guì zhī	1.2g	Ramulus Cinnamomi
熟石膏(打)	shú shí gāo	9g	Gypsum Fibrosum Praeparatum (crushed)
鲜竹茹	xiān zhú rú	6g	Caulis Bambusae in Taenia (fresh)

桑枝	sāng zhī	12g	Ramulus Mori
指迷茯苓丸(包)	Zhǐ Mí Fú Líng Wán	24g	(wrapped)

【Third Visit】

The condition showed slight improvement. The following formula was prescribed:

桂枝	guì zhī	1.2g	Ramulus Cinnamomi
熟石膏(打)	shú shí gāo	9g	Gypsum Fibrosum Praeparatum (crushed)
防风	fáng fēng	3g	Radix Saposhnikoviae
生赤芍	shēng chì sháo	6g	Radix Paeoniae Rubra (raw)
蚕沙	cán shā	9g	Faeces Bombycis
姜黄	jiāng huáng	2.4g	Rhizoma Curcumae Longae
茯苓	fú líng	1.5g	Poria
荆芥穗	jīng jiè suì	3g	Spica Schizonepetae
大贝母	bèi mŭ	9g	Bulbus Fritillaria
海桐皮	hăi tóng pí	9g	Cortex Erythrinae
丝瓜络	sī guā luò	12g	Retinervus Luffae Fructus

【Fourth Visit】

The condition showed some improvement. The following formula was prescribed:

桂枝	guì zhī	1.2g	Ramulus Cinnamomi
熟石膏(打)	shú shí gāo	15g	Gypsum Fibrosum Praeparatum (crushed)
防风	fáng fēng	3g	Radix Saposhnikoviae
生赤芍	shēng chì sháo	6g	Radix Paeoniae Rubra (raw)
秦艽	qín jiāo	3g	Radix Gentianae Macrophyllae
白薇	bái wēi	6g	Radix et Rhizoma Cynanchi Atrati
半夏	bàn xià	6g	Rhizoma Pinelliae
海桐皮	hăi tóng pí	9g	Cortex Erythrinae
桑枝	sāng zhī	12g	Ramulus Mori
蚕沙	cán shā	9g	Faeces Bombycis
姜黄	jiāng huáng	2.4g	Rhizoma Curcumae Longae
贝母	bèi mŭ	9g	Bulbus Fritillaria

茺蔚子	chōng wèi zǐ	9g	Fructus Leonuri
指迷茯苓丸(包)	Zhǐ Mí Fú Líng Wán	24g	(wrapped)

【Fifth Visit】

The pain was relieved by 70%-80%. There was still swelling and poor mobility of the joints. The following formula was prescribed:

全当归	quán dāng guī	6g	Radix Angelica Sinensis (whole)
丹参	dān shēn	6g	Radix et Rhizoma Salviae Miltiorrhizae
茺蔚子	chōng wèi zǐ	9g	Fructus Leonuri
赤芍	chì sháo	6g	Radix Paeoniae Rubra
蚕沙	cán shā	9g	Faeces Bombycis
生草节	shēng cǎo jié	1.8g	Glycyrrhizae Radix Resinosa Cruda
忍冬藤	rěn dōng téng	12g	Caulis Lonicerae Japonicae
海桐皮	hǎi tóng pí	9g	Cortex Erythrinae
大贝母	bèi mǔ	9g	Bulbus Fritillaria
炙僵蚕	zhì jiāng cán	9g	Bombyx Batryticatus (liquid-fried)
红花	hóng huā	2.4g	Flos Carthami
桑枝	sāng zhī	12g	Ramulus Mori
指迷茯苓丸(包)	Zhǐ Mí Fú Líng Wán	24g	(wrapped)

(2) Dampness Entering the Collaterals with Concurrent Blood Stasis

Patient: Yang You; adult female; peasant.

【Initial Visit】

The patient complained of numbness, swelling, and pain in the hands and feet with tenderness. She could not raise her hand nor move her feet. The symptoms had started 2 months prior to the visit. She also had scanty urine, dry stool, a red-margined tongue with yellow and glossy coating, and a wiry, rapid pulse.

【Pattern Differentiation】

Dampness entering the collaterals with concurrent blood stasis.

【Treatment Principle】

Clear heat, dispel wind, unblock the collaterals, and relieve pain.

【Prescription】

羚羊片	líng yáng piàn	3g	Cornu Saigae Tataricae (decocted first)
鲜石斛	xiān shí hú	9g	Caulis Dendrobii (fresh)
白薇	bái wēi	4. 5g	Radix et Rhizoma Cynanchi Atrati (fresh)
生赤芍	shēng chì sháo	6g	Radix Paeoniae Rubra (raw)
生甘草	shēng gān cǎo	1. 5g	Radix et Rhizoma Glycyrrhizae (raw)
茺蔚子	chōng wèi zǐ	6g	Fructus Leonuri
鲜竹茹	xiān zhú rú	6g	Caulis Bambusae in Taenia (fresh)
丝瓜络	sī guā luò	6g	Retinervus Luffae Fructus
忍冬藤	rěn dōng téng	12g	Caulis Lonicerae Japonicae
夜交藤	yè jiāo téng	12g	Caulis Polygoni Multiflori
桑枝	sāng zhī	12g	Ramulus Mori
大地龙(酒洗)	dì lóng	6g	Pheretima (washed in wine)

【Second Visit】

After taking 10 batches of the above formula, the numbness and pain in the hands and feet were relieved by 60%-70%. The swelling had also decreased. The patient still could not raise the limbs. Her tongue was red with no coating, and her pulse was less rapid. She had thirst with scanty urine and dry stool. The same formula was prescribed with the removal of *dì lóng* (Pheretima) and the addition of *tiān huā fěn* (Radix Trichosanthis).

After taking another 10 batches, the numbness and pain ceased. The patient only experienced fatigue in the four limbs. The previous prescription was modified by removing *líng yáng piàn* (Cornu Saigae Tataricae), *bái wēi* (Radix et Rhizoma Cynanchi Atrati), and *shí hú* (Caulis Dendrobii).

生赤芍	shēng chì sháo	6g	Radix Paeoniae Rubra (raw)
生甘草	shēng gān cǎo	1. 5g	Radix et Rhizoma Glycyrrhizae (raw)
茺蔚子	chōng wèi zǐ	6g	Fructus Leonuri
鲜竹茹	xiān zhú rú	6g	Caulis Bambusae in Taenia (fresh)
丝瓜络	sī guā luò	6g	Retinervus Luffae Fructus

忍冬藤	rěn dōng téng	12g	Caulis Lonicerae Japonicae
夜交藤	yè jiāo téng	12g	Caulis Polygoni Multiflori
桑枝	sāng zhī	12g	Ramulus Mori
大地龙(酒洗)	dì lóng	6g	Pheretima (washed in wine)
天花粉	tiān huā fěn	12g	Radix Trichosanthis
紫丹参	zī dān shēn	6g	Radix et Rhizoma Salviae Miltiorrhizae
全当归	quán dāng guī	9g	Radix Angelica Sinensis (whole)
西秦艽	xī qín jiāo	4.5g	Radix Gentianae Macrophyllae
怀牛膝	huái niú xī	6g	Radix Achyranthis Bidentatae

[Ding Gan-ren. *Further Case Studies of Ding Gan-ren* (丁甘仁医案续编). Shanghai Science and Technology Publishing House.1989]

4. Zhu Liang-chun's Case Study: Yang Qi Depletion with Cold-damp Invasion and Binding Obstruction of Phlegm and stasis

Patient: Zhao; 59 year-old female; peasant.

【Initial Visit】

December 20th 1982: The patient had RA for over 3 years. After taken glucocorticoids (20mg GC each time, 3 times a day), the swelling and pain was relieved to some extent. The swelling of the wrists and fingers were still present. She also had sensations of stiffness and heaviness in the knee, ankle, and hip joints. Because of the long-term use of glucocorticoids, she developed Cushing's syndrome. The patient came to our hospital for medicinal therapy.

Present symptoms: Articular symptoms as described above, accompanied by facial edema, distress, fatigue, a pale tongue with thin greasy coating, and a thready, wiry pulse. X-ray showed narrowing of the joint spaces of the fingers and deformity of the digital bones with osteoporosis in both hands. ESR: 76 mm/h, RF (-).

【Pattern Differentiation】

Yang qi depletion with cold-damp invasion and binding obstruction of phlegm and stasis.

【Treatment Principle】

Boost the kidney, strengthen the governing vessel, alleviate *bi*, unblock the collaterals, and warm and transform phlegm-stasis.

【Prescription】

Yì Shèn Juān Bì Wán (益肾蠲痹丸): 250g, 6g each time, two times a day, taken after meals.

【Second Visit】

January 10th, 1983: 3 weeks after taking the pills, the swelling and pain did not show any change, and the tongue and pulse manifestations were the same as before. This was due not to wrong treatment, but to inadequate dosage. The patient was advised to take larger doses of the pills.

【Third Visit】

February 10th, 1983: The wrist and finger pain was relieved, and the pain on the back of the palm gradually improved. The stiffness and pain of the ankle, knee, and wrist joints also improved. The patient could walk with the assistance of a cane and was in better spirits. Her tongue was wet with thin and white coating, and her pulse was thready. The pills proved to be effective, so they were prescribed again.

【Fourth Visit】

March 1st, 1983: The swelling and pain in the finger, wrist, ankle, and hip joints began to disappear. The dose of glucocorticoids was raised to 15mg each time, 3 times a day. The tongue was pale with thin and white coating. And the pulse was thready. The same pills were prescribed, and the patient was advised to gradually wean off the glucocorticoids.

【Fifth Visit】

March 20th, 1983: After 3 months of taking the pills, the swelling and pain had ceased. The glucocorticoids had been withdrawn completely. ESR was 12 mm/h. The patient was basically cured.

[Wang Ying-mo. Zhu Liang-chun's Experience in the Treatment of *Bi*

Syndromes (朱良春老中医治疗痹病的经验). *Zhejiang Journal of Chinese Medicine* (浙江中医杂志). 1983,18(12): 540-542.]

5. Zhao Shao-qin's Case Study: Dampness Transforming into Heat and Phlegm-Stasis Obstructing the Collaterals

Patient: Zhang; 29 year-old female.

【Initial Visit】

After two years of the onset of disease, the patient had pain in the finger joints that was aggravated by cold. In recent years, the joints were swollen and distended, particularly the joints of index finger, middle finger, and fourth finger. The finger joints exhibited fusiform shape with pain upon touch, darkening of the skin, and inhibited bending and stretching. RF (+). The patient was diagnosed with RA. The pulse was wiry, slippery, and rapid. The tongue was red with white greasy coating.

【Pattern Differentiation】

Dampness transforming into heat and phlegm-stasis obstructing the collaterals.

【Treatment Principle】

Clear heat, dispel dampness, remove phlegm, and disperse swelling.

【Prescription】

大豆卷	dà dòu juǎn	10g	Semen Sojae Germinatum
秦艽	qín jiāo	10g	Radix Gentianae Macrophyllae
威灵仙	wēi líng xiān	10g	Radix et Rhizoma Clematidis
苏子	sū zǐ	10g	Fructus Perillae
莱菔子	lái fú zǐ	10g	Semen Raphani
白芥子	bái jiè zǐ	6g	Semen Sinapis
冬瓜子	dōng guā zǐ	10g	Semen Benincasae
皂角子	zào jiǎo zǐ	5g	Semen Gleditsiae
桑枝	sāng zhī	10g	Ramulus Mori
丝瓜络	sī guā luò	10g	Retinervus Luffae Fructus

7 batches were prescribed.

【Second Visit】

After taking the medicinals, the pain was relieved, but the swelling remained. The prolonged course of disease led to the severe obstruction of the collaterals and vessels which requires at least 10 days of therapy to produce a noticeable improvement. The pulse was still deep and slippery which indicated phlegm constraint. The treatment strategies of removing phlegm and unblocking the collaterals were continued. 7 batches of the following medicinals were prescribed:

苏子	sū zǐ	10g	Fructus Perillae
莱菔子	lái fú zǐ	10g	Semen Raphani
白芥子	bái jiè zǐ	6g	Semen Sinapis
冬瓜子	dōng guā zǐ	10g	Semen Benincasae
皂角	zào jiǎo	6g	Spina Gleditsiae
丝瓜络	sī guā luò	10g	Retinervus Luffae Fructus
桑枝	sāng zhī	10g	Ramulus Mori
海风藤	hǎi fēng téng	10g	Caulis Piperis Kadsurae
络石藤	luò shí téng	10g	Caulis Trachelospermi
天仙藤	tiān xiān téng	10g	Herba Aristolochiae
片姜黄	piàn jiāng huáng	6g	Rhizoma Wenyujin Concisum

【Third Visit】

The joint swelling began to dissipate. The pain was relieved tremendously. The tongue was white with a moist coating. 7 batches of the following medicinals were prescribed:

苏子	sū zǐ	10g	Fructus Perillae
莱菔子	lái fú zǐ	10g	Semen Raphani
白芥子	bái jiè zǐ	6g	Semen Sinapis
冬瓜子	dōng guā zǐ	10g	Semen Benincasae
皂角	zào jiǎo	6g	Spina Gleditsiae
生薏苡仁	shēng yì yǐ rén	30g	Semen Coicis (raw)
丝瓜络	sī guā luò	10g	Retinervus Luffae Fructus

桑枝	sāng zhī	10g	Ramulus Mori
海风藤	hǎi fēng téng	10g	Caulis Piperis Kadsurae
络石藤	luò shí téng	10g	Caulis Trachelospermi
天仙藤	tiān xiān téng	10g	Herba Aristolochiae
焦三仙	jiāo sān xiān	10g each	Fructus Crataegi, Fructus Hordei Germinatus, and Massa Medicata Fermentata (scorch-fried)
水红花子	shuǐ hóng huā zǐ	10g	Fructus Polygoni Orientalis

【Fourth Visit】

The pain of the joints was relieved by 50%. The pulse was soft and slippery, and the tongue was white with a moist coating. 7 batches of the following medicinals were prescribed:

苏子	sū zǐ	10g	Fructus Perillae
莱菔子	lái fú zǐ	10g	Semen Raphani
白芥子	bái jiè zǐ	6g	Semen Sinapis
冬瓜子	dōng guā zǐ	10g	Semen Benincasae
皂角	zào jiǎo	6g	Spina Gleditsiae
生薏苡仁	shēng yì yǐ rén	30g	Semen Coicis (raw)
丝瓜络	sī guā luò	10g	Retinervus Luffae Fructus
桑枝	sāng zhī	10g	Ramulus Mori
海风藤	hǎi fēng téng	10g	Caulis Piperis Kadsurae
络石藤	luò shí téng	10g	Caulis Trachelospermi
焦三仙	jiāo sān xiān	10g each	Fructus Crataegi, Fructus Hordei Germinatus, and Massa Medicata Fermentata (scorch-fried)

[Peng Jian-zhong. *Discussions on the Essentials of Ancient and Modern Chinese Medical Case Studies* (中医古今医案精粹选评). Beijing: Xueyuan Publishing House.1998]

6. Gao Hui-yuan's Case Study: Disharmony of the Nutritive and Defense and of Qi and Blood, with Obstruction of the Collaterals by Wind-cold-damp

Patient: Shen; 40 year-old female.

【Initial Visit】

December 6th, 1997: The patient complained of recurrent pain in the joints of the limbs for 4 years with pronounced morning stiffness and fear of wind and cold. The swelling and pain of the wrists and ankles were worse in the last 3 months, and was accompanied by a poor appetite. The ESR was 40 mm/h, RF (+) 1:80. The patient had taken drugs (e.g., indomethacin) without any improvement. The tongue was pale with white greasy coating, and the pulse was deep and thready.

【Pattern Differentiation】

Disharmony of the nutritive and defense and of qi and blood, with obstruction of the collaterals by wind-cold-damp.

【Treatment Principle】

Boost qi, fortify the spleen, eliminate dampness, warm the channels, invigorate blood, and unblock the collaterals.

【Prescription】

黄芪	huáng qí	15g	Radix Astragali
赤芍	chì sháo	10g	Radix Paeoniae Rubra
白术	bái zhú	10g	Rhizoma Atractylodis Macrocephalae
防己	fáng jǐ	10g	Radix Stephaniae Tetrandrae
太子参	tài zǐ shēn	10g	Radix Pseudostellariae
木瓜	mù guā	10g	Fructus Chaenomelis
生薏苡仁	shēng yì yǐ rén	15g	Semen Coicis (raw)
桑枝	sāng zhī	15g	Ramulus Mori
桂枝	guì zhī	8g	Ramulus Cinnamomi
炙甘草	zhì gān cǎo	5g	Radix et Rhizoma Glycyrrhizae Praeparata cum Melle

After taking 24 batches of the prescribed formula, the joint pain improved significantly, and the swelling gradually dissipated. The ESR was 29 mm/h, RF (+) 1:40. After the patient took 36 more batches of the formula, the swelling and pain disappeared, and the ESR was 20 mm/h, RF (+) 1:16. The patient's condition was stabilized.

[Peng Jian-zhong. *Discussions on the Essentials of Ancient and Modern Chinese Medical Case Studies* (中医古今医案精粹选评). Beijing: Xueyuan Publishing House.1998]

7. Zhang Bo-yu's Case Study: Long-term Obstruction of the Vessels and Collaterals by Wind-cold-damp Complicated by Stasis Binding

Patient: Shang; 56 year-old male.

【Initial Visit】

April 22nd, 1976: The patient suffered from RA for over 3 years. His fingers and toes were swollen, painful, and deformed. Accompanying signs and symptoms: fear of cold, fatigue, a deep and thready pulse, and a thin white tongue coating.

【Pattern Differentiation】

Long-term obstruction of the vessels and collaterals by wind cold damp complicated by stasis bind.

【Treatment Principle】

Dispel wind, eliminate dampness, transform stasis, and unblock the collaterals.

【Prescription】

制川乌(先煎)	zhì chuān wū	9g	Radix Aconiti Praeparata (decocted first)
制草乌(先煎)	zhì cǎo wū	9g	Radix Aconiti Kusnezoffii Praeparata (decocted first)
生黄芪	shēng huáng qí	15g	Radix Astragali (raw)
麻黄	má huáng	6g	Herba Ephedrae
全当归	quán dāng guī	9g	Radix Angelica Sinensis (whole)
细辛	xì xīn	3g	Radix et Rhizoma Asari
生甘草	shēng gān cǎo	9g	Radix et Rhizoma Glycyrrhizae (raw)
炒赤芍	chì sháo	9g	Radix Paeoniae Rubra
炒白芍	bái sháo	9g	Radix Paeoniae Alba
桃仁	táo rén	9g	Semen Persicae
红花	hóng huā	6g	Flos Carthami

蕲蛇	qí shé	6g	Agkistrodon
全蝎粉	quán xiē fěn	1.2g	Scorpio (powdered)
纯蜜(冲)	chún mì	15g	pure honey (to be dissolved in decoction)

More than 30 batches of this formula were prescribed, with slight modifications according to the presenting signs and symptoms.

【Second Visit】

May 28th, 1976: The swelling and pain in the toes and fingers were relieved, but the fear of cold remained. The pulse was deep and thready, and the tongue coating was thin and white. The following medicinals were prescribed:

制川乌(先煎)	zhì chuān wū	9g	Radix Aconiti Praeparata (decocted first)
制草乌(先煎)	zhì cǎo wū	9g	Radix Aconiti Kusnezoffii Praeparata (decocted first)
生黄芪	shēng huáng qí	18g	Radix Astragali (raw)
麻黄	má huáng	6g	Herba Ephedrae
桂枝	guì zhī	9g	Ramulus Cinnamomi
细辛	xì xīn	3g	Radix et Rhizoma Asari
炒赤芍	chǎo chì sháo	9g	Radix Paeoniae Rubra
炒白芍	bái sháo	9g	Radix Paeoniae Alba
熟附片(先煎)	shú fù piàn	9g	Radix Aconiti Lateralis Praeparata (decocted first)
生甘草	shēng gān cǎo	9g	Radix et Rhizoma Glycyrrhizae (raw)
全当归	quán dāng guī	15g	Radix Angelica Sinensis (whole)
露蜂房	lù fēng fáng	9g	Nidus Vespae
蕲蛇	qí shé	9g	Agkistrodon
全蝎粉	quán xiē fěn	1.2g	Scorpio (powdered)
纯蜜(冲)	chún mì	15g	pure honey (to be dissolved in decoction)

【Third Visit】

June 22nd, 1976: The swelling and pain in the toes ceased. The pain and deformity of the fingers were also relieved. The pulse was thready, and the tongue coating was white. Medicinals that tonify qi and nourish blood were added. 14 batches were prescribed.

制川乌(先煎)	zhì chuān wū	9g	Radix Aconiti Praeparata (decocted first)
制草乌(先煎)	zhì cǎo wū	9g	Radix Aconiti Kusnezoffii Praeparata (decocted first)
熟附片(先煎)	shú fù piàn	9g	Radix Aconiti Lateralis Praeparata (decocted first)
全当归	quán dāng guī	15g	Radix Angelica Sinensis (whole)
桂枝	guì zhī	9g	Ramulus Cinnamomi
细辛	xì xīn	3g	Radix et Rhizoma Asari
熟地	shú dì	15g	Radix Rehmanniae Praeparata
炙黄芪	zhì huáng qí	15g	Radix Astragali (honey-fried)
炒赤芍	chǎo chì sháo	9g	Radix Paeoniae Rubra (dry-fried)
炒白芍	chǎo bái sháo	9g	Radix Paeoniae Alba (dry-fried)
炒川芎	chǎo chuān xiōng	6g	Rhizoma Chuanxiong (dry-fried)
鹿角片	lù jiǎo piàn	9g	Cornu Cervi
全蝎粉(分吞)	quán xiē fěn (swallowed separately)	1.2g	Scorpio (powdered)
蕲蛇	qí shé	9g	Agkistrodon
纯蜜(冲)	chún mì (to be dissolved in decoction)	15g	pure honey

[Zhang Bo-yu. *Zhang Bo-yu's Case Studies* (张伯臾医案). Shanghai Science and Technology Publishing House.1979]

8. Hu Zhen-ya's Case Study: Cold Evil Obstructing the Collaterals and Liver and Kidney Depletion

Patient: Guang; 22 year-old male.

【Initial Visit】

January 9th, 1978: The patient complained of recurrent swelling and pain in the knee and ankle joints for more than 2 years. The symptoms gradually worsened over time. He had loss of mobility in the joints, muscle atrophy and weakness of the lower limbs, and occasionally, inability to walk. In the winter of 1976, his hands and feet were swollen and painful from frostbite. He was diagnosed with frostbite and was given no treatment. In the winter of 1977, his right foot began to swell and hurt, and he was unable to walk. He was diagnosed with RA at a hospital. After being treated with anti-rheumatoid drugs and glucocorticoids, the symptoms were relieved and he was able to walk with a cane. However, he still suffered from recurrent joint swelling and pain. On January 2nd, 1978, the patient exhibited redness, swelling, and severe pain in the right knee and ankle after catching a cold and developing a fever. He visited the hospital and was diagnosed with RA (confirmed by X-ray and blood test). After receiving ineffective drug therapy, he finally decided to try Chinese medicine.

Present symptoms: A thin and weak body, deficiency puffiness of the face and eyes, muscle atrophy of the lower limbs with sensations of heaviness and fatigue (more severe in the left limbs), swelling of the knees and ankles, marked deformity of the index fingers and the big toes, severe pain, inability to walk without assistance, aching pain of the lumbar spine with inability to turn sides, fear of cold and preference for warmth, night fever, vexation, poor appetite, sloppy stool (with 2-3 bowel movements a day), scanty and turbid urine, a pale tongue with white glossy coating, and a deep, wiry, and thready pulse.

【Pattern Differentiation】

Cold evil obstructing the collaterals and liver and kidney depletion.

【Treatment Principle】

Warm the kidney, disperse cold, scatter wind, transform dampness, regulate qi and blood, and unblock the channels and collaterals.

【Prescription】

干地黄	gān dì huáng	40g	Radix Rehmanniae
全当归	quán dāng guī	30g	Radix Angelica Sinensis (whole)
透骨草	tòu gǔ cǎo	25g	Caulis Impatientis
防己	fáng jǐ	15g	Radix Stephaniae Tetrandrae
白芍	bái sháo	12g	Radix Paeoniae Alba

赤芍	chì sháo	12g	Radix Paeoniae Rubra
酒地龙	jiǔ dì lóng	12g	Pheretima (prepared with wine)
威灵仙	wēi líng xiān	15g	Radix et Rhizoma Clematidis
炙山甲	zhì shān jiǎ	9g	Squama Manis (liquid-fried)
木瓜	mù guā	12g	Fructus Chaenomelis
炙鳖甲	zhì biē jiǎ	12g	Carapax Trionycis (liquid-fried)
炒白芥子	bái jiè zǐ	10g	Semen Sinapis (dry-fried)
桂枝	guì zhī	10g	Ramulus Cinnamomi
生麻黄	shēng má huáng	10g	Herba Ephedrae (raw)
连皮茯苓	lián pí fú líng	30g	Poria (with skin)
全蝎	quán xiē	6g	Scorpio
制附子	zhì fù zǐ	12g	Radix Aconiti Lateralis Praeparata (pre-decocted for 20-40 minutes)

【Second Visit】

January 16th, 1978: After taking 6 batches of the medicinal formula, the swelling and pain of the joints showed slight improvement. His fear of cold and generalized fever were gone. The lower limbs were still unable to flex or extend, and the lumbus was still painful. He had sloppy diarrhea, 1-2 times a day. His urine was less turbid (the dampness was expelled through the urine). His tongue was pale with a white greasy coating, and his pulse was deep, tight, and weak. Medicinals that tonify the kidney, assist yang, replenish essence, tonify marrow, and secure the root were added.

干地黄	gān dì huáng	50g	Radix Rehmanniae
补骨脂	bǔ gǔ zhī	30g	Fructus Psoraleae
当归	dāng guī	30g	Radix Angelica Sinensis
透骨草	tòu gǔ cǎo	30g	Caulis Impatientis
防己	fáng jǐ	15g	Radix Stephaniae Tetrandrae
白芍	bái sháo	10g	Radix Paeoniae Alba
威灵仙	wēi líng xiān	15g	Radix et Rhizoma Clematidis
炙山甲	zhì shān jiǎ	12g	Squama Manis (liquid-fried)
木瓜	mù guā	12g	Fructus Chaenomelis

独活	dú huó	10g	Radix Angelicae Pubescentis
桂枝	guì zhī	10g	Ramulus Cinnamomi
生麻黄	shēng má huáng	10g	Herba Ephedrae (raw)
连皮茯苓	lián pí fú líng	20g	Poria (with skin)
全蝎	quán xiē	6g	Scorpio
炒白芥子	bái jiè zĭ	12g	Semen Sinapis (dry-fried)
制附子	zhì fù zĭ	15g	Radix Aconiti Lateralis Praeparata (pre-decocted for 20-40 minutes)

【Third Visit】

January 27th, 1978: The above formula was prescribed 12 more times, with modifications where necessary. The swelling in the joints improved. There was still soreness and weakness of the lumbus and knees with difficulty in walking, which is attributed to kidney deficiency. The stool was still loose but less frequent. The frequency of urination was increased, with occasional turbidity. The tongue and pulse manifestations were the same as those of the previous visit. 10 more batches of the previous formula were prescribed.

【Fourth Visit】

February 12th, 1978: The patient's limbs felt more relaxed and slightly stronger. His appetite improved and he was sleeping better. The swelling and pain of the knees decreased, and he was able to walk with the assistance of a cane. He still had loose stool. The tongue was pale with white and glossy coating, the pulse was deep, wiry, and thready. The following medicinals were prescribed:

干地黄	gān dì huáng	60g	Radix Rehmanniae
补骨脂	bŭ gŭ zhī	40g	Fructus Psoraleae
当归	dāng guī	30g	Radix Angelica Sinensis
透骨草	tòu gŭ căo	30g	Caulis Impatientis
炙山甲	zhì shān jiă	15g	Squama Manis (liquid-fried)
防己	fáng jĭ	12g	Radix Stephaniae Tetrandrae
威灵仙	wēi líng xiān	12g	Radix et Rhizoma Clematidis

独活	dú huó	10g	Radix Angelicae Pubescentis
桂枝	guì zhī	10g	Ramulus Cinnamomi
生麻黄	shēng má huáng	12g	Herba Ephedrae (raw)
鲜桑枝	sāng zhī	60g	Ramulus Mori (fresh)
全蝎	quán xiē	8g	Scorpio
连皮茯苓	fú líng	20g	Poria (with skin)
炒白芥子	bái jiè zǐ	12g	Semen Sinapis (dry-fried)
制附子	zhì fù zǐ	25g	Radix Aconiti Lateralis Praeparata

【Fifth Visit】

March 5th, 1978: After taking 20 batches of the medicinal formula, all the symptoms improved. The patient could walk slowly without a cane. His knees and ankles were still swollen but less painful and no longer red, and he was able to flex and extend the limbs. The toe joints were still deformed but less stiff. The stool and the urine were normal. The tongue was pale with white glossy coating, and the pulse was deep and wiry. The following formula was prescribed in the form of pills (the patient requested to take pills since he was unable to decoct the medicinals):

干地黄	gān dì huáng	300g	Radix Rehmanniae
补骨脂	bǔ gǔ zhī	200g	Fructus Psoraleae
炒白芥子	chǎo bái jiè zǐ	90g	Semen Sinapis (dry-fried)
鸡血藤	jī xuè téng	90g	Caulis Spatholobi
穿山甲	chuān shān jiǎ	60g	Squama Manis
蕲蛇	qí shé	60g	Agkistrodon
蜈蚣	wú gōng	30g	Scolopendra
龟板胶	guī bǎn jiāo	60g	Colla Carapax et Plastrum Testudinis
茜草	qiàn cǎo	75g	Radix et Rhizoma Rubiae
川乌	chuān wū	60g	Radix Aconiti
制草乌	zhì cǎo wū	30g	Radix Aconiti Kusnezoffii Praeparata
生麻黄	shēng má huáng	30g	Herba Ephedrae (raw)
皂刺	zào cì	60g	Spina Gleditsiae
肉桂	ròu guì	40g	Cortex Cinnamomi
全蝎	quán xiē	15g	Scorpio

蜂房	fēng fáng	90g	Nidus Vespae
鹿角胶	lù jiăo jiāo	90g	Colla Cornus Cervi
甘草	gān căo	150g	Radix et Rhizoma Glycyrrhizae
蛤蚧	gé jiè	4g	Gecko

Preparation method: All the medicinals were dry-fried together except for *guī jiă jiāo* (Colla Carapax et Plastrum Testudinis) and *lù jiăo jiāo* (Colla Cornus Cervi). *Guī jiă jiāo* (Colla Carapax et Plastrum Testudinis) and *lù jiăo jiāo* (Colla Cornus Cervi) were fried together with *gé jiè* (Gecko) powder to form beads. All the medicinals were ground into a fine powder and made into pills (of 6g each) by mixing with honey. 2 pills were taken with yellow rice wine each time, 3 times a day. The patient was advised to avoid cold and sweet foods and to avoid exposure to wind and cold. He was instructed to exercise often and massage the affected areas of the body, thereby facilitating recovery.

After taking the pills for 4 months, the patient was cured. A follow-up visit a year later revealed that the illness did not recur, and the patient was able to perform light labor and exercise.

(Editorial Board of *Anthology of the Experiences of Beijing Chinese Medicine Doctors*: *Anthology of the Experiences of Beijing Chinese Medicine Doctors – Second Volume*. 1986)

9. Guo Qian-heng's Case Study: Blood Deficiency and Wind Invasion Obstructing the Channels and Collaterals

Patient: Li; 41 year-old female.

【Initial Visit】

August 21st, 1985: The patient complained of pain and deformity for 12 years and was diagnosed with RA. Long-term use of medicinals and modern drugs produced no effect. She once visited our hospital for the redness, swelling, and pain of the joints in 1977. The condition was diagnosed as damp-heat, and she was given *Sān Miào Săn* (三妙散)

along with other medicinals to dispel wind-damp, clear heat, invigorate blood, and unblock the collaterals. After taking 10 batches, the swelling and pain had been relieved. Then, she discontinued with the therapy, and 2 months later, the condition got worse and she began to take ibuprofen and piroxicam. The condition alternated between improvement and exacerbation. She complained of poor appetite with occasional stomachaches.

Physical examination: deformity with stiffness and pain in the fingers, toes, wrists, ankles, hips and elbows. The patient had difficulty in raising the limbs and walking. She had to move with the support of a cane or wall. There was wandering pain in the upper and lower limbs, with no apparent connection to climate changes. The patient had a poor appetite and weak body. Her stool and urine were normal. The tongue was dusky and red with slightly greasy coating, and the pulse was deep and wiry.

【Pattern Differentiation】

Blood deficiency and wind invasion obstructing the channels and collaterals.

【Treatment Principle】

Nourish blood, track down evils, disperse stasis, unblock the collaterals, and eliminate *bi*.

【Prescription】

Líng Shé Tòu Gŭ Dān (灵蛇透骨丹), an empirical formula:

生地	shēng dì	24g	Radix Rehmanniae Recens
当归	dāng guī	12g	Radix Angelica Sinensis
防风	fáng fēng	9g	Radix Saposhnikoviae
威灵仙	wēi líng xiān	9g	Radix et Rhizoma Clematidis
透骨草	tòu gŭ căo	9g	Caulis Impatientis
白花蛇	bái huā shé	1	Agkistrodon
鸡血藤	jī xuè téng	12g	Caulis Spatholobi
丹参	dān shēn	15g	Radix et Rhizoma Salviae Miltiorrhizae

姜黄	jiāng huáng	6g	Rhizoma Curcumae Longae
川牛膝	chuān niú xī	6g	Radix Cyathulae

The medicinals were decocted in 500ml of water until reduced to 150ml of liquid. After filtering out the decoction and putting it aside, 400ml of water was added to the dregs and decoct again to obtain 120ml of liquid. The decoction was filtered and mixed with the previous decoction. Each batch was divided into portions and taken warm every 6 hours. The patient was taken off the modern drugs.

【Second Visit】

September 30th, 1985: After taking 30 batches of the medicinal formula, the pain was relieved and the functions of the limbs were restored. The patient could squat by herself. The large joints were no longer stiff and the small joints were less swollen with pain only upon movement. The following medicinals were prescribed in the form of pills:

【Prescription】

生地	shēng dì	300g	Radix Rehmanniae Recens
当归	dāng guī	90g	Radix Angelica Sinensis
威灵仙	wēi líng xiān	180g	Radix et Rhizoma Clematidis
白花蛇	bái huā shé	14	Agkistrodon
透骨草	tòu gŭ căo	90g	Caulis Impatientis
秦艽	qín jiāo	90g	Radix Gentianae Macrophyllae
防风	fáng fēng	90g	Radix Saposhnikoviae
地鳖虫	tŭ biē chóng	90g	Eupolyphaga seu Steleophaga
血竭	xuè jié	90g	Sanguis Draconis
丹参	dān shēn	120g	Radix et Rhizoma Salviae Miltiorrhizae
姜黄	jiāng huáng	45g	Rhizoma Curcumae Longae
鸡血藤	jī xuè téng	120g	Caulis Spatholobi
千年健	qiān nián jiàn	90g	Rhizoma Homalomenae
牛膝	niú xī	45g	Radix Achyranthis Bidentatae
甘草	gān căo	45g	Radix et Rhizoma Glycyrrhizae
夜交藤	yè jiāo téng	90g	Caulis Polygoni Multiflori

The medicinals were ground into a fine powder and made into pills. A dose of 4g was taken each time, 2 times a day, with warm water.

【Third Visit】

April 1st, 1987: After taking the pills in 1985, the patient was able to walk at a normal pace. The swelling of the joints were relieved. The lower limbs were no longer hyperextended. The patient could stand by herself without a cane. She had a dry mouth, gingival atrophy, toothache, numbness of the tongue and lip (relieved by the withdrawl of the medicine), occasional dizziness, poor sleep, and dry stool. Her tongue was red with no coating, and her pulse was weak, thready, and rapid. (The wind-dispelling medicinals damaged the yin fluids, hence medicinals that nourish stomach and kidney yin were added.)

生地	shēng dì	15g	Radix Rehmanniae Recens
元参	yuán shēn	9g	Radix Scrophulariae
麦冬	mài dōng	9g	Radix Ophiopogonis
秦艽	qín jiāo	9g	Radix Gentianae Macrophyllae
玉竹	yù zhú	12g	Rhizoma Polygonati Odorati
沙参	shā shēn	12g	Radix Glehniae/Adenophorae
花粉	huā fěn	9g	Radix Trichosanthis
石斛	shí hú	12g	Caulis Dendrobii

【Fourth Visit】

August 29th,1987: After taking the formula in April, the dry mouth was relieved. The patient still had slight dizziness and palpitation with insomnia and numbness on the lips and tongue. The tongue was dusky and red, and the pulse was weak and thready. The following prescription was made into pills and taken to nourish yin and calm the heart:

熟地	shú dì	90g	Radix Rehmanniae Praeparata
山药	shān yào	90g	Rhizoma Dioscoreae
山萸肉	shān yú ròu	30g	Fructus Corni
丹皮	dān pí	30g	Cortex Moutan

茯苓	fú líng	50g	Poria
泽泻	zé xiè	30g	Rhizoma Alismatis
白术	bái zhú	40g	Rhizoma Atractylodis Macrocephalae
枸杞	gǒu qǐ	40g	Fructus Lycii
玉竹	yù zhú	40g	Rhizoma Polygonati Odorati
木瓜	mù guā	30g	Fructus Chaenomelis
麦冬	mài dōng	40g	Radix Ophiopogonis
菊花	jú huā	30g	Flos Chrysanthemi
莲子	lián zǐ	50g	Semen Nelumbinis
枣仁	zǎo rén	40g	Semen Ziziphi Spinosae
甘草	gān cǎo	30g	Radix et Rhizoma Glycyrrhizae

The ingredients were ground into a fine powder and made into pills of 12g each. 1 pill was taken every night with warm water.

【Fifth Visit】

September 18th, 1987: After taking the pills for 10 days, the numbness on the lips and tongue, dizziness, and palpitation had all vanished. The patient was advised to continue taking the formula to consolidate the treatment effects as well as nourish the heart and kidney to strengthen the root.

[Qiu De-wen, Sha Feng-tong. *A Compilation of the Academic Experience of China's Famous Doctors of Chinese Medicine* (中国名老中医药专家学术经验集). Guizhou Technology Publishing House.1995]

Discussions

1. Jiao Shu-de Discusses the Etiology and Pathomechanism of Lame *Bi* and Creates an Empirical Formula for its Treatment

The concept of "*lame bi* (尪痹; *wāng bì*)" was first introduced by Jiao Shu-de of the China-Japan Friendship Hospital in Beijing. Dr. Jiao holds that lame *bi* falls under the scope of *bi* syndromes, and thus the general rule that "the three evils--wind, cold, and dampness--combine to form *bi*" also applies to its chief pathomechanism. In addition, lame *bi* also possesses the following characteristics:

(1) Constitutional Kidney Deficiency

If the kidney is deficient, marrow cannot be filled and true qi is debilitated. Prevalence of cold-damp will take advantage of this deficiency and invade the kidney, causing obstruction to the waterways. The evil penetrates deeply into the bones to block up the channels and collaterals. As a result, the flow of qi and blood is disrupted, the joints become inflexible, and the sinews and bones lose their nourishment. Gradually, there will also be spasms of the sinews, joint deformity, and inhibited bending and stretching.

(2) In the Winter, There is Prevalence of Cold

When combined with wind, cold, and dampness invading the kidney, there will be heaviness of the bones with soreness and inability to lift objects. Over a long period of time, deformity of the limbs, which is one of the more difficult-to-treat symptoms of lame *bi*, may arise.

(3) Repeated Contractions of Wind, Cold, and Dampness Affecting the Liver and Kidney

The liver governs the sinews and the kidney governs the bones. A prolonged course of *bi* syndrome with repeated contractions of wind, cold, and dampness will severely and adversely affect the liver and kidney. Disease of the sinews and the bones will arise, eventually giving way to spasms of the sinews, loss of bone density, and joint deformity.

Dr. Jiao holds that the pathomechanism of lame *bi* is more complex and severe than common wind-cold-damp *bi*. The three evils, wind, cold and dampness enter the bone marrow and damage the liver and kidney, causing bone destruction and sinew spasms. Over time, cold-damp, wind evil, phlegm-turbidity, and stasis combine to obstruct the flow of qi and blood and congest the channels and collaterals, further aggravating the condition. Dr. Jiao created three commonly used formulas: *Bǔ Shèn Qū Hán Zhì Wāng Tāng* (补肾祛寒治尪汤) for kidney deficiency with cold exuberance; *Jiā Jiǎn Bǔ Shèn Zhì Wāng Tāng* (加减补肾治尪汤) for the milder pattern of kidney deficiency with branch heat excess; and *Bǔ Shèn Qīng Rè Zhì Wāng Tāng* (补肾清热治尪汤) for the more severe pattern of kidney deficiency with branch heat predominance. Observation of the clinical effects and laboratory tests prove that these formulas effectively strengthen the immune system and restore normal joint function.

[Jiao Shu-de. *Essentials of Jiao Shu-de's Clinical Experience* (焦树德临床经验辑要). Beijing: China Medical Science and Technology Publishing House. 2001. 6]

2. Lou Duo-feng Uses Effective Medicinals and Formulas in Accordance with Differential Diagnosis and Disease Location

The *bi* patterns seen in the clinic are often closely related to right qi deficiency, external evils, and static blood. These three factors influence one other and are inseparable. The invading evils are the external pathogens, while deficiency and stasis are the internal pathogens. Only when mixed with the internal pathogens can the external pathogens induce illness. As for the pathomechanism, long-term retention of evils and stasis can lead to deficiency, and severe deficiency makes it more difficult to rid of the evils and stasis.

Pattern differentiation of *bi* syndromes are based on the quality of the pain, the disease location, the disease history, and any concurrent diseases that the patient might have in addition to this condition. During treatment, emphasis is placed on coursing and unblocking the channels and collaterals and smoothing the flow of qi and blood, hence common primary treatment principles include dispelling evils, invigorating blood, and unblocking the collaterals. For those with excess, attacking the evils is the main strategy; for those with deficiency, the simultaneous application of attack and tonification should be adopted.

(1) Wind-cold-damp Pattern

Dispel wind, unblock the collaterals, dissipate cold, eliminate dampness, and invigorate and tonify the blood using *Tōng Bì Tāng* (通痹汤).

当归	dāng guī	18g	Radix Angelica Sinensis
丹参	dān shēn	18g	Radix et Rhizoma Salviae Miltiorrhizae
鸡血藤	jī xuè téng	21g	Caulis Spatholobi
海风藤	hǎi fēng téng	18g	Caulis Piperis Kadsurae
透骨草	tòu gǔ cǎo	21g	Caulis Impatientis
独活	dú huó	18g	Radix Angelicae Pubescentis
钻地风	zuān dì fēng	18g	Schizophragma integrifolium Oliv
香附	xiāng fù	21g	Rhizoma Cyperi

【Modifications】

➢ For exuberant wind, add *fáng fēng* (Radix Saposhnikoviae), *qiāng huó* (Rhizoma et Radix Notopterygii), and *wēi líng xiān* (Radix et Rhizoma Clematidis).

➢ For exuberant cold, add *zhì chuān wū* (Radix Aconiti Praeparata), *zhì cǎo wū* (Radix Aconiti Kusnezoffii Praeparata), *guì zhī* (Ramulus Cinnamomi), and *xì xīn* (Radix et Rhizoma Asari).

➢ For exuberant dampness, add *yì yǐ rén* (Semen Coicis) and *bì xiè* (Rhizoma Dioscoreae Hypoglaucae).

➢ For qi deficiency, add *huáng qí* (Radix Astragali) and *bái zhú* (Rhizoma Atractylodis Macrocephalae).

➢ For yang deficiency, add *yín yáng huò* (Herba Epimedii) and *xiān máo* (Rhizoma Curculiginis)

(2) Wind-damp-heat Pattern

Dispel wind, eliminate dampness, invigorate blood, and unblock the collaterals with *Qīng Bì Tāng* (清痹汤).

忍冬藤	rěn dōng téng	60g	Caulis Lonicerae Japonicae
败酱草	bài jiàng cǎo	30g	Herba Patriniae
络石藤	luò shí téng	18g	Caulis Trachelospermi
青风藤	qīng fēng téng	60g	Caulis Sinomenii
土茯苓	tǔ fú líng	21g	Rhizoma Smilacis Glabrae
老鹳草	lǎo guàn cǎo	30g	Herba Erodii or Herba Geranii
丹参	dān shēn	30g	Radix et Rhizoma Salviae Miltiorrhizae
香附	xiāng fù	15g	Rhizoma Cyperi

【Modifications】

➢ For exterior wind heat, add *lián qiào* (Fructus Forsythiae) and *gé gēn* (Radix Puerariae Lobatae).

➢ For excessive heat in the qi level, add *shí gāo* (Gypsum Fibrosum) and *zhī mŭ* (Rhizoma Anemarrhenae).

➢ For heat entering the nutrient-blood level, add *shēng dì huáng* (Radix Rehmanniae recens), *dān pí* (Cortex Moutan), and *yuán shēn* (Radix Scrophulariae).

➢ For exuberant damp-heat, add *fáng jĭ* (Radix Stephaniae Tetrandrae) and *bái huā shé shé cǎo* (Herba Hedyotis Diffusae).

➢ For internal heat from yin deficiency, add *shēng dì huáng* (Radix Rehmanniae), *bái sháo* (Radix Paeoniae Alba), and *zhī mŭ* (Rhizoma Anemarrhenae).

(3) Static Blood Pattern

Invigorate blood, transform stasis, move qi, and unblock the collaterals with *Huà Yū Tōng Bì Tāng* (化瘀通痹汤):

当归	dāng guī	18g	Radix Angelica Sinensis
丹参	dān shēn	18g	Radix et Rhizoma Salviae Miltiorrhizae
鸡血藤	jī xuè téng	21g	Caulis Spatholobi
制乳香	zhì rŭ xiāng	9g	Olibanum (prepared)
制没药	zhì mò yào	9g	Myrrha (prepared)
元胡	yuán hú	12g	Rhizoma Corydalis

香附	xiāng fù	12g	Rhizoma Cyperi
透骨草	tòu gŭ căo	18g	Caulis Impatientis

【Modifications】

- For exuberant cold, add *guì zhī* (Ramulus Cinnamomi), *zhì chuān wū* (Radix Aconiti Praeparata), *zhì căo wū* (Radix Aconiti Kusnezoffii Praeparata), and *xì xīn* (Radix et Rhizoma Asari).
- For exuberant heat, add *bài jiàng căo* (Herba Patriniae) and *dān pí* (Cortex Moutan).
- For qi deficiency, add *huáng qí* (Radix Astragali).
- For chronic *bi* with swollen, enlarged, and deformed joints, add *chuān shān jiă* (Squama Manis), *wū shāo shé* (Zaocys), *dì lóng* (Pheretima), *wú gōng* (Scolopendra), *quán xiē* (Scorpio), and *zhì mă qián zĭ* (Semen Strychni Praeparata).

When administering medicinal therapy, pay attention to the following 3 points:

A. While dispelling evils and invigorating blood, do not forget to boost qi and nourish blood.

The qi and blood that circulate in the channels are important nutrients in the body. Chronic *bi* with lingering evils invariably leads to qi and blood deficiency. Unfortunately, medicinals that treat *bi* are often acrid and drying, and thus their long-term use can consume qi and impair blood. Add *huáng qí* (Radix Astragali) and *bái zhú* (Rhizoma Atractylodis Macrocephalae) to boost qi and fortify the spleen. In the case of blood deficiency, the vessels are dry and rough and blood flow is impaired; this can be likened to a boat getting stuck in a shallow river. Consequently, the disease evil and static blood become difficult to eliminate. During treatment, emphasis should be placed on nourishing the blood. Select medicinals that can dispel evils and invigorate and nourish blood, i.e., *dāng guī* (Radix Angelicae Sinensis), *dān shēn* (Radix et Rhizoma Salviae

Miltiorrhizae), and *jī xuè téng* (Caulis Spatholobi). For blood deficiency, add *bái sháo* (Radix Paeoniae Alba). For yin deficiency, increase the dosage of *shēng dì huáng* (Radix Rehmanniae Recens) to increase body fluid and thereby relieve constipation, alleviate spasms, and counteract the acrid and drying nature of the other medicinals. If too much attention is paid to expelling evils and invigorating blood while neglecting to boost qi and nourish blood, one cannot achieve the optimum curative effects and the condition may worsen. Do not forget to boost qi and nourish blood while expelling evils and invigorating blood.

B. If the right qi can withstand it, use large dosages of medicinals to expel evils.

For those with strong right qi, large dosages of medicinals that expel evils should be used (start with small dosages and increase gradually). Reactions will vary according to the differences in constitution and medicinal tolerance. Sudden increases in dosage should be avoided to prevent adverse reactions. The application of large dosages is based on the logic that since the pathological changes of *bi* syndromes are located in the skin, flesh, channels and collaterals, it is difficult for small dosages of medicinals to reach the location of the disease. *Bi* syndromes are caused by obstruction due to evils and static blood, and therefore, only medicinals prescribed in large dosages are able to unblock the channels, collaterals, and blood vessels.

Pain is the main complaint of patients suffering from *bi* syndromes, so the immediate goal is to relieve pain. Small dosages have a slow analgesic effect. In the initial stages of the illness, right qi is still sufficient and the evils are excessive; large dosages of medicinals can quickly expel evils. Otherwise, if the evils linger for a long period of time, the right qi will be impaired, and the condition will become chronic and difficult to treat.

Large dosages of medicinals can induce mild symptoms of the gastrointestinal tract in patients during the initial phase of administration. Generally, patients will adapt after 3 doses and the adverse reactions will disappear. If the reactions continue, instruct the patient to take the medicinals after meals.

C. During treatment, it is important to understand the nature of the disease.

Bi syndrome is not an urgent and violent disease. It is relatively stable and its pathological changes and development of symptoms are fairly slow. Particularly in patients with chronic *bi*, even the most appropriate formula may not produce any effect initially. In some patients, symptoms might actually get worse after taking the first few doses; this must be realized as a good sign, one that means right qi is fighting with the evils. If the practitioner does not know this general rule of disease progression and gives in to the patient's demand for rapid improvement, the formula is altered frequently and thus all previous efforts would have been wasted. However, sticking to a base formula does not mean to prescribe the same exact formula every time without any modifications at all. The ingredients should be modified according to symptom manifestation, so as to not "take measures without regard to changes in circumstances (刻舟求剑 ; a Chinese idiom)."

[Lou Duo-feng. *Experience in the Treatment of Bi Syndromes* (痹证治验). Henan Science and Technology Publishing House.1983]

3. Wang Wei-lan Divides RA into Acute Episodes and Chronic Remission

Acute attacks can be classified into heat and cold patterns. This is commonly seen in the early and middle stages of RA.

(1) Heat Prevalence

This pattern presents with redness, swelling, and pain in the small joints of the hands and feet. The involved joints are hot and red with impaired mobility and difficulty in walking or holding objects. Other accompanying symptoms include low grade fever (or a sensation of fever), thirst, sweating, a red face, a red tongue with thin white coating, and a wiry, slippery and rapid pulse. This pattern is caused by the constraint of latent evil. These pathogens turn into toxins and impair *yíng wèi* (营卫; nutritive and defense), sinews, and vessels; when combined with qi stagnation and blood stasis, the pathogens give rise to joint dysfunction. Treatment principles: clear heat, resolve toxins, unblock the channels, transform stasis, and dispel evils from the collaterals.

【Basic Prescription】

桑枝	sāng zhī	30g	Ramulus Mori
忍冬藤	rěn dōng téng	30g	Caulis Lonicerae Japonicae
丹参	dān shēn	15g	Radix et Rhizoma Salviae Miltiorrhizae
丹皮	dān pí	10g	Cortex Moutan
生白芍	shēng bái sháo	15g	Radix Paeoniae Alba (raw)
甘草	gān cǎo	10g	Radix et Rhizoma Glycyrrhizae
赤芍	chì sháo	10g	Radix Paeoniae Rubra
黄柏	huáng bǎi	10g	Cortex Phellodendri Chinensis
地龙	dì lóng	12g	Pheretima
银花	yín huā	15g	Flos Lonicerae Japonicae
连翘	lián qiào	10g	Fructus Forsythiae

【Modifications】

➢ For excessive heat of the qi level, add *shēng shí gāo* (raw Gypsum Fibrosum) and *zhī mǔ* (Rhizoma Anemarrhenae).

➢ For excessive heat of the nutrient-blood level, add *shēng dì huáng* (Radix Rehmanniae Recens) and *shuǐ niú jiǎo* (Cornu Bubali).

➢ For severe heat with blood stasis, add *táo rén* (Semen Persicae) and *yán hú suǒ* (Rhizoma Corydalis).

➢ For severe heat with phlegm stasis, add *dǎn nán xīng* (Arisaema cum Bile) and *zhú rú* (Caulis Bambusae in Taenia).

- For severe heat with obstruction in the collaterals, add *sī guā luò* (Retinervus Luffae Fructus) and *wáng bù liú xíng* (Semen Vaccariae).
- For severe heat with swelling, add *fáng jǐ* (Radix Stephaniae Tetrandrae) and *fú líng pí* (Cutis Poriae).
- For severe heat with constipation, add *dà huáng* (Radix et Rhizoma Rhei) and *xuán míng fěn* (Natrii Sulfas Exsiccatus).
- For severe pain, add *wēi líng xiān* (Radix et Rhizoma Clematidis) and *luò shí téng* (Caulis Trachelospermi).
- For stiff joints, add *zào jiǎo cì* (Spina Gleditsiae) and *quán xiē* (Scorpio).

(2) Cold Prevalence

This pattern presents with swelling and deformity of the small joints of the hands and feet; stiffness, numbness, and inhibited movement; local aversion to wind; cold limbs; subjective feeling of an outward emission of wind throughout the body; a pale tongue with thin white coating, and a deep, thready pulse. Other possible symptoms include scorching heat, swelling, and deformity of the small joints of the hands and feet with fear of cold. Symptoms may vary from patient to patient.

This pattern has a high recurrence rate, caused by exposure to cold and dampness or to excessive physical labor.

Treatment principles: warm the channels, disperse cold, unblock the collaterals, transform phlegm, and dispel evils from the collaterals.

【Basic Prescription】

熟地	shú dì	30g	Radix Rehmanniae Praeparata
鹿角胶	lù jiǎo jiāo	10g	Colla Cornus Cervi
麻黄	má huáng	5g	Herba Ephedrae
肉桂	ròu guì	5g	Cortex Cinnamomi
姜黄	jiāng huáng	5g	Rhizoma Curcumae Longae
炒白芥子	bái jiè zǐ	10g	Semen Sinapis (dry-fried)
炮附子	páo fù zǐ	10g	Radix Aconiti Lateralis (blast-fried)
鸡血藤	jī xuè téng	20g	Caulis Spatholobi

甘草	gān cǎo	3g	Radix et Rhizoma Glycyrrhizae
全蝎	quán xiē	6g	Scorpio
蜈蚣	wú gōng	2 pieces	Scolopendra

【Modifications】

➢ For exuberant cold evils, add *xì xīn* (Radix et Rhizoma Asari) and *fù zǐ* (Radix Aconiti Lateralis).

➢ For yang deficiency, add *ròu guì* (Cortex Cinnamomi), *lù jiǎo jiāo* (Colla Cornus Cervi), and *bái jiè zǐ* (Semen Sinapis).

➢ For pronounced cold with blood stasis, add *dāng guī* (Radix Angelicae Sinensis), *chuān xiōng* (Rhizoma Chuanxiong), and *shuǐ zhì* (Hirudo).

➢ For exuberant cold obstructing the collaterals, add *zhì chuān wū* (Radix Aconiti Praeparata) and *zhì cǎo wū* (Radix Aconiti Kusnezoffii Praeparata).

➢ For joint stiffness and deformity, add *chǎo shān jiǎ* (dry-fried Squama Manis), *zào jiǎo cì* (Spina Gleditsiae), and *fēng fáng* (Nidus Vespae).

(3) Cold-heat Complex

This pattern is caused by the combination of cold and heat. The evils lie latent in the sinews and vessels, causing obstruction and stagnation in the collaterals and inhibiting the joints. Treatment principles: Clear heat, disperse cold, unblock the channels, relieve pain, and dispel evils from the collaterals.

桂枝	guì zhī	10g	Ramulus Cinnamomi
白芍	bái sháo	15g	Radix Paeoniae Alba
赤芍	chì sháo	15g	Radix Paeoniae Rubra
知母	zhī mǔ	10g	Rhizoma Anemarrhenae
白术	bái zhú	10g	Rhizoma Atractylodis Macrocephalae
麻黄	má huáng	9g	Herba Ephedrae
附子	fù zǐ	10g	Radix Aconiti Lateralis Praeparata
防风	fáng fēng	10g	Radix Saposhnikoviae

甘草	gān cǎo	9g	Radix et Rhizoma Glycyrrhizae
生姜	shēng jiāng	6g	Rhizoma Zingiberis Recens

(4) Chronic Remission

Seen in the advanced stages of RA. Clinical manifestations include severe joint destruction with stiffness and deformity or dysfunction of the limbs and spine. The overall symptoms are relieved, and the joints are neither red nor swollen, or only swollen with no red skin or local heat. Parts of the joints are painful. The condition is comparatively stable, with normal tongue and pulse manifestations. It is caused by excessive evils combined with right qi deficiency. Simultaneous application of tonifying and purging should be administered to strengthen the kidney, fortify the bones, nourish blood, relax the sinews, dispel phlegm, transform stasis, disperse swelling, relieve pain, and dispel evils from the collaterals.

【Basic Prescription】

当归	dāng guī	30g	Radix Angelicae Sinensis
熟地	shú dì	60g	Radix Rehmanniae Praeparata
鹿角胶	lù jiǎo jiāo	30g	Colla Cornus Cervi
龟板胶	guī bǎn jiāo	30g	Colla Carapax et Plastrum Testudinis
炒山甲	chuān shān jiǎ	25g	Squama Manis (dry-fried)
皂刺	zào cì	25g	Spina Gleditsiae
乳香	rǔ xiāng	25g	Olibanum
没药	mò yào	25g	Myrrha
麻黄	má huáng	20g	Herba Ephedrae
炒白芥子	chǎo bái jiè zǐ	60g	Semen Sinapis (dry-fried)
鸡血藤	jī xuè téng	60g	Caulis Spatholobi
赤芍	chì sháo	30g	Radix Paeoniae Rubra

【Modifications】

➢ For exuberant phlegm-damp, add *dǎn nán xīng* (Arisaema cum Bile), *fǎ bàn xià* (Rhizoma Pinelliae Praeparatum), and *bái jiè zǐ* (Semen Sinapis).

- For blood stasis with stabbing pain, add *shuǐ zhì* (Hirudo) and *tǔ biē chóng* (Eupolyphaga seu Steleophaga).
- For yin deficiency with hot pain, add *qín jiāo* (Radix Gentianae Macrophyllae) and *dì lóng* (Pheretima).
- For yang deficiency with cold pain, add *chuān wū* (Radix Aconiti Praeparata) and *cǎo wū* (Radix Aconiti Kusnezoffii Praeparata).
- For spleen deficiency, add *dǎng shēn* (Radix Codonopsis), *bái zhú* (Rhizoma Atractylodis Macrocephalae), *fú líng* (Poria), *gān cǎo* (Radix et Rhizoma Glycyrrhizae), and *huáng qí* (Radix Astragali).
- For liver blood deficiency, add *dāng guī* (Radix Angelicae Sinensis), *bái sháo* (Radix Paeoniae Alba), *chuān xiōng* (Rhizoma Chuanxiong), *shú dì huáng* (Radix Rehmanniae Praeparata), and *gǒu qǐ* (Fructus Lycii).
- For kidney yin deficiency, add *shú dì huáng* (Radix Rehmanniae Praeparata), *shān yú ròu* (Fructus Corni), *shān yào* (Rhizoma Dioscoreae), *gǒu qǐ* (Fructus Lycii), *huái niú xī* (Radix Achyranthis Bidentatae), combined with herbs for tonifying yang.
- For kidney yang deficiency, add *tù sī zǐ* (Semen Cuscutae), *páo fù zǐ* (blast-fried Radix Aconiti Lateralis Praeparata), *ròu guì* (Cortex Cinnamomi), *gǒu jǐ* (Rhizoma Cibotii), *dù zhòng* (Cortex Eucommiae), and *xiān líng pí* (Herba Epimedii), along with herbs that nourish yin.
- For depletion of essence and marrow, add *zhū jǐ suǐ* (Suis Spinae Medulla), *shān yú ròu* (Fructus Corni), *gǒu qǐ* (Fructus Lycii), *ē jiāo* (Colla Corii Asini), *shā yuàn zǐ* (Semen Astragali Complanati), *yú biāo jiāo* (Colla Piscis), *lù róng* (Cornu Cervi Pantotrichum), and *rén shēn* (Radix Ginseng).

[*An Anthology of the Experiences of Beijing Chinese Medicine Doctors* (北京市老中医经验选编). Beijing Publishing House, 1980]

4. Lu Zhi-zheng Emphasizes the Following Points

(1) Wind medicinals should not be used alone for *bi* syndromes:

Overdose of wind herbs can consume the right qi, transform the wind evil into fire, transform cold into heat, or change an excess pattern into a deficiency pattern, thereby aggravating the illness.

(2) Pay close attention to phlegm, stasis, dryness and toxins:

Phlegm and dampness are of the same origin. Before the dampness transforms into phlegm, the joints are swollen and soft. If the dampness transforms into phlegm, the joint texture becomes hard with local subcutaneous nodules. If there is internal stasis, the local skin is dark with stasis macules, and the tongue is purple and dusky. If there is dryness, the joint pain is accompanied by manifestations of the notion "when dryness prevails, there is aridity," i.e., dry mouth, scanty saliva, and dry eyes. Dr. Lu proposed the term "dryness *bi*" according to the signs and symptoms of this pattern. (Refer to the chapter of "dryness syndrome"). *Bi* syndromes with internal heat toxins can manifest in the joints as red skin with sensations of scorching heat, diffuse swelling and severe pain. Accompanying symptoms include fever, thirst, and vexation.

(3) Pay attention to the spleen and stomach during the treatment of *bi* syndromes:

(4) Utilize combined therapies:

I.e., hot compresses, external application, steams and washes, local rubbing, and acupuncture.

(5) Acupuncture for joint deformity:

Needle from the two sides of the deformed joints, directing the needle towards the joints with medium stimulation. Retain the needles for 15-20 minutes. Use rapid insertion to bleed both sides of the toe nail distal to the affected joint. Administer treatment once every other day.

[Lu Zhi-zheng. *A Compendium of Lu zhi-zheng's Clinical Experience* (路志正医林集腋). Beijing: People's Medical Publishing House.1990]

5. Xie Hai-zhou Discusses the 3 Essentials and 4 Rules in the Treatment of *Bi* Syndromes

The three essential points are (1) supporting the right qi and consolidating the root, (2) dispelling dampness and fortifying the spleen, and (3) freeing the joints and resolving toxins.

The four rules are: (1) warming the kidney to treat cold *bi*, (2) nourishing yin to treat heat *bi*, (3) unblocking obstruction to treat cold-heat complex, and (4) invigorating blood and weeding out pathogens to treat chronic illness entering the collaterals.

Dr. Xie uses pairs and groups of medicinals to effectively relieve pain. *Chuān shān lóng* (Dioscoreae Nipponicae Rhizoma) and *xú cháng qīng* (Radix et Rhizoma Cynanchi Paniculati) disperse cold and relieve pain. *Qīng fēng téng* (Caulis Sinomenii), *hǎi fēng téng* (Caulis Piperis Kadsurae), *jī xuè téng* (Caulis Spatholobi), and *rěn dōng téng* (Caulis Lonicerae Japonicae), which are moistening and therefore not drying, are often used to warm, unblock, and lift; they unblock the collaterals and reach the limbs. *Zhuī dì fēng* (Cortex Illicii) and *qiān nián jiàn* (Rhizoma Homalomenae) dispel wind-damp and strengthen the sinews and bones. *Sāng zhī* (Ramulus Mori) and *guì zhī* (Ramulus Cinnamomi) unblock the collaterals and relieve pain. *Rǔ xiāng* (Olibanum) and *mò yào* (Myrrha) disperse swelling and relieve pain. *Qín jiāo* (Radix Gentianae Macrophyllae) and *wēi líng xiān* (Radix et Rhizoma Clematidis) clear heat and unblock the collaterals.

[Lou Yu-qian. *A Compendium of Bi Syndromes* (中国痹病大全). Beijing: Chinese Science and Technology Publishing House. 1993]

6. Hu Qiao-wu Divides *Bi* Syndrome into Three Stages

(1) In the early stages, the disease is in the channels; treat the qi.

Wǔ Jī Sǎn (五积散) is selected. The formula contains medicinals that resolve the exterior and disperse cold, dispel wind and transform dampness, and warm yang and harmonize the nutritive qi. It is the best formula for the early stages of RA (which are caused by wind, cold, and dampness evils). If wind and damp are predominant, add *qiāng huó* (Rhizoma et Radix Notopterygii), *dú huó* (Radix Angelicae Pubescentis), *fáng fēng* (Radix Saposhnikoviae), and *yì yǐ rén* (Semen Coicis). If wind and cold are predominant, add *cǎo wū* (Radix Aconiti Kusnezoffii Praeparata), *chuān wū* (Radix Aconiti Praeparata), and *xì xīn* (Radix et Rhizoma Asari). If there is heat evil, add *zhī mǔ* (Rhizoma Anemarrhenae), *shí gāo* (Gypsum Fibrosum), and *qín jiāo* (Radix Gentianae Macrophyllae). If there is qi deficiency, add *huáng qí* (Radix Astragali). If there is exterior yang deficiency, add *fù zǐ* (Radix Aconiti Lateralis). After the symptoms have been relieved, use *Huáng Qí Guì Zhī Wǔ Wù Tāng* (黄芪桂枝五物汤) or *Guì Zhī Jiā Fù Zǐ Tāng* (桂枝加附子汤) to consolidate the treatment effect.

(2) Chronic illness enters the collaterals; treat the blood.

Use medicinals that nourish and enrich yin, i.e., *shēng dì* (Radix Rehmanniae Recens), *shú dì huáng* (Radix Rehmanniae Praeparata), *gǒu qǐ* (Fructus Lycii), *hé shǒu wū* (Radix Polygoni Multiflori), and *ē jiāo* (Colla Corii Asini). Add *jī xuè téng* (Caulis Spatholobi), *lù xián cǎo* (Herba Pyrolae), *xī xiān cǎo* (Herba Siegesbeckiae), and *yè jiāo téng* (Caulis Polygoni Multiflori) to unblock the collaterals and harmonize blood. If there is cold-damp or damp-heat evil, select the appropriate herbs to dispel the evil. If there is blood stasis obstructing the collaterals, add insect medicinals to invigorate blood and unblock the collaterals while nourishing yin and tonifying blood. For instance, add *hóng huā* (Flos Carthami), *dān shēn* (Radix et Rhizoma Salviae Miltiorrhizae), *zé lán* (Herba Lycopi), *shuǐ zhì* (Hirudo), *méng chóng* (Tabanus), *wú gōng* (Scolopendra), *quán xiē* (Scorpio), *chán yī* (Periostracum Cicadae), and *jiāng cán* (Bombyx Batryticatus) to *Sì Wù Tāng* (四物汤) for better results. While treating the blood, tonifying qi and warming yang should also be considered. Mildly acrid and moistening herbs such as *tù sī zǐ* (Semen Cuscutae), *yín yáng huò* (Herba Epimedii), *ròu cōng róng* (Herba Cistanches), *tài zǐ shēn* (Radix Pseudostellariae), and *huáng qí* (Radix Astragali) can be added to promote the generation of both yin and yang.

(3) In the late stage, there is bone destruction; treat the bone.

Large dosages of medicinals are used to tonify the liver and kidney, thereby nourishing essence and replenishing marrow. Medicinals that warm and nourish original yang include *shú dì huáng* (Radix Rehmanniae Praeparata), *shān yú ròu* (Fructus Corni), *bā jǐ tiān* (Radix Morindae Officinalis), *bǔ gǔ zhī* (Fructus Psoraleae), *ròu guì* (Cortex Cinnamomi), *zǐ hé chē* (Placenta Hominis), and *lù jiǎo jiāo* (Colla Cornus Cervi). Medicinals that replenish and tonify true yin include *ē jiāo* (Colla Corii Asini), *shēng dì* (Radix Rehmanniae Recens), *gǒu qǐ zǐ* (Fructus Lycii), *shā yuàn zǐ* (Semen Astragali Complanati), *huái niú xī* (Radix Achyranthis Bidentatae), *zhū jǐ suǐ* (Suis Spinae Medulla), *guī jiǎ jiāo* (Colla Carapax et Plastrum Testudinis), and *biē jiǎ jiāo* (Carapax Trionycis). Dr. Hu advocates that while tonifying the liver and kidney, one should also eliminate the lingering evils. Insect medicinals are necessary for this purpose, in addition to medicinals that clear heat, dispel damp, disperse cold, dispel wind, unblock the collaterals, transform phlegm, and expel stasis.

[Shan Shu-jian, Chen Zi-hua. *The Golden Mirror of the Clinical Experience of Famous Ancient and Modern Physicians* (古今名医临证金鉴). Beijing: China Publishing House of Chinese Medicine.1999]

7. Zhang Pei-qiu Divides *Bi* Syndrome into Heat and Cold Patterns and Uses Insect Medicinals to Treat Chronic *Bi*

Dr. Zhang believes that all *bi* syndromes can be attributed to wind, cold, and dampness, and although it is hard to separate the three evils, it is possible to determine which evil is more predominant. The key to differentiation is to distinguish between cold and heat. Dr. Zhang divides the syndrome into damp-heat and cold-damp.

➢ For mild damp-heat with a concurrent exterior pattern, use *Má Huáng Lián Qiào Chì Xiăo Dòu Tāng* (麻黄连翘赤小豆汤):

净麻黄	má huáng	5g	Herba Ephedrae
连翘	lián qiào	15g	Fructus Forsythiae
赤小豆	chì xiăo dòu	30g	Semen Phaseoli
防风	fáng fēng	10g	Radix Saposhnikoviae
桂枝	guì zhī	5g	Ramulus Cinnamomi
赤芍	chì sháo	10g	Radix Paeoniae Rubra
生甘草	shēng gān căo	3g	Radix et Rhizoma Glycyrrhizae (raw)
忍冬藤	rĕn dōng téng	30g	Caulis Lonicerae Japonicae
川羌活	qiāng huó	15g	Rhizoma et Radix Notopterygii
生姜	shēng jiāng	3 pieces	Rhizoma Zingiberis Recens

➢ Once the exterior pattern has been resolved, if there is still joint swelling and pain, use *Guī Sháo Xī Căo Tāng* (归芍　草汤):

当归	dāng guī	15g	Radix Angelicae Sinensis
赤芍	chì sháo	15g	Radix Paeoniae Rubra
白芍	bái sháo	15g	Radix Paeoniae Alba
豨莶草	xī xiān căo	30g	Herba Siegesbeckiae
秦艽	qín jiāo	10g	Radix Gentianae Macrophyllae
伸筋草	shēn jīn căo	15g	Herba Lycopodii
威灵仙	wēi líng xiān	15g	Radix et Rhizoma Clematidis
地龙	dì lóng	10g	Pheretima
防风	fáng fēng	10g	Radix Saposhnikoviae
生地	shēng dì	30g	Radix Rehmanniae Recens
制乳香	zhì rŭ xiāng	6g	Olibanum (prepared)
制没药	zhì mò yào	6g	Myrrha (prepared)
桑枝	sāng zhī	10g	Ramulus Mori
炙马钱子	zhì mă qián zĭ	0.5g	Semen Strychni (liquid-fried)

➢ For severe damp-heat, use *Shí Gāo Jiā Guì Zhī Tāng* (石膏加桂枝汤):

桂枝	guì zhī	5g	Ramulus Cinnamomi
知母	zhī mŭ	10g	Rhizoma Anemarrhenae
生石膏	shēng shí gāo	30g	Gypsum Fibrosum (raw)
黄芩	huáng qín	15g	Radix Scutellariae
黄连	huáng lián	5g	Rhizoma Coptidis
黄柏	huáng băi	10g	Cortex Phellodendri Chinensis
络石藤	luò shí téng	30g	Caulis Trachelospermi
地龙	dì lóng	10g	Pheretima
桑枝	sāng zhī	30g	Ramulus Mori
忍冬藤	rěn dōng téng	30g	Caulis Lonicerae Japonicae
川羌活	qiāng huó	15g	Rhizoma et Radix Notopterygii
甘草	gān căo	5g	Radix et Rhizoma Glycyrrhizae

➢ For cold-damp obstructing the collaterals, use *Dà Wū Tóu Jiān* (大乌头煎) plus *Dāng Guī Sì Nì Tāng* (当归四逆汤):

制川乌(先煎)	zhì chuān wū	9g	Radix Aconiti Praeparata(decocted first)
制草乌(先煎)	zhì căo wū	9g	Radix Aconiti Kusnezoffii Praeparata (decocted first)
黄芪	huáng qí	15g	Radix Astragali
细辛	xì xīn	3g	Radix et Rhizoma Asari
麻黄	má huáng	6g	Herba Ephedrae
桂枝	guì zhī	6g	Ramulus Cinnamomi
当归	dāng guī	10g	Radix Angelicae Sinensis
白术	bái zhú	10g	Rhizoma Atractylodis Macrocephalae
羌活	qiāng huó	15g	Rhizoma et Radix Notopterygii
独活	dú huó	15g	Radix Angelicae Pubescentis
威灵仙	wēi líng xiān	15g	Radix et Rhizoma Clematidis
蕲蛇	qí shé	10g	Agkistrodon
炙全蝎	zhì quán xiē	5g	Scorpio (liquid-fried)
炙马钱子	zhì mă qián zĭ	1.5g	Semen Strychni (liquid-fried)

➢ For chronic *bi* with phlegm and stasis, add insect medicinals to penetrate the bones and track down and dispel evils from the collaterals while simultaneously tonifying qi and nourishing blood.

乌梢蛇	wū shāo shé	Zaocys
蕲蛇	qí shé	Agkistrodon
全蝎	quán xiē	Scorpio
蜈蚣	wú gōng	Scolopendra
地龙	dì lóng	Pheretima

[Jiao Shu-de. The Treatment of Bi Syndromes (痹证论治). *Journal of Chinese Medicine* (中医杂志).1989, 30 (4): 4-10]

8. Zhang Ming-he Emphasizes the Expulsion of Evils in the Treatment of RA

Dr. Zhang believes that the formation of joint disease is associated with a weak constitution and insufficiency of right qi (internal factors), and is attributed to the contraction of wind, cold, dampness, and heat (external factors). The external evils stir up the internal evils; the two types of evils combine and give rise to illness. The key pathogenesis is erosion of the bones by damp-heat toxins that pour into the channels and collaterals and form blood stasis and toxic heat. The primary treatment principle is to dispel the evils; the methods include clearing heat, resolving toxins, draining dampness, invigorating blood, and unblocking the collaterals. *Jīn yín huā* (Flos Lonicerae Japonicae), *pú gōng yīng* (Herba Taraxaci), *zǐ huā dì dīng* (Herba Violae), *bái huā shé shé cǎo* (Herba Hedyotis Diffusae), *huáng bǎi* (Cortex Phellodendri Chinensis), and *bǎn lán gēn* (Radix Isatidis) are selected to clear heat and resolve toxins. *Tǔ fú líng* (Rhizoma Smilacis Glabrae), *yì yǐ rén* (Semen Coicis), and *tǔ bèi mǔ* (Rhizoma Bolbostematis) are used to drain dampness and disperse swelling. *Táo rén* (Semen Persicae), *hóng huā* (Flos Carthami), *tǔ biē chóng* (Eupolyphaga seu Steleophaga), *fēng fáng* (Nidus Vespae), and *quán xiē* (Scorpio) are used to invigorate blood and unblock the collaterals. All of the above are used during the active stage of RA.

(Shan Shu-jian, Chen Zi-hua. *The Golden Mirror of the Clinical Experience of Famous Ancient and Modern Physicians* (古今名医临证金鉴). Beijing: China Publishing House of Chinese Medicine.1999)

9. Wu Sheng-nong Advocates the Four Methods of Expelling Evils to Treat RA

(1) Cool blood and resolve toxins

For heat *bi* with red, swollen, and hot joints, marked tenderness, no fever or unsurfaced generalized fever, a rapid, wiry, and thready pulse, and a red tongue with thin coating, use modified *Xī Jiăo Săn* (犀角散):

犀角	xī jiăo	5g	Cornu Rhinocerotis
生地	shēng dì	20-30g	Radix Rehmanniae Recens
鸡血藤	jī xuè téng	20-30g	Caulis Spatholobi
油松节	yóu sōng jié	10-15g	Lignum Pini Nodi
忍冬藤	rĕn dōng téng	12-30g	Caulis Lonicerae Japonicae
虎杖	hŭ zhàng	12-20g	Rhizoma et Radix Polygoni Cuspidati
寻骨风	xún gŭ fēng	10-20g	Herba Aristolochiae Mollissimae
白花蛇舌草	bái huā shé shé căo	10-20g	Herba Hedyotis Diffusae
海桐皮	hăi tóng pí	10-15g	Cortex Erythrinae

【Modifications】

➢ For pronounced heat, add *dān pí* (Cortex Moutan) 12g and *fáng jĭ* (Radix Stephaniae Tetrandrae) 6-9g.

➢ For stasis, add *liú jì nú* (Herba Artemisiae Anomalae) 10-15g, *é zhú* (Rhizoma Curcumae) 10-15g, and *Xiăo Huó Luò Wán* (小活络丸) [4.5g, mixed with water].

➢ For severe pain, add *Xiē Wú Piàn* (蝎蜈片) [4 tablets, 3 times a day].

(2) Invigorate blood and transform stasis

Static blood obstructing the collaterals manifests as fixed and stabbing pain, swollen joints or bluish-purple joints, stiffness, thin fingertips, inhibited bending and stretching, a slow and deep or slow and rough pulse, and a purple tongue with stasis macules or distended sublingual veins. Use modified *Bŭ Yáng Huán Wŭ Tāng* (补阳还五汤):

黄芪	huáng qí	15-60g	Radix Astragali
桂枝	guì zhī	9-12g	Ramulus Cinnamomi
赤芍	chì sháo	9-12g	Radix Paeoniae Rubra
当归尾	dāng guī wěi	9-12g	Radix Angelicae Sinensis (tail)
鸡血藤	jī xuè téng	20-30g	Caulis Spatholobi
寻骨风	xún gŭ fēng	10-15g	Herba Aristolochiae Mollissimae
姜黄	jiāng huáng	10-15g	Rhizoma Curcumae Longae

【Modifications】

➢ For pronounced dampness, add *shēng dì* (Radix Rehmanniae Recens) 15-30g, *shú dì huáng* (Radix Rehmanniae Praeparata) 15-30g, and *yì yĭ rén* (Semen Coicis).

➢ For external contraction, add *má huáng* (Herba Ephedrae) 3-6g.

➢ For severe pain, add *Xiē Wú Piàn* (蝎蜈片) [4 tablets, 3 times a day].

(3) Warm the channels and unblock the collaterals:

This treatment principle is used for RA due to cold-damp binding and causing stasis obstruction in the channels and collaterals which collects and lingers in the joints. If not treated, over time this can give rise to heavy limbs with inability to raise, cold pain with distention, a slow and soft pulse, and a pale, dusky tongue with thin white greasy coating or distended sublingual veins. Use modified *Wū Tóu Tāng* (乌头汤):

制川乌(先煎)	zhì chuān wū	9-12g	Radix Aconiti Praeparata (decocted first)
制草乌(先煎)	zhì căo wū	9-12g	Radix Aconiti Kusnezoffii Praeparata (decocted first)
黄芪	huáng qí	9-12g	Radix Astragali
桂枝	guì zhī	4-6g	Ramulus Cinnamomi

北细辛	běi xì xīn	3-6g	Radix et Rhizoma Asari
麻黄	má huáng	9-12g	Herba Ephedrae
生薏苡仁	shēng yì yǐ rén	15-30g	Semen Coicis (raw)
地龙	dì lóng	9-15g	Pheretima

【Modifications】

➢ For severe pain in the upper limbs, add *sāng zhī* (Ramulus Mori) 15-20g.

➢ For pain in the lower limbs, add *huái niú xī* (Radix Achyranthis Bidentatae) 9g and *mù guā* (Fructus Chaenomelis) 9g.

➢ For severe pain, add *Xiē Wú Piàn* (蝎蜈片) [4 tablets, 3 times a day].

(4) Support the right qi and dispel evils

Chronic *bi* manifests as fatigue, weakness, lassitude, and aching of the entire body; swollen and enlarged joints or dcformity of the small joints; a pale and lusterless face; a thready and weak pulse; and a pale, enlarged tooth-marked tongue with thin white coating. Use modified *Huáng Qí Guì Zhī Wŭ Wù Tāng* (黄芪桂枝五物汤):

黄芪	huáng qí	12-30g	Radix Astragali
芍药	sháo yào	9-12g	Radix Paeoniae Alba
生姜	shēng jiāng	12-15g	Rhizoma Zingiberis Recens
寻骨风	xún gŭ fēng	12-15g	Herba Aristolochiae Mollissimae
姜黄	jiāng huáng	9-12g	Rhizoma Curcumae Longae
鸡血藤	jī xuè téng	10-20g	Caulis Spatholobi

【Modifications】

➢ For external contraction, add *qiāng huó* (Rhizoma et Radix Notopterygii) 9-12g.

➢ For concurrent dampness, add *yì yĭ rén* (Semen Coicis) 10-30g and *fáng jĭ* (Radix Stephaniae Tetrandrae) 9-12g.

➢ For blood stasis, add *liú jì nú* (Herba Artemisiae Anomalae) 15-20g and *dāng guī* (Radix Angelicae Sinensis) 15-20g.

➢ For yin deficiency, add *shēng dì huáng* (Radix Rehmanniae) 15-20g.

[Shan Shu-jian, Chen Zi-hua. *The Golden Mirror of the Clinical Experience of Famous Ancient and Modern Physicians* (古今名医临证金鉴). Beijing: China Publishing House of Chinese Medicine.1999]

10. Chen Xiang-jun Treats RA by Tonifying Qi and Warming Yang

Chen Xiang-jun believes that RA is most prevalent among young to middle-aged females. The disease has a tendency to relapse and become chronic. It is characterized by local swelling and pain, stiffness, and possible deformity and progressive rigidity. Accompanying symptoms include general fear of cold, a pale facial complexion, fatigue, shortness of breath, poor appetite, loose stool, a pale red tongue with thin white coating, and a weak, thready pulse. The condition is attributed to yang qi deficiency leading to the local accumulation of excess evils (i.e., cold congealing, damp obstruction, heat congestion, and blood stasis). The main treatment principle is to boost qi and warm yang, assisted by dispelling wind, dispersing cold, transforming dampness, unblocking the collaterals, and invigorating blood.

【Modifications】

生黄芪	shēng huáng qí	30-60g	Radix Astragali (raw)
桂枝	guì zhī	6g	Ramulus Cinnamomi
制川乌	zhì chuān wū	9g	Radix Aconiti Praeparata
当归	dāng guī	9g	Radix Angelicae Sinensis
巴戟天	bā jǐ tiān	12g	Radix Morindae Officinalis
乳香	rǔ xiāng	6g	Olibanum
没药	mò yào	6g	Myrrha
泽泻	zé xiè	30g	Rhizoma Alismatis
青风藤	qīng fēng téng	15g	Caulis Sinomenii
忍冬藤	rěn dōng téng	30g	Caulis Lonicerae Japonicae
骨碎补	gǔ suì bǔ	9g	Rhizoma Drynariae

红花	hóng huā	6g	Flos Carthami
甘草	gān cǎo	6g	Radix et Rhizoma Glycyrrhizae

[Zhou Shi-gao. Professor Chen Xiang-jun's Experience in the Use of Chinese Medicinals to Treat Rheumatism (陈湘君教授运用中医中药治疗风湿病的经验). *Asia Journal of Chinese Medicine* (亚洲中医杂志). 1999, 1: 19]

11. Wang Shi-fu on the Use of Large Dosages in the Treatment of the Early, Middle, and Late Stages of *Bi* Syndromes

In the early stage of *bi* syndromes, determine if the pathogen is wind, cold, dampness and/or heat. Use large dosages of medicinals to quickly dispel the evils. In the middle stage, if the evils have not yet been expelled, add a small dosage of medicinals that tonify the right qi, e.g., *huáng qí* (Radix Astragali), *dāng guī* (Radix Angelicae Sinensis), *sāng jì shēng* (Herba Taxilli), and *bái zhú* (Rhizoma Atractylodis Macrocephalae). Long-term accumulation of evils in the channels and collaterals disturb the normal circulation of qi and blood and turns the pattern into one of deficiency, particularly blood deficiency. In this case, it is necessary to nourish and tonify the blood, and thus *Dú Huó Jì Shēng Tāng* (独活寄生汤) is the most effective formula for the late stage of *bi* syndromes.

For heat *bi*, herbs like *niú bàng zǐ* (Fructus Arctii), *jīng jiè suì* (Spica Schizonepetae), and *lián qiào* (Fructus Forsythiae) can be used to clear heat and resolve toxins. If there is severe pain accompanied by a thick, white and glossy tongue coating, add *dú huó* (Radix Angelicae Pubescentis) 60g to dispel wind, transform dampness, and relieve pain. To clear heat, prescribe a large dose of *Bái Hǔ Tāng* (白虎汤). If the pulse is large, increase the dosage of *shí gāo* (Gypsum Fibrosum) to 120g-250g. To resolve toxins, use *bái huā shé shé cǎo* (Herba Hedyotis Diffusae) 30g, *rěn dōng téng* (Caulis Lonicerae Japonicae) 30g, and *jīn yín huā* (Flos Lonicerae Japonicae) 30g. After the high fever has subsided, if there is intermittent low fever with redness, swelling, and pain of the joints, add *shēng dì* (Radix Rehmanniae Recens), *xuán shēn* (Radix Scrophulariae), *dān pí* (Cortex Moutan), *chì sháo* (Radix Paeoniae Rubra), and *shān chuān liǔ* (Cacumen Tamaricis) 15-20g to the previous formula to clear heat from the nutritive level.

In chronic *bi*, the toxic heat binds together with phlegm-turbidity and static blood, obstructing the collaterals and causing redness, swelling, and pain of the joints, and in severe cases, stiffness and deformity, which are the most difficult to treat. Add *shān cí gū* (Pseudobulbus Cremastrae seu Pleiones) 10-15g, *hóng yá dà jǐ* (Radix Knoxiae) 6-12g, and insect medicinals to resolve toxins. For swollen, enlarged joints with hypertonicity and deformity due to the administration of large doses of excessively hot and acrid formulas or to long-term lapse in treatment, *Sì Wù Tāng* (四物汤), *Zēng Yè Tāng* (增液汤), and *Hǔ Qiǎn Wán* (虎潜丸) can be taken to nourish blood, strengthen the Kidney, and boost essence.

Cold *bi* is often treated with *Wū Tóu Tāng* (乌头汤) plus *Sì Wù Tāng* (四物汤). First, decoct *chuān wū* (Radix Aconiti Praeparata) 30g, *cǎo wū* (Radix Aconiti Kusnezoffii Praeparata) 30g, and *shēng gān cǎo* (Radix et Rhizoma Glycyrrhizae) 30g for one hour; then, add the other medicinals. Stop administration of the formula after it has taken effect. Dr. Wang believes that those who are too afraid to use large dosages of *chuān wū* (Radix Aconiti Praeparata) and *cǎo wū* (Radix Aconiti Kusnezoffii Praeparata) because of their highly toxic nature often end up using smaller dosages over a longer period of time. This method, however, is indeed what allows the toxic qualities of the two herbs to harm the body. Therefore, Dr. Wang advocates using large dosages of the two herbs over a short period of time.

Fixed *bi* (着痹; *zhuó bì*) is treated with *Zhǐ Mí Fú Líng Wán* (指迷茯苓丸), a formula created by Zhu Dan-xi. It can dry dampness and eliminate phlegm. Increase the dosages of *bàn xià* (Rhizoma Pinelliae) to

60g and *dǎn nán xīng* (Arisaema cum Bile) to 60g in order to effectively eliminate phlegm and relieve pain.

[Shan Shu-jian, Chen Zi-hua. *The Golden Mirror of the Clinical Experience of Famous Ancient and Modern Physicians* (古今名医临证金鉴). Beijing: China Publishing House of Chinese Medicine.1999]

PERSPECTIVES OF INTEGRATIVE MEDICINE

The multiple damage and stubborn nature of the clinical manifestations of RA present as formidable challenges in the treatment of RA. Modern medical research indicates that 2 years after the onset of RA, the disease enters the stage of joint deformity and bone damage, manifestations that cannot be reversed. For this reason, early treatment should be advocated to control the progression of the disease.

1. The Integration of Internal and External Treatment to Replace or Reduce the Use of NSAIDs

During attack episodes of RA, the main symptoms are joint pain, swelling, and morning stiffness. In the clinic, NSAIDs and glucocorticoids are often used. NSAIDs such as indometacin, ibuprofen, and diclofenac produce side effects such as serious gastrointestinal tract impairment and bone depression, as well as liver and kidney toxicity. Glucocorticoids can rapidly relieve the clinical symptoms, but they can neither slow the progression of the disease nor reverse bone destruction, and their long-term use can induce osteoporosis, diabetes mellitus, and decreased immunity. Therefore, glucocorticoids are not suitable for long-term use. To reduce the dose of NSAIDs, Chinese medicinals such as insect or vine medicinals can be added to track down and remove wind from the collaterals and relieve pain. If NSAIDs are used, a proton pump inhibitor should be prescribed to protect the stomach, or Chinese medicinals that fortify the spleen and harmonize the stomach can be administered along with the other medicinals.

RA is a systemic autoimmune disease. However, in the end, it manifests as local pathological changes of the joints. Chinese medicine holds that the articular pain is due to external evils lingering in the collaterals and vessels, which, over time, impede the circulation of qi and blood and produce phlegm-turbidity and blood stasis, giving rise to obstruction of the channels and collaterals and hence pain. Apart from internal medicinal treatment, external treatment can also be employed to treat RA. Clinical research shows that the integration of internal and external treatment can enhance the effects of relieving pain, dispersing swelling, and improving articular function. Chinese medicine offers highly effective external treatment modalities such as acupuncture, moxibustion, massage, tui na, external application of medicinals, and bee acupuncture.

2. Early Application of Slow-acting Drugs (Combined with Chinese Medicinals to Reduce Side Effects)

DMARDs (disease-modifying anti-rheumatic drugs) act slower than NSAIDs. Generally, it requires at least 2-3 months or, in most cases, up to half a year to exert their effects. This category of drugs has no analgesic or anti-inflammatory effects, and it produces side effects such as impairment of liver and kidney function or bone marrow depression. Clinical experiments indicate that DMARDs can improve the disease condition and slow its progression. Therefore, according to the biomedical treatment principles, most RA patients should be treated with a combination of slow-acting drugs as early as possible. To reduce their the side effects, *Liù Wèi Dì Huáng Wán* (六味地黄丸) or medicinals that tonify the kidney and invigorate blood can be prescribed (according to pattern differentiation). Vascular proliferation accompanied by pannus formation is a predominant characteristic of RA synovitis. Patients may also develop an accumulation of complementary compound particles, which induce the cells to release various types of protease that activates blood clotting. Rheumatoid factor complexes also form a viscous aggregate, often accompanied by an increased platelet count. Deposits of fibrin and fibrinogen in the synovium are the main cause of chronic synovitis and fibrosis. Suppression of fiber coagulation and promotion of fiber dissolution can stop the progression of RA synovitis. Studies have proved that Chinese medicinals that invigorate blood and transform stasis can strengthen fiber dissolution. In addition, the large number of free radicals in RA joint cavities promote the infestation of cartilage and sclerotin. Many medicinals that invigorate blood, transform stasis, and tonify the kidney can remove free radicals, and thus they are useful in the treatment of RA. These medicinals can also increase the therapeutic effects of tripterygium glycosides and methotrexate, as well as reduce their toxicity.

3. Use Hormones with Caution (Chinese Medicinals can counteract the Misuse or Abuse of Hormone Therapy)

Glucocorticoids have a powerful anti-inflammatory effect, and can rapidly reduce joint pain and swelling. For acute attacks or for severe cases affecting the heart, lungs, eyes, and nervous system, glucocorticoids can be administered in doses that correspond to the severity of the illness. Long-term use of glucocorticoids can lead to many serious side effects. There are still controversies regarding the use of low-dose glucocorticoid therapy in the rheumatology field. We believe that most RA patients should limit or avoid the use of glucocorticoids because they have a tendency to cause yin deficiency. Patients that misuse or abuse the use of glucocorticoids should gradually decrease the dose (not suddenly). When yin deficiency arises, prescribe *Liù Wèi Dì Huáng Wán* (六味地黄丸) to clear heat and nourish yin.

In addition, among the new medicinals used for treating RA, some biological agents approved by the Food and Drug Administration Bureau of the United States are quick-acting and produce few side effects with no general immunosuppression. However, biological agents also have their disadvantages, i.e., non-oral route of administration, transfusion-related toxic reaction, immunogenicity-related rapid tolerance in few cases, and high cost. Furthermore, biological agents are not effective for all cases of RA, and they cannot cure RA. After discontinuing their use, RA can still recur. Studies have shown that some patients who did not respond to the biological agents initially can obtain partial relief by taking the biological agents together with medicinals that tonify the kidney and invigorate blood.

Challenges and Solutions

RA is a stubborn disease that is difficult to treat. Although it mainly presents with articular symptoms, it is frequently complicated by other systemic or organ diseases. The manifestations are varied among patients. The development of the illness primarily takes the form of progression, and few cases actually show reversal. It is difficult to effectively treat the disease with one therapeutic regimen, and the efficacy of long-term combination therapy is uncertain. At the same time, a certain number of patients withdraw from the drugs because of intolerance to their side effects.

Challenge 1: How to Diagnose the Disease as Early as Possible

To form a diagnosis early on and administer prompt treatment has been the focus of research all over the world. Since single or nonsymmetrical arthritis involving the big joints with possible RF (-) do not meet the standards of the diagnostic criteria of RA, and the joint symptoms (including joint destruction) get progressively worse, early diagnosis appears to be even more important. It is not difficult to diagnose typical cases based on the classification criteria set forth by the ARA (American Rheumatism Association). In the early stage of RA, when there are slight and atypical symptoms, correct diagnosis depends on the doctor's vigilance and ability to differentiate, the necessary lab tests (i.e., RA-related antibodies, autoimmune antibodies, and radiological tests), and the objective analysis of these tests. It is easy to make a wrong diagnosis when there are symptoms of the internal organs or systems without any disease involvement of the small joints of the hands and no clear-cut clues from joint X-rays. CT, MRI, synovial biopsy, synovianalysis, and/or seroimmunity tests can be performed if necessary. Joint puncture for synovial fluid tests and biopsy under the arthroscope are both helpful to the diagnosis of atypical arthritis. Despite this, sensitive and specific methods have not yet been found for an early diagnosis of RA. Doctors should closely monitor RA patients and take corresponding measures to treat the manifestations of the disease. Correct diagnosis is the key to providing appropriate treatment.

Although RA falls under the category of *bi* syndromes, it is different from general *bi* syndromes. It is caused by wind cold damp lingering in the liver and kidney and invading the sinews and bones, and therefore requires special medicinals and treatment strategies. Diagnosis of early stage RA mainly depends on the combination of complaints, signs, laboratory results and radiology tests.

Challenge 2: How to Promptly Control the Symptoms

Prompt management of the symptoms and rapid alleviation of the patients' suffering are beneficial to ameliorating the illness and strengthening therapeutic effects. In Chinese medical treatment of RA, the principle of tonifying the kidney and dispersing cold is adopted.

Based on this principle, use the appropriate vine and insect medicinals to dispel wind, disperse cold, eliminate dampness, and transform phlegm and stasis. Morning stiffness is the first symptom in RA patients, and occurs even before joint pain. Morning stiffness is equivalent to the concept of "spasms" or "rigidity" in classical texts of Chinese medicine. Morning stiffness refers to pronounced stiffness in the morning. The evils involved are cold-damp or damp-heat, phlegm, and stasis in the channels, collaterals, and joints that obstruct the circulation of qi and blood. During the night, the limbs are resting and thus the obstruction is aggravated, leading to pronounced stiffness upon awakening in the morning.

Use *chuān wū* (Radix Aconiti Praeparata), *gān jiāng* (Rhizoma Zingiberis), *táo rén* (Semen Persicae), *jiāng cán* (Bombyx Batryticatus), and *jiāng huáng* (Rhizoma Curcumae Longae) to disperse cold, transform dampness, and unblock the channels and collaterals. Internal medicinal therapy can be combined with external application and exercise. For symmetrical joint swelling and pain involving the metacarpophalangeal, wrist, shoulder, interphalangeal, ankle, and knee joints, or for redness, swelling, heat, and pain of the joints with decreased mobility, treatment is mainly focused on unblocking the collaterals, tonifying qi, and nourishing blood. According to the nature of the pain, it can be divided into categories of wind pain, cold pain, damp pain, heat pain, and stasis pain. Wind pain is wandering; dispel wind and unblock the collaterals with *dú huó* (Radix Angelicae Pubescentis), *qí shé* (Agkistrodon), and *hǎi fēng téng* (Caulis Piperis Kadsurae). Cold pain is aggravated by cold or by flexion and extension, and relieved by heat; warm the channels, disperse cold, and relieve spasms with hot herbs such as *chuān wū* (Radix Aconiti Praeparata), *cǎo wū* (Radix Aconiti Kusnezoffii Praeparata), *fù zǐ* (Radix Aconiti Lateralis), and *xì xīn* (Radix et Rhizoma Asari). Damp pain is represented by sensations of heaviness and numbness; fortify the spleen, transform dampness, and warm yang with the appropriate medicinals. Heat pain usually occurs during acute attacks of *bi* syndromes or in chronic illness where evils bind together and transform into heat. It is represented by reddening of the skin and swelling of the joints with hot pain that is relieved by cold. Accompanying signs and symptoms include fever, dry mouth, a yellow tongue coating, and a rapid pulse. Treat by clearing heat, dispersing swelling, and relieving pain. Stasis pain occurs during long-term and unresolved *bi* syndromes. It is represented by chronic joint pain with functional impairment, and is caused by the binding of evils with stasis in the channels and collaterals. Common medicinals may not have an effect on stasis pain. Use medicinals that can track down phlegm and stasis in the channels and collaterals, penetrate the bones, and eliminate phlegm and stasis, such as *wú gōng* (Scolopendra), *quán xiē* (Scorpio), *jiāng cán* (Bombyx Batryticatus), *dì biē chóng* (Eupolyphaga seu Steleophaga), and *tiān nán xīng* (Rhizoma Arisaematis). In reference to the pathomechanism of RA, tonification of the liver and kidney is a necessary and important part of the treatment strategy. *Dù zhòng* (Cortex Eucommiae), *xù duàn* (Radix Dipsaci), *sāng jì shēng* (Herba Taxilli), *bǔ gǔ zhī* (Fructus Psoraleae), *tù sī zǐ* (Semen Cuscutae), *xiān líng pí* (Herba Epimedii), and *gǒu jǐ* (Rhizoma Cibotii) can be selected according to the nature and location of the disease influence.

If at the time of the first visit, the disease has already caused damage to target organs, e.g., heart involvement, distal end vasculitis, skin ulcer, peripheral neuropathy, pericarditis, arteritis of internal organs such as the heart, lungs, intestinal tract, spleen, pancreas, kidneys, lymph nodes or testes, careful differentiation is required to determine if the pathogen is one of cold or heat, and of deficiency or excess. The chief contradiction of the illness is the target of treatment.

Challenge 3: How to Effectively Stop Progression

According to the latest EBM research, bone destruction in RA is most serious in the first 3 months. If diagnosis can be made during this stage followed by active therapy, the progression of the disease can be delayed to the point of stabilization or long-term remission. But how to achieve an early diagnosis is a big challenge to both Chinese medicine and biomedicine. Since there is no radical cure for RA, the goal of both Chinese medical and biomedical treatments is to prevent joint destruction, protect joint function, and improve the patients' life quality. The present biomedical treatment strategies and medication can barely improve the pathological changes of the sclerotin or reverse the disease progression to be of long-term use.

Chinese medicine believes that the kidney governs the bones and produces marrow (the kidney stores essence, which produces marrow). Marrow is stored in the bones to nourish the skeleton and promote its growth, development, and recovery. This is what the saying "the kidney governs the bones" refers to. Many Chinese medicinals that are beneficial to the kidney, e.g., *bǔ gǔ zhī* (Fructus Psoraleae), tonify the kidney, strengthen yang, and secure essence. Modern pharmacological studies have shown that the medicinal has estrogen-like effects. It can slow down bone metabolism and reduce bone loss to prevent and treat osteoporosis. *Gǔ suì bǔ* (Rhizoma Drynariae) can alter the function of chondrocytes, delay the development of degenerative bone diseases, and reduce the occurrence of bone disorders. Some studies show that *yín yáng huò* (Herba Epimedii) has a notable effect on strengthening the bones. It can promote DNA synthesis of bone marrow cells, promote bone growth, and increase bone density. Formulas that tonify the kidney, e.g., *Liù Wèi Dì Huáng Wán* (六味地黄丸) or *Yòu Guī Wán* (右归丸), can relieve the manifestations of secondary osteoporosis to some extent by: (1) regulating the metabolism of calcium and phosphate to increase the concentration of blood calcium, (2) increasing the regional BMD of the weight-bearing femur bone and lumbar vertebrae, and (3) increasing the weight-bearing capacity of bone. Chinese medicinals that tonify the kidney can prevent and treat osteoporosis possibly via the following mechanisms of action: regulating the metabolism of sex hormones, correcting ACH-induced hypocalcemia, increasing the calcium and phosphate content in the blood, preventing hypocalcemia-induced secondary hyperparathyroidism, and prohibiting the active factors (IL-1, IL-6) from absorbing bone. When comparing Chinese medicinals with Western pharmaceutical drugs during the course of half a year, studies show that the former is better than the latter in preventing bone destruction. Therefore, Chinese medicine can effectively prevent the progression of RA, and thus, should be used to its full potential.

Challenge 4: How to Prevent the Side Effects of Western Pharmaceutical Drugs

The combination of Western pharmaceutical drugs with Chinese medical pattern differentiation and treatment can facilitate the relief of RA symptoms and control the disease condition. Some adverse effects of the Western drugs can severely influence the management of RA, and under certain circumstances, the side effects may even exceed their therapeutic effects. For some underlying diseases such as digestive tract ulcer and anemia, the side effects may be serious. Thus, how to prevent the side effects of Western drugs is a problem that requires special attention.

Chinese medicinal therapy can reduce the adverse effects of the drugs, which include but are not limited to nausea, vomiting, and poor appetite. Long-term use of NSAIDs can easily induce symptoms of the digestive system, e.g., dyspepsia and digestive tract ulcer (digestive system symptoms occur in 10%-25% patients with long-term use of NSAIDs). Furthermore, it can lead to side effects of the nervous and vascular systems. Chinese medicine believes that the spleen and stomach are the root of acquired constitution, and are the source of qi and blood production. The essence of the kidney and the yin and blood of the liver all rely on the constant generation, ripening and transformation of the essence of water and grain. If the spleen and stomach are fortified, qi and blood are vigorous, the circulation of qi and blood is smooth, and nutritive and defensive qi are in harmony; there will be no place for the evil to stay. Moreover, the essence and blood of the kidney and liver will be vigorous, the sinews and bones will be well nourished and strong. If the spleen and stomach are impaired, food and medication cannot be absorbed. Therefore, protecting the spleen and stomach is an important point that cannot be ignored.

Rén shēn (Radix Ginseng), *dǎng shēn* (Radix Codonopsis), *huáng qí* (Radix Astragali), *bái zhú* (Rhizoma Atractylodis Macrocephalae), *fú líng* (Poria), *biǎn dòu* (Semen Lablab Album), *shān yào* (Rhizoma Dioscoreae), and *gān cǎo* (Radix et Rhizoma Glycyrrhizae) can tonify the spleen and stomach to reduce the side effects of Western pharmaceutical drugs. Modern studies indicate that these Chinese medicinals can improve the immune function to prevent and treat the illness by tonifying the spleen and stomach. Chinese medicinals that tonify qi and nourish blood, e.g., *dǎng shēn* (Radix Codonopsis), *dāng guī* (Radix Angelicae Sinensis), *ē jiāo* (Colla Corii Asini), and *shú dì huáng* (Radix Rehmanniae Praeparata) can significantly increase the body's resistance and detoxification function and improve the functioning of the vascular system (to raise the body's functional capacity), thereby counteracting DMARD-induced bone marrow depression. In addition, studies show that *shé chuáng zǐ* (Fructus Cnidii), *dōng chóng xià cǎo* (Cordyceps), *hé shǒu wū* (Radix Polygoni Multiflori), *rén shēn* (Radix Ginseng), *sān qī* (Radix et Rhizoma

Notoginseng), *nǚ zhēn zǐ* (Fructus Ligustri Lucidi), *lú sǔn* (Cacumen Asparagi), *lù róng* (Cornu Cervi Pantotrichum), *gé jiè* (Gecko), *ē jiāo* (Colla Corii Asini), *lóng yǎn ròu* (Arillus Longan), the polysaccharides of *huái shān yào* (Rhizoma Dioscoreae), tea polysaccharides, β- carotene, the total flavonoids of the stem and leaf of *mó jiá huáng qí* (Astragalus Membranaceus), polysaccharides of *xī yáng shēn* (Radix Panacis Quinquefolii), and the polysaccharides of *gǒu qǐ zǐ* (Fructus Lycii) can all enhance immune function. More importantly, Chinese medicinals can not only reduce the side effects of Western drugs, but can also increase the therapeutic effect, relieve the patients' suffering, and reduce the necessary dose of Western drugs (especially hormones).

Insight from Empirical Wisdom

1. Understanding the Characteristics of the Disease, Accurately Identifying the Pattern, and Sticking to Medicinal Therapy

The core of Chinese medical treatment of RA is pattern differentiation. Clinically, the disease can be divided into 3 stages: early, middle, and late. In the early stage, the evil is in the superficial aspect of the body, and primarily manifests as signs and symptoms of excess evil. In the middle stage, the disease condition is prolonged and manifests as a deficiency-excess complex. In the late stage, the evil is in the interior aspect of the body, and primarily manifests as either right qi deficiency or right qi deficiency with abiding evil. In all three stages, the condition may alternate between periods of attack and relief. Generally speaking, after treatment during acute attacks, the condition shifts into remission and is relatively stable, or the joints may be deformed but without pain, swelling, or obvious signs of cold and heat, which makes pattern differentiation difficult. The illness is caused by the combination of internal and external evils, with right qi deficiency as the underlying root cause and excess evil as the resulting branch manifestation. Right qi deficiency first manifests as liver and kidney depletion, and over time, the internal generation of phlegm-turbidity and static blood forms the basis of the disease onset. The external evils involved are mainly cold combined with wind and damp. Long-term phlegm-damp obstruction in the joints causes swelling. Phlegm-damp and stasis stagnation in the channels and vessels causes joint enlargement and deformity. Phlegm-damp and phlegm constraint in the skin causes heavy, cumbersome limbs with puffy swelling (superficial edema). In chronic illness, the evils enter the interior, shifting the condition from mild to severe. Static blood obstructs the channels and collaterals. Phlegm-turbidity binds together with static blood and causes the illness to be prolonged and difficult to treat. Treatment, therefore, becomes much more troublesome, since the condition may give rise to other syndromes that further complicate the original disease, and lead to joint deformity and local disability. In this case, careful pattern differentiation is required to identify the cause of the complex signs and symptoms and plan the appropriate treatment strategy.

In the early and middle stages, excess evils are the main manifestation. To dispel the evils, use the methods of coursing wind, dispersing cold, clearing heat, draining dampness, moving qi, and invigorating blood. In the late stage, there are excess evils with right qi deficiency. To treat this stage, support the right qi and dispel the evils by regulating and tonifying the liver and kidney, boosting qi, and invigorating blood.

RA is a chronic and difficult-to-treat disease. Even when the condition is stabilized, Chinese medicinals or patent medicine should be taken to regulate yin, yang, qi and blood, expel the lingering evils, prolong stabilization, and reduce the rate of relapse. One medicinal formula that supports right qi and treats the root, and one patent formula that dispels wind-damp are commonly chosen. Particularly in the case of lame *bi*, which has a long and severe course, it is necessary to stick with long-term medicinal therapy in order to see improvement. Do not be too quick to change the formula frequently. Provided there are no adverse effects, a formula based on accurate pattern differentiation requires 50-100 daily doses to produce noticeable therapeutic effects. After long-term administration of medicinal therapy, if the disease shows significant improvement (most of the symptoms are relieved), modify the formula accordingly, then grind all the ingredients into a powder and take them with warm water or yellow rice wine, twice a day over a long period of time, to consolidate the treatment effects.

2. Tonify the Kidney, Disperse Cold, Transform Stasis, and Eliminate Phlegm Throughout the Entire Course of the Disease

Judging from its pathogenesis, clinical characteristics, and progression, lame *bi* is considered more complex and serious than other common wind cold damp *bi* syndromes. Wind cold damp evils, particularly cold and dampness, deeply invade the kidney and affect the liver, causing bone damage and sinew spasms. The long-term stagnation of evils transforms into heat and makes the condition more complicated. Wind, cold, dampness, and heat lingering in the channels and collaterals eventually lead to the generation of stasis, phlegm, and turbidity, which penetrate deep into the bones and sinews and cause joint stiffness and deformity. Cold and dampness entering the kidney and affecting the liver is the difference between lame *bi* and other *bi* syndromes, and therefore the treatment principle is to tonify the kidney, disperse cold, transform dampness, course wind, invigorate stasis, unblock the collaterals, and strengthen the sinews and bones. The kidney's functions of governing the bones and engendering marrow have a close connection with the modern medical concept of immunology, since it plays an important role in maintaining immunological homeostasis. The kidney is the viscus of water and fire; it stores true yin and houses original yang. Tonifying the kidney not only nourishes essence, engenders marrow, and strengthens the bones, but also makes qi and blood plentiful; it not only enriches and nourishes congenital essence to promote the growth and development, but also improves the absorption and transformation of acquired essence.

3. Choose Appropriate Vine and Insect Medicinals to Strengthen the Effects of Tracking Down Wind and Scraping Evils from the Collaterals

RA is a serious disease. Its prolonged disease course leads to the obstruction of the channels and collaterals by static blood and phlegm-turbidity, which congeal together and are difficult to disperse. Treatment requires strong vine and insect medicinals to track down wind and scrape the collaterals. The commonly used medicinals are as follows:

(1) Vine Medicinals

Most of these medicinals have the effects of unblocking the channels, quickening the collaterals, soothing the sinews, and relieving pain. After identifying the correct pattern, choose one or two vine medicinals based on their properties, the channels that the medicinals enter, and their indications. These medicinals act as envoys to the corresponding channels and reach the location of the disease, thereby increasing the therapeutic effect. Vine medicinals are light and quick. They can easily unblock the joints and reach the four limbs. Medicinals in this category include *luò shí téng* (Caulis Trachelospermi), *rěn dōng téng* (Caulis Lonicerae Japonicae), *hǎi fēng téng* (Caulis Piperis Kadsurae), and *shí nán téng* (Caulis Photiniae). *Rěn dōng téng* (Caulis Lonicerae Japonicae) is an ideal herb for treating acute RA, particularly in cases of hot, red joints with inhibited bending and stretching; as long as there are heat signs, it can be used, regardless of deficiency or excess. *Luò shí téng* (Caulis Trachelospermi) is commonly used for wind damp heat *bi*; it is especially effective for unblocking the joints, relieving pain, soothing the sinews, and alleviating spasms. It can also unblock the collaterals and is suitable for treating wind-damp *bi* of the liver and kidney. *Hăi fēng téng* (Caulis Piperis Kadsurae) excels at expelling wind from the collaterals to relieve wandering pain. It is commonly used to treat wind-damp *bi* that presents with aching pain and spasms of the sinews. Among the vine medicinals, *jī xuè téng* (Caulis Spatholobi) is the only one that can tonify and invigorate blood, dispel wind and resolve toxins, and disperse swelling and relieve pain; thus it is suitable for treating cold, heat, deficiency, and excess patterns of all types of *bi* syndromes.

(2) Insect Medicinals

This category of medicinals can track down wind and scrape them from the collaterals. Ye Tian-shi of the Qing dynasty said, "Those that fly ascend, and those that walk descend. Blood is not congealed, qi can perfuse normally. No other medicinals are more effective than insect medicinals for tracking down and expelling evils from the channels and collaterals to treat wind, dampness, phlegm, and stasis." (俾飞者升，走者降，血无凝者，气可宣通，搜剔经络之风湿痰瘀莫如虫类。) Insect medicinals can be divided into 3 groups, according to their properties: 1) those that warm yang, dispel wind, and unblock the collaterals, e.g., *wū shāo shé* (Zaocys), *bái huā shé* (Agkistrodon), *quán xiē* (Scorpio), *wú gōng* (Scolopendra), and *fēng fáng* (Nidus Vespae); 2) those that clear heat, dispel wind, and unblock the collaterals, e.g., *dì lóng* (Pheretima) and *jiāng cán* (Bombyx Batryticatus); 3) those that break stasis and expel phlegm, e.g., *dì biē chóng* (Eupolyphaga seu Steleophaga), *chuān shān jiă* (Squama Manis), *méng chóng* (Tabanus), and *shuĭ zhì* (Hirudo). The clinical integration of the properties of different categories of medicinals are applied according to pattern differentiation. For example, *wú gōng* (Scolopendra) is quick-acting and excels at tracking down wind and scraping it from the collaterals; *quán xiē* (Scorpio) is good at treating wind phlegm, dispelling cold, and breaking stasis; and *jiāng cán* (Bombyx Batryticatus) can treat morning stiffness and severe joint swelling. However, insect medicinals are usually toxic, and thus their long-term use has the tendency to break qi and consume blood. Only 1 or 2 different insect medicinals should be used at a time, in appropriate dosages. Use *yù zhú* (Rhizoma Polygonati Odorati) and *huái shān yào* (Rhizoma Dioscoreae) to prevent the impairment of yin and enhance the effect of tracking down and expelling evils.

Chinese medicine holds that a certain medicinal can affect one or several channels and has little or even no effect on other channels; this is called channel tropism, or channel entry (归经; *guī jīng*). In clinical application, if the *bi* is located in the upper limbs, add *jiāng huáng* (Rhizoma Curcumae Longae), *guì zhī* (Ramulus Cinnamomi), and *sāng zhī* (Ramulus Mori); if the *bi* is in the lower limbs, add *huái niú xī* (Radix Achyranthis Bidentatae), *fáng jǐ* (Radix Stephaniae Tetrandrae), *mù guā* (Fructus Chaenomelis), and *dú huó* (Radix Angelicae Pubescentis); for back pain, use *gé gēn* (Radix Puerariae Lobatae) or *lù jiǎo jiāo* (Colla Cornus Cervi); for lumbar pain, add *shú dì huáng* (Radix Rehmanniae Praeparata), *dù zhòng* (Cortex Eucommiae), *xù duàn* (Radix Dipsaci), *gǒu jǐ* (Rhizoma Cibotii), *gǒu qǐ zǐ* (Fructus Lycii), *nǚ zhēn zǐ* (Fructus Ligustri Lucidi), and *hú táo ròu* (Semen Juglandis). These envoys guide the actions of the medicinals directly to the disease location, thereby strengthening the treatment effect.

4. Protect the Right Qi at All Times to Reduce the Risk of External Evil Invasion

Modern researchers believe that the onset of RA may be due to an "activated chain reaction" initiated by certain antigens. Infection and autoimmune reactions are the key factors of the onset and progression of

RA, while other factors (i.e., endocrine, hereditary, and environmental) increase one's susceptibility to the disease. The onset and progression of RA are also connected to external environmental factors (cold, dampness, excessive physical labor, trauma, infection, and malnutrition) as well as to constitutional deficiencies due to hereditary, autoimmune, and endocrine factors. Chinese medicine considers the cause of lame *bi* to be congenital deficiency and right qi deficiency combined with the invasion of wind, cold, dampness, and/or heat. The evils linger in the muscles, joints, and channels and collaterals, and impair the flow of qi and blood. Over time, they damage the liver and kidney and weaken the sinews and bones, thereby inducing the onset of RA. Only strong right qi can resist the invasion of external evils or prevent the condition from getting worse. Protecting the right qi is an important part of the treatment and prevention of RA.

The following suggestions should be heeded:

(1) Diet

There are no dietary restraints and food preferences required. Certain foods should be limited, but there is no need to abstain from them. Eat foods that are nutritious (contain vitamins and protein). Avoid alcohol and coffee. Refrain from smoking and avoid second-hand smoke. Alcohol, coffee, and smoking can aggravate the arthritis.

(2) Living Environment

The living space should face the sun and should be well ventilated, dry, and fresh. The bed should be clean and flat. Patients should try to stay warm and avoid cold drafts, as well as wear clothes that are appropriate to the different seasons and climates. In the case of acute attacks, patients should rest an additional 2 weeks after most of the objective and subjective symptoms are relieved. Afterwards, physical exercise can be gradually increased. It is also beneficial to establish a daily exercise routine.

(3) Emotional Health

Ancient physicians realized the close connection between mental activity and illness. Modern studies show that psychological stress lead to disorders of the endocrine and immune systems. The emotions have a direct relationship with the development of many diseases. Patients should try to be optimistic and cooperate with their healthcare providers by maintaining compliance with the treatment.

5. Refer the Patient to Biomedical Care if Necessary

If any of the following conditions occur, refer the patient to biomedical care:

(1) Acute and severe attacks involving multiple joints accompanied by a high titer of RF, bone destruction, or severe systemic symptoms such as fever, anemia, and fatigue.

(2) Severe complications such as pericardial effusion, severe eye disorders, cerebrovascular disease leading to disorders of the central nervous system, severe anemia, recurrent fever, joint pain and swelling, and a greatly elevated ESR.

(3) In the case of severe joint deformity and bone destruction up to 3-4 degrees (as confirmed by radiological examination), surgery for joint replacement or removal of the synovial membrane is necessary.

Summary

Rheumatoid arthritis is a chronic, progressive autoimmune disease. In biomedicine, the etiology of RA is still unclear, and thus there is no efficient therapy aiming at the "onset factor" of the disease. The current first-line, second-line, third-line, and immunoregulating drugs can only treat the clinical manifestations during the various stages of the disease course, reduce patient suffering, and treat concurrent diseases and complications. They cannot control the disease as a whole, and they invariably have certain (and sometimes severe) side effects.

Of the Western pharmaceutical drugs, NSAIDs, slow-acting antirheumatic medication, glucocorticoids, and biological agents can be selected. Western pharmaceuticals are apparently more effective for relieving pain and improving clinical symptoms. However, severe side effects adversely affect the management of rheumatoid arthritis, and under some circumstances, particularly in patients with concurrent underlying diseases, the side effects are much greater than the benefits.

The treatment of RA with Chinese medicine is based on pattern differentiation. Chinese medicine has a long history of preventing the onset of *bi* syndromes; certain formulas have been adopted for certain patterns, and emphasis has been placed on holism. Chinese medicine has the advantages of actively relieving suffering, preventing recurrent attacks, prolonging remission, and strengthening resistance to disease. Early prevention and treatment are also stressed in order to protect joint function and prevent bone destruction and deformity.

When the therapeutic effects of Western pharmaceutical drugs on RA turn out to be less than ideal, we can utilize Chinese medical therapies (i.e., Chinese medicinals, acupuncture, massage, and medicinal steams and washes). The integration of Chinese medicine and biomedicine can be applied when necessary to make up for each other's shortcomings, thereby increasing the clinical efficacy and improving patients' quality of life. If there are any serious complications such as hydropericardium, nephrotic syndrome, CVD, or severe deformity which calls for plastic surgery, refer the patient immediately to the appropriate specialist.

SELECTED QUOTES FROM CLASSICAL TEXTS

Yellow Emperor's Inner Classic: Basic Questions - Treatise on *Bi* Syndromes (黄帝内经素问 · 痹论篇 , *Huáng Dì Nèi Jīng Sù Wèn - Bì Lùn Piān*):

"风寒湿三气杂至，合而为痹也。其风气胜者行痹，寒气胜者为痛痹，湿气胜者为着痹。"

"The three evils, i.e., wind, cold, and dampness, combine and form *bi*. When wind is predominant, it is called moving *bi*; when cold is predominant, it is called painful *bi*; when dampness is predominant, it is called fixed *bi*."

"以冬遇此者为骨痹，以春遇此者为筋痹，以夏遇此者为脉痹，以至阴遇此者为肌痹，以秋遇此者为皮痹。"

"If it is encountered in the winter, it is called bone *bi*; if it is encountered in the spring, it is called sinew *bi*; if it is encountered in the summer, it is called vessel *bi*; if it is encountered during late summer, it is called flesh *bi*; if it is encountered in the autumn, it is called skin *bi*."

"五藏皆有合，病久而不去者，内舍于其合也。故骨痹不已，复感于邪，内舍于肾……所谓痹者，各以其时重感于风寒湿之气也。"

"The five viscera all have their connections [referring to the exterior-interior relationship with the five body constituents]. Chronic and unresolved disease [evil] will linger in these connections. Thus, if bone *bi* is not treated, repeated contraction of evils will enter the body and reside in the kidney…That which is called *bi*, is the repeated contraction of wind, cold, and damp evil."

"其风气胜者，其人易已也。"

"If wind evil is predominant, the patient can easily recover."

"其入藏者死，其留连筋骨间者疼久，其留皮肤间者易已。"

"When the evils enter the viscera, the disease is fatal; when the evils linger in the sinews and bones, there will be chronic pain; when the evils invade the skin, the disease is easy to treat."

“痹……痛者，寒气多也，有寒故痛也。其不痛不仁者，病久入深，营卫之行涩，经络时疏，故不痛，皮肤不营，故为不仁。其寒者，阳气少，阴气多，与病相益，故寒也；其热者，阳气多，阴气少，病气胜阳乘阴，故为痹热，其多汗而濡者，此其逢湿甚也，阳气少，阴气盛，两气相感，故汗出而濡也。”

“The pain of *bi* syndrome is usually caused by cold. In those with numbness but no pain, the evils have entered deep into the body, the flow of nutritive and defensive qi are rough, and the channels and collaterals are obstructed; yet, there is no pain. The skin is not nourished, hence there is numbness. The cold *bi* is due to decreased yang and increased yin, which further aggravates the condition. In heat *bi*, there is increased yang and decreased yin; heat evil dominates in this condition, and yang subjugates yin, giving rise to heat *bi*. Profuse sweating and a soft pulse is due to decreased yang, increased yin and prevalence of dampness evil.”

Yellow Emperor's Inner Classic: Basic Questions - Treatise on Needling Joints (素问 · 长刺节论 , *Sù Wèn - Cháng Cì Jié Lùn*):

“病有筋，筋挛节痛，不可以行，名曰筋痹。……病在肌肤，肌肤尽痛，名曰肌痹，……病在骨，骨重不可举，骨髓酸痛，寒气至，名曰骨痹。”

“If the disease involves the sinews, there is hypertonicity of the sinews with joint pain and inability to walk; this is called sinew *bi*…if the disease is in the skin and flesh, there is generalized pain of the skin and flesh; this is called flesh *bi*…if the disease is in the bones, there is heaviness of the bones with inability to lift, and soreness of the bone and marrow upon exposure to cold; this is called bone *bi*.”

Prescriptions of Essentials from the Golden Cabinet - The Pulse, Patterns, and Treatment of Wind Strike and Joint-running Wind (金匮要略方论 · 中风历节病脉证并治 , *Jīn Guì Yào Lüè Fāng Lùn - Zhòng Fēng Lì Jié Bìng Mài Zhèng Bìng Zhì*):

“营气不通，卫不独行，营卫俱微，三焦无所御，四属断绝，身体羸瘦，独足肿大，黄汗出，胫冷。假令发热，便为历节也。”

“Impaired flow of the nutritive qi and defensive qi makes them both debilitated; the *san jiao* loses its resistance function, and the four limbs lose their nourishment, giving rise to a thin body, swollen feet, yellowish sweat, and a cold sensation in the lower legs. If accompanied by fever, this condition is called joint-running [disease].”

“病历节不可屈伸疼痛，乌头汤主之。”

"Those suffering from joint-running disease have pain and inability to bend and stretch; *Wū Tóu Tāng* (乌头汤) is indicated."

Prescriptions of Essentials from the Golden Cabinet - The Pulse, Patterns, and Treatment of Blood *Bi* and Deficiency Taxation (金匮要略方论 · 血痹虚劳病脉证并治 , *Jīn Guì Yào Lüè Fāng Lùn - Xuè Bì Xū Láo Bìng Mài Zhèng Bìng Zhì*):

“血痹……夫尊荣人 , 骨弱肌肤甚 , 重因疲劳汗出 , 卧不时动摇 , 加被微风 , 遂得之。”

“Blood *bi*…those of high with honor and prestige do little work, and thus their bones and flesh are very weak. When subjected to heavy labor, they become fatigued and sweaty; they will shake when lying down, and have aversion to mild wind even if covered with blankets; this is how they acquire this disease.”

“血痹，阴阳俱微，寸口关上微，尺中小紧，外证身体不仁，如风痹状，黄芪桂枝五物汤主之。”

"In blood *bi*, yin and yang are both debilitated, while the *guan* pulse is faint and *chi* pulse is slightly tight in the *cun kou* (radial pulse). External symptoms include numbness of the whole body which resembles that of wind *bi*. *Huáng Qí Guì Zhī Wǔ Wù Tāng* (黄芪桂枝五物汤) can treat this condition."

Central Treasury Canon, Treatise on *Bi* Syndromes (中藏经·论痹, *Zhōng Zàng Jīng, Lùn Bì*):

"痹者，风寒暑湿之气中于脏腑之为也。入腑则病浅易治，入脏腑则病深难治。"

"*Bi* is caused by invasion of the viscera and bowels by wind, cold, and dampness. If the evils enter the bowels, the disease is superficial and easy to treat; if the evils enter the viscera, the disease is deep and hard to treat."

Teachings of Zhu Dan-xi - Painful Wind and Pain in the Joints of the Limbs (丹溪心法·痛风附肢节痛, *Dān Xī Xīn Fǎ - Tòng Fēng Fù Zhī Jié Tòng*):

"四肢关节走痛是也，他方谓之白虎历节风证。大率有病、风热、风湿、血虚。因于风者，小续命汤。因于湿者，苍术、白术之类，佐以竹沥。因于痰者，二陈汤加酒炒黄芩，羌活、苍术。因于血虚者，用芎、归之类，佐以红花，桃仁。大法之方，苍术、川芎、白芷、南星、当归、酒黄芩。在上者，加羌活、威灵仙、桂枝；在下者，加牛膝、防己、木通、黄柏。血虚，《格致余论》评言，多用川芎、当归、佐以桃仁、红花、薄桂、威灵仙。"

"Wandering pain in the joints of the four limbs is called white tiger joint-running wind syndrome. The disease is usually due to wind-heat, wind-damp, and blood deficiency. If the disease is caused by wind, use *Xiǎo Xù Mìng Tāng* (小续命汤). If it is caused by dampness, use medicinals like *cāng zhú* (Rhizoma Atractylodis) and *bái zhú* (Rhizoma Atractylodis Macrocephalae), assisted by *zhú lì* (Succus Bambusae). If it is caused by phlegm, use *Èr Chén Tāng* (二陈汤) plus *huáng qín* (Radix Scutellariae), *qiāng huó* (Rhizoma et Radix Notopterygii), and *cāng zhú* (Rhizoma Atractylodis). If it is caused by blood deficiency, use medicinals like *chuān xiōng* (Rhizoma Chuanxiong) and *dāng guī* (Radix Angelicae Sinensis), assisted by *hóng huā* (Flos Carthami) and *táo rén* (Semen

Persicae). The main formula consists of *cāng zhú* (Rhizoma Atractylodis), *chuān xiōng* (Rhizoma Chuanxiong), *bái zhǐ* (Radix Angelicae Dahuricae), *nán xīng* (Rhizoma Arisaematis), *dāng guī* (Radix Angelicae Sinensis), and *huáng qín* (Radix Scutellariae). If the disease affects the upper body, add *qiāng huó* (Rhizoma et Radix Notopterygii), *wēi líng xiān* (Radix et Rhizoma Clematidis), and *guì zhī* (Ramulus Cinnamomi); if it affects the lower body, add *huái niú xī* (Radix Achyranthis Bidentatae), *fáng jǐ* (Radix Stephaniae Tetrandrae), *mù tōng* (Caulis Akebiae), and *huáng bǎi* (Cortex Phellodendri Chinensis). For blood deficiency, use *chuān xiōng* (Rhizoma Chuanxiong) and *dāng guī* (Radix Angelicae Sinensis), aided by *táo rén* (Semen Persicae), *hóng huā* (Flos Carthami), *bó guì* ([thin] Ramulus Cinnamomi), and *wēi líng xiān* (Radix et Rhizoma Clematidis)."

"瘦人肢节痛，是血虚，宜四物加防风、羌活。"

"Limb pain in a thin body is caused by blood deficiency; use *Sì Wù Tāng* (四物汤) plus *fáng fēng* (Radix Saposhnikoviae) and *qiāng huó* (Rhizoma et Radix Notopterygii)."

Medical Principles (医学统旨, *Yī Xué Tǒng Zhǐ*):

"热痹者脏腑移热，复遇外邪，客搏经络，留而不行，阳遭其阴，故瘅痹熻然而闷，肌肉热极，体上如鼠走样状，唇口反裂。皮肤色变，宜升麻汤。"

"In heat *bi*, the heat spreads to the *zang-fu*. Repeated contraction of external evils linger in the channels and collaterals while yang and yin fight with each other, resulting in the burning of lame *bi*. The flesh feels extremely hot, as if a mouse is crawling on the skin; the lips and mouth become cracked; and the skin changes color. *Shēng Má Tāng* (升麻汤) is appropriate for this condition."

Indispensable Tools for Pattern Treatment - Moving *Bi* (证治准绳·行痹, *Zhèng Zhì Zhǔn Shéng - Xíng Bì*):

"骨碎补丸，治走注疼痛。骨碎补一两半，威灵仙、草乌头（炒）各一两，天南星（姜制）、木鳖子（去壳）、枫香脂（另研）、自然铜（醋淬）、地龙（去土炒）各一两，没药（另研）、乳香（另研）各半两。上为细末，同研合匀，醋煮面糊为丸如梧子大。每服五丸，加玉十丸，用温酒下，不拘时候，日进二服。”

"*Gŭ Suì Bŭ Wán*（骨碎补丸）treats traveling influx pain. The formula consists of *gŭ suì bŭ* (Rhizoma Drynariae) 45g, *wēi líng xiān* (Radix et Rhizoma Clematidis) 30g, *chăo căo wū tóu* (dry-fried Radix Aconiti Kusnezoffii) 30g, *jiāng zhì tiān nán xīng* (Rhizoma Arisaematis, processed with ginger) 30g, *mù biē zĭ* (Semen Momordicae, hulled) 30g, *fēng xiāng zhĭ* (Resina Ferulae, ground separately) 30g, *zì rán tóng* (Pyritum, dipped in vinegar) 30g, *chăo dì lóng* (dry-fried Pheretima) 30g, *mò yào* (Myrrha, ground separately) 15g, and *rŭ xiāng* (Olibanum, ground separately) 15g. The above medicinals are ground into a fine powder and mixed together, then decocted with vinegar and mixed with flour and water paste to form pills the size of parasol seeds. For each dose, take 5 pills with *Yù Shí Wán*（玉十丸）and warm wine, any time. Take twice a day."

Collected Treatises of Zhang Jing-yue, Wind *Bi*（景岳全书·风痹，*Jĭng Yuè Quán Shū, Fēng Bì*):

“观《痹论》曰：风寒湿三气杂至，合而为痹。而《寿夭刚柔篇》又曰：在阳者命曰风，在阴者命曰痹。何也？盖三气之合，乃专言痹证之所固也。曰在阳为风，在阴为痹，又分言表里之有殊也。……若既受寒邪而初无发热头痛，及延绵久不能愈，而外无表证之见者，是皆无形之谓。此以阴邪直在阴分，即诸痹之属也，故病在阴者命曰痹。其或既有表证，而疼痛又不能愈，此即平表平里，阴阳俱病之证，故阴阳俱命曰风痹。此所以风病在阳，而痹病在阴也。然则诸痹者皆在阴分，亦总由真阳衰弱，精血亏损，故三气得以乘之，而为此诸症。经曰：邪入于阴则痹，正谓此也，是以治痹之法，最宜峻补真阴，使血气流行，则寒邪随去。若过用风湿痰滞等药，而再伤阴气，必反增其病矣。”

"*Yellow Emperor's Inner Classic: Basic Questions*, Treatise on *Bi*

Syndromes (黄帝内经素问 · 痹论篇, *Huáng Dì Nèi Jīng Sù Wèn, Bì Lùn*) mentions: 'The three evils, i.e., wind, cold, and dampness, combine and form *bi*.' *Yellow Emperor's Inner Classic: Divine Pivot - Treatise on Length of Life and Toughness and Softness* (黄帝内经灵枢 · 寿夭刚柔篇, *Huáng Dì Nèi Jīng Líng Shū - Shòu Yāo Gāng Róu Piān*) states: 'if the evil is in the yang aspect of the body, the condition is called wind; if the evils lies in the yin aspect of the body, the condition is called *bi*.' Why? The combination of the three evils refers specifically to the *bi* pathogens, and distinguishing the evils as being in the yang aspect or the yin aspect refers to the difference between exterior and interior conditions… If one contracts cold evil but does not exhibit the initial symptoms of fever or headache, and the course of illness is prolonged and without exterior signs and symptoms, this is due to yin evil directly entering the yin aspect of the body. The condition is called *bi*, since the evil is in the yin aspect of the body. If the condition exhibits exterior symptoms with unremitting pain, then the condition lies between the exterior and the interior, and both yin and yang are affected. Since the evil is in both the yin and yang aspects, the condition is then called wind *bi*. Thus, it has been established that wind disease is in the yang aspect, and *bi* disease is in the yin aspect. All *bi* syndromes are located in the yin aspect of the body; they are caused by deficiency of true yang and depletion of essence and blood, which allow the three evils to invade the body and become *bi*. The classics say: 'Evil entering the yin aspect causes *bi*,' and it is so. To treat *bi*, the most appropriate method is to drastically tonify true yin and allow qi and blood to flow smoothly; the cold evil will then leave the body. However, excessive use of medicinals that dispel wind-damp and phlegm stagnation will damage yin and qi, and further exacerbate the disease."

Collected Treatises of Zhang Jing-yue - Joint-running Wind Pain (景岳全书 · 历节风痛, *Jǐng Yuè Quán Shū - Lì Jié Fēng Tòng*):

“大都痛痹之证，多有昼轻而夜重者，正阴邪之在阴分也。其有遇风雨阴晦而甚者，此正阴邪侮阳主证也。或得暖遇热而甚者，此湿热伤阴之火证也。有火者宜从清凉，有寒者宜从温热。若筋脉拘滞，伸缩不利者，此血虚、血燥证也，非养血养气不可。”

"Painful *bi* is often mild during the day and severe at night; this is because yin evil is in the yin aspect during the night. If the disease is exacerbated by exposure to windy, rainy, and cloudy weather, it is a sign of yin evil rebelling against yang qi. If the disease is exacerbated by heat and warmth, it is a sign of damp-heat damaging the yin. If there is fire, use clearing and cooling methods; if there is cold, use warming and heating methods. If there is hypertonicity of the sinews with inhibited bending and stretching, this is due to blood deficiency and blood dryness; it is imperative to nourish blood and qi."

Ye's Selection of Medical Discussions - Discussion on the Analysis of Bi Syndromes (叶选医衡 · 痹证析微论 ,*Yè Xuǎn Yī Héng - Bì Zhèng Xī Wēi Lùn*):

“至于治痹之要，治行痹者散风为主，祛寒湿仍入可废，大抵参以治血之药，盖治风先治血，血行风自灭也。治痛痹者散寒为主，疏风燥湿仍不可缺，大抵参以补火之剂，非大辛大温不能释其凝寒为害也。治著痹者利湿为主，祛风解寒仍不可少，大抵参补脾补气之剂，盖土强可以制湿而气自足，自无顽麻也。然痹而因三气者治之宜然。若邪郁病久，风变为火，寒变为热，湿变为痰，即当易辄寻之，以降火清热豁痰为主，参以通经活血，流散邪滞之剂，安可全作正气治哉。”

“The treatment of *bi* is as follows: Moving *bi* is treated primarily by dispersing wind, in addition to dispelling cold-damp, and assisted by medicinals that invigorate blood, following the concept that in order to treat wind, first treat the blood and the wind will naturally be extinguished. The main treatment method for painful *bi* is to disperse cold, which must be combined with coursing wind and drying dampness. Generally speaking, formulas that tonify fire are used, because without highly acrid and highly warm medicinals, the damage induced by congealing cold cannot be resolved. The main treatment method for fixed *bi* is to drain dampness, which must be combined with dispelling wind and resolving cold. Generally, formulas that tonify the spleen and qi are used, because if Earth is strengthened, dampness is controlled, qi is naturally sufficient, and there is no stubborn numbness. These treatment principles are suitable for *bi* syndromes caused by the three evils. If the evils linger in the body for a long period of time, the wind transforms into fire, the cold transforms into heat, and the dampness transform into phlegm. The main treatment strategy is to downbear fire, clear heat, and sweep phlegm, assisted by formulas that unblock the collaterals, invigorate blood, and course and disperse evil stagnation, thereby treating the right qi."

The Essentials of Medicine According to the Masters - Wind Bi Atrophy (医学从众录 · 风痹痿 , *Yī Xué Cóng Zhòng Lù - Fēng Bì Wěi*):

"至久痛必入络，如木通，刺蒺藜、红花、金银花、钩藤之类最能通络，可随宜加入。久痛必挟郁，郁而成热，热盛则生痰，如南星、半夏、瓜蒌根、黄柏、郁金、川贝、竹沥、姜汁之类俱能解郁清热化痹，可随宜加入。多用桑枝，桑寄生及虎骨者，亦达支节及以骨治骨之义也。用乌附辛桂之药而不效者，宜用葳蕤、麦冬、桑叶、升麻、生黄芪、菊花、蒺藜、阿胶、甘草之类，为膏滋养阳明，亦是柔润熄肝风之法。"

"Enduring pain invariably enter the collaterals; add medicinals that are most effective for unblocking the collaterals, e.g., *mù tōng* (Caulis Akebiae), *cì jí lí* (Fructus Tribuli), *hóng huā* (Flos Carthami), *jīn yín huā* (Flos Lonicerae Japonicae), and *gōu téng* (Ramulus Uncariae Cum Uncis). Enduring pain is invariably complicated by constraint, and constraint transforms into heat; heat exuberance leads to the generation of phlegm. Add medicinals that resolve constraint, clear heat, and transform *bi*, e.g., *dǎn nán xīng* (Arisaema cum Bile), *bàn xià* (Rhizoma Pinelliae), *tiān huā fěn* (Radix Trichosanthis), *huáng bǎi* (Cortex Phellodendri Chinensis), *yù jīn* (Radix Curcumae), *chuān bèi mǔ* (Bulbus Fritillariae Cirrhosae), *zhú lì* (Succus Bambusae), and ginger juice. Use *sāng zhī* (Ramulus Mori), *sāng jì shēng* (Herba Taxilli), and *hǔ gǔ* (Os Tigris); they reach the joints and follow the principle of using bones to treat bones. If using *wū tóu* (Radix Aconiti), *fù zǐ* (Radix Aconiti Lateralis Praeparata), *xì xīn* (Radix et Rhizoma Asari), and *guì zhī* (Ramulus Cinnamomi) produce no effects, use *wēi ruí* (Rhizoma Polygonati Odorati), *mài dōng* (Radix Ophiopogonis), *sāng yè* (Folium Mori), *shēng má* (Rhizoma Cimicifugae), *shēng huáng qí* (raw Radix Astragali), *jú huā* (Flos Chrysanthemi), *jí lí* (Fructus Tribuli), *ē jiāo* (Colla Corii Asini), and *gān cǎo* (Radix et Rhizoma Glycyrrhizae) to nourish the yang and yin. This is applying the method of moistening the liver to extinguish wind."

Collected Writings of Medicine Organized by Category - Category of Bi Disease (医钞类编 · 痹病门 , *Yī Chāo Lèi Biān - Bì Bìng Mén*):

"治痹病当分新久之法。新痛为寒，宜辛温药；久痛属热，宜清凉药。河间所谓暴痛非热，久痛非寒是也。大法宜顺气清痰，搜风散湿，养血祛瘀为要。"

"To treat *bi* syndromes, one should differentiate between acute and chronic. Acute pain is attributed to cold, and requires acrid and warm medicinals. Chronic pain is attributed to heat, and requires heat-clearing and cool medicinals. Liu He-jian holds that sudden, violent pain is not caused by heat, and that chronic pain is not caused by cold. The main treatment principle is to normalize qi, clear phlegm, track down wind, disperse dampness, nourish blood, and dispel stasis."

Systematized Patterns with Clear-cut Treatments - Bi Syndromes (类证治裁 · 痹证 , *Lèi Zhèng Zhì Cái - Bì Zhèng*):

"……三痹各有所胜，用药以胜者为主，而兼者辅之，治行痹散风为主，兼祛寒利湿，参以补血，……防风汤。治痛痹温寒为主。兼疏风胜湿，参以益火。……加减五积散。治著痹利湿为主，兼祛风逐寒，参以补脾补气，……川芎茯苓汤加芪、术。其症有风湿，羌活胜湿汤、史公酒；有寒湿，苡仁汤、三痹汤。痹而身寒，为从水中出者，属寒湿，附子丸。有湿热，加味二妙散，苍术散。肩背沉重，肢节疼痛，下注足胫，属湿热，当归拈痛散。……有冷痹，风冷顽麻，巴戟天汤。有热痹，热毒流注骨节，《千金》犀角散。有营热，四物汤去川芎，加钩藤、丹皮。有营虚，当归建中汤。有卫虚，防己黄芪汤。有气痹，痹在气分，蠲痹汤。有血痹，痹在血分，因劳汗出，卧被风吹，血凝于肤，黄芪桂枝五物汤加当归。有瘀血，散血入络，桃红散煎成入麝香。有停痰，遍身走痛，二陈汤加羌活、白芥子、风化硝，姜汁泛丸。有支饮，臂痛不举，眩冒麻痹，指迷茯苓丸。有在经，木防己汤。有入络，活络饮加桑寄生、威灵仙，钩藤、牛膝、或活络丹。治法总以补助真元，宣通脉络，如活血丹合续断丹，或人参散之类，使气血流畅，则痛自已。”

"…For prevalence of any of the three types of *bi*, use the corresponding medicinals to treat the prevalence, in conjunction with assistant herbs. When treating moving *bi*, the main treatment principle is to dissipate wind, in conjunction with dispelling cold and draining dampness, assisted by tonifying the blood…use *Fáng Fēng Tāng* (防风汤). When treating painful *bi*, the main treatment principle is to warm the cold, in conjunction with coursing wind and overcoming dampness, and assisted by boosting Fire…use *Jiā Jiăn Wŭ Jī Săn* (加减五积散). When treating fixed *bi*, the main treatment principle is to drain dampness, in conjunction with dispelling wind and expelling cold, and assisted by tonifying the spleen and tonifying the qi…use *Chuān Xiōng Fú Líng Tāng* (川芎茯苓汤) plus *huáng qí* (Radix Astragali) and *bái zhú* (Rhizoma Atractylodis Macrocephalae). For wind-damp, use *Qiāng Huó Shèng Shī Tāng* (羌活胜湿汤) and *Shĭ Gōng Jiŭ* (史公酒). For cold-damp, use *Yĭ Rén Tāng* (苡仁汤) and *Sān Bì Tāng* (三痹汤). If the body is cold, as if one just emerged from water, this is attributed to cold-damp; use *Fù Zĭ Wán* (附子丸). For damp-heat, use *Jiā Wèi Èr Miào Săn* (加味二妙散) and *Cāng Zhú Săn* (苍术散). Heaviness of the shoulder and back with pain in the joints of the limbs that pours down to the lower legs and feet is attributed to damp-heat; use *Dāng Guī Niān Tòng Săn* (当归拈痛散)……For cold *bi*, use *Bā Jĭ Tiān Tāng* (巴戟天汤). For heat *bi*, use *Xī Jiăo Săn* (犀角散) of *Important Formulas Worth a Thousand Gold Pieces* (千金要方, *Qiān Jīn Yào Fāng*). For heat in the nutritive level, use *Sì Wù Tāng* (四物汤); remove *chuān xiōng* (Rhizoma Chuanxiong) and add *gōu téng* (Ramulus Uncariae Cum Uncis) and *dān pí* (Cortex Moutan). For nutritive qi deficiency, use *Dāng Guī Jiàn Zhōng Tāng* (当归建中汤). For defensive qi deficiency, use *Fáng Jĭ Huáng Qí Tāng* (防己黄芪汤). For qi *bi*, use *Juān Bì Tāng* (蠲痹汤). For blood *bi* caused by sweating after physical labor and then being exposed to wind when lying down, use *Huáng Qí Guì Zhī Wŭ Wù Tāng* (黄芪桂枝五物汤) plus *dāng guī* (Radix Angelicae Sinensis). For blood stasis entering the collaterals, use *Táo Hóng Săn* (桃红散) with *shè xiāng* (Moschus). For retention of phlegm with generalized wandering pain, use *Èr Chén Tāng* (二陈汤) plus *qiāng huó* (Rhizoma et Radix Notopterygii), *bái jiè zĭ* (Semen Sinapis), *fēng huà xiāo* (Natrii Sulfas Exsiccatus), and ginger juice. For propping rheum that manifests as arm pain with inability to lift the arm, veiling dizziness, and paralysis, use *Zhĭ Mí Fú Líng Wán* (指迷茯苓丸). For evils in the channels, use *Mù Fáng Jĭ Tāng* (木防己汤). For evils in the collaterals, use *Huó Luò Yĭn* (活络饮) plus *sāng jì shēng* (Herba Taxilli), *wēi líng xiān* (Radix et Rhizoma Clematidis), *gōu téng* (Ramulus Uncariae Cum Uncis), and *huái niú xī* (Radix Achyranthis Bidentatae), or *Huó Luò Dān* (活络丹). The treatment principle is to tonify and assist the true origin and diffuse and unblock the vessels and collaterals with formulas such as *Huó Luò Dān* (活络丹) combined with *Xù Duàn Dān* (续断丹), or *Rén Shēn Săn* (人参散), to promote the smooth flow of qi and blood, thereby allowing the pain to dissipate on its own."

MODERN RESEARCH

Clinical Research

1. Treatment Principles and Methods

(1) Tonify the Kidney and Invigorate Blood

Yu Jiang-di[1] used *lù jiăo piàn* (Cornu Cervi), *yín yáng huò* (Herba Epimedii), and *xiān máo* (Rhizoma Curculiginis) to tonify the kidney and regulate the autoimmune function; *sān qī* (Radix et Rhizoma Notoginseng), *dān shēn* (Radix et Rhizoma Salviae Miltiorrhizae), *chuān xiōng* (Rhizoma Chuanxiong), *bái sháo* (Radix Paeoniae Alba), and *hóng huā* (Flos Carthami) to invigorate blood, dispel stasis, improve microcirculation, enhance the tonification of the kidney, and promote the regeneration of the tissues in the joints; *wū shāo shé* (Zaocys), black ants, and *wú gōng* (Scolopendra) to track down wind, expel stasis, resolve toxins, discharge turbidity, disperse swelling, and relieve pain; *dăn nán xīng* (Arisaema cum Bile), *bàn xià* (Rhizoma Pinelliae), and *bái jiè zĭ* (Semen Sinapis) to dispel phlegm, unblock the collaterals, and eliminate dampness; *huá shí* (Talcum), *yì yĭ rén* (Semen Coicis), *fáng jĭ* (Radix Stephaniae Tetrandrae), and *léi gōng téng* (Tripterygium Wilfordii) to disperse swelling, relieve pain, soften hardness, and dissipate nodules.

Ji Hai-wang[2] treated 43 cases of RA by tonifying the kidney and invigorating blood (total efficacy: 90%).

(2) Enrich Yin and Unblock the Collaterals

Zhou Xue-ping[3] created *Shū Guān Chōng Jì* (舒关冲剂) to enrich the kidney, clear heat, disperse phlegm, and transform stasis. He used this formula to treat 46 cases of RA of the yin deficiency type during the middle and late stages, and compared the results with those of the control group, which consisted of 41 patients treated with *Wāng Bì Chōng*

Jì (尪痹冲剂). Treatment group: excellent improvement = 54.35%, total efficacy = 91.3%. Control group: excellent improvement = 29.27%, total efficacy = 73.17%.

(3) Clear Heat and Resolve Toxins

Ying Sen-lin[4] created a formula to clear heat, eliminate dampness, cool blood, resolve toxins, unblock the collaterals, and relieve pain. The formula consists of *tǔ fú líng* (Rhizoma Smilacis Glabrae) 60g, *jīn yín huā* (Flos Lonicerae Japonicae) 30g, *shēng dì* (Radix Rehmanniae Recens) 30g, *táo rén* (Semen Persicae) 30g, *fáng jǐ* (Radix Stephaniae Tetrandrae) 20g, *qín jiāo* (Radix Gentianae Macrophyllae) 20g, *chì sháo* (Radix Paeoniae Rubra) 15g, *sāng zhī* (Ramulus Mori) 15g, *mǎ biān cǎo* (Herba Verbenae) 15g, *zhī zǐ* (Fructus Gardeniae) 15g, *bái huā shé shé cǎo* (Herba Hedyotis Diffusae) 15g, and *gān cǎo* (Radix et Rhizoma Glycyrrhizae) 10g.

Modifications: for redness, swelling, and hot pain of the joints, or fever, *shēng shí gāo* (Gypsum Fibrosum) 30g and *zhī mǔ* (Rhizoma Anemarrhenae) 15g were added; for severe pain with afternoon fever, *dì gǔ pí* (Cortex Lycii) 15g and *dān pí* (Cortex Moutan) 10g were added; for marked swelling, *chē qián cǎo* (Herba Plantaginis), *zé xiè* (Rhizoma Alismatis), and *tōng cǎo* (Medulla Tetrapanacis) were added; for joint deformity or subcutaneous nodules, *yuán shēn* (Radix Scrophulariae) 15g, *zào jiǎo cì* (Spina Gleditsiae) 10g, and *shān jiǎ zhū* (Squama Manis) 10g were added. Among 26 patients treated with this formula and the above modifications, 8 were stabilized, 10 showed excellent improvement, 6 showed some improvement, and 2 showed no improvement. Total efficacy = 92.31%.

(4) Clear Heat and Invigorate Blood

Wang Zhen-qing[5] created *Xiāo Bì Wán* (消痹丸), which consists of *shuǐ zhì* (Hirudo) 300g, *yán hú suǒ* (Rhizoma Corydalis) 200g, *dān shēn* (Radix et Rhizoma Salviae Miltiorrhizae) 200g, *hóng huā* (Flos Carthami)

150g, *chuān shān jiă* (Squama Manis) 150g, *pú gōng yīng* (Herba Taraxaci) 300g, *zĭ huā dì dīng* (Herba Violae) 300g, *jīn yín huā* (Flos Lonicerae Japonicae) 300g, *niú bàng zĭ* (Fructus Arctii) 300g, *huáng băi* (Cortex Phellodendri Chinensis) 150g, *qín jiāo* (Radix Gentianae Macrophyllae) 150g, and *cāng zhú* (Rhizoma Atractylodis) 150g. Of 202 patients treated with this formula, 124 (61.38%) showed significant improvement, 56 (27.72%) showed some improvement, and 22 (10. 89%) showed no improvement. Total efficacy = 89.1%.

(5) Eliminate Dampness and Unblock *Bi*

Huang Lie-sheng[6] successfully treated RA with this formula: *sāng jì shēng* (Herba Taxilli) 15g, *xù duàn* (Radix Dipsaci) 15g, *huáng qí* (Radix Astragali) 15g, *dāng guī* (Radix Angelicae Sinensis) 9g, *jī xuè téng* (Caulis Spatholobi) 12g, *dú huó* (Radix Angelicae Pubescentis) 12g, *qín jiāo* (Radix Gentianae Macrophyllae) 10g, *qiāng huó* (Rhizoma et Radix Notopterygii) 10g, *fú líng* (Poria) 10g, *chuān xiōng* (Rhizoma Chuanxiong) 10g, and *bái sháo* (Radix Paeoniae Alba) 10g. For neck pain, he added *gé gēn* (Radix Puerariae Lobatae); for pain of the upper limbs, he added *guì zhī* (Ramulus Cinnamomi) and *sāng zhī* (Ramulus Mori); for discomfort of the lumbus and back, he added *gŏu jĭ* (Rhizoma Cibotii) and *dù zhòng* (Cortex Eucommiae); for pain of the lower limbs, he added *niú xī* (Radix Achyranthis Bidentatae) and *mù guā* (Fructus Chaenomelis); for *bi* in the joints of the far extremities, he added *hăi fēng téng* (Caulis Piperis Kadsurae) and *rĕn dōng téng* (Caulis Lonicerae Japonicae); for heat signs, he removed *huáng qí* (Radix Astragali) and added *shí gāo* (Gypsum Fibrosum), *huáng băi* (Cortex Phellodendri Chinensis), and *fáng jĭ* (Radix Stephaniae Tetrandrae). The medicinals were decocted with water, and one batch was prescribed per day.

(6) Invigorate Blood and Transform Stasis

Chen Xiao-zhen[7] treated 168 cases of RA with this method. The basic formula consisted of *huáng qí* (Radix Astragali) 30g, *dāng guī* (Radix Angelicae Sinensis washed in wine) 30g, *fáng fēng* (wine-fried Radix Saposhnikoviae) 20g, *qiāng huó* (Rhizoma et Radix Notopterygii) 20g, *dú huó* (Radix Angelicae Pubescentis) 20g, *shú dì huáng* (Radix Rehmanniae Praeparata) 20g, *sāng jì shēng* (wine-fried Herba Taxilli) 20g, *yán shuǐ chǎo dù zhòng* (fried with saltwater Cortex Eucommiae) 20g, *tù sī zǐ* (wine-fried Semen Cuscutae), *nǚ zhēn zǐ* (Fructus Ligustri Lucidi) 20g, *chuān niú xī* (fried with saltwater Radix Cyathulae) 15g, *gǒu jǐ* (Rhizoma Cibotii) 15g, *bǔ gǔ zhī* (fried with saltwater Cortex Eucommiae Fructus Psoraleae) 12g, *gǔ suì bǔ* (Rhizoma Drynariae) 12g, *guì zhī* (Ramulus Cinnamomi) 12g, *bái sháo* (wine-fried Radix Paeoniae Alba) 12g, *zhì fù zǐ* (Radix Aconiti Lateralis Praeparata) 12g, *wēi líng xiān* (wine-fried Radix et Rhizoma Clematidis) 9g, *qín jiāo* (Radix Gentianae Macrophyllae) 9g, *cāng zhú* (Rhizoma Atractylodis) 9g, *rén shēn* (Radix Ginseng) 6g, and *gān cǎo* (Radix et Rhizoma Glycyrrhizae) 6g. For yang deficiency, *bā jǐ tiān* (wine-fried Radix Morindae Officinalis) 20g, *gǒu qǐ* (wine-fried Fructus Lycii) 12g, *shān yú ròu* (Fructus Corni) 12g, *lù róng* (wine-fried Cornu Cervi Pantotrichum) 6g, and *ròu guì* (Cortex Cinnamomi) 6g were added; for severe pain, *fēng téng* (Caulis Piperis Kadsurae) 12g, *shēn jīn cǎo* (Herba Lycopodii) 12g, *mù guā* (Fructus Chaenomelis) 9g, *mù fáng jǐ* (Radix Cocculi) 9g, and *mù xiāng* (Radix Aucklandiae) 9g were added. For blood stasis, *dān shēn* (Radix et Rhizoma Salviae Miltiorrhizae) 20g, *sān qī* (Radix et Rhizoma Notoginseng) 12g, and *hóng huā* (Flos Carthami) 12g were added. The medicinals were decocted with water to obtain 1000ml of liquid decoction. 200ml were taken each time, 3 times a day. 50ml of yellow rice wine were added to the remaining decoction, which was used to wash the affected parts of the body for 30 minutes each time, two times a day. Results: Of the 168 patients treated, the symptoms of 25 patients were controlled, 50 showed excellent improvement, 75 showed some improvement, and 18 showed no change. Total efficacy = 82.9%.

(7) Transform Stasis, Unblock the Collaterals, and Disperse Nodules

Wang Yong-jun[8] devised the following formula to treat RA: *dān shēn* (Radix et Rhizoma Salviae Miltiorrhizae) 30g, *mù guā* (Fructus Chaenomelis) 30g, *dāng guī* (Radix Angelicae Sinensis) 20g, *chuān niú xī* (Radix Cyathulae) 20g, *shēng huáng qí* (raw Radix Astragali) 20g, *dì lóng* (Pheretima) 15g, *quán xiē* (Scorpio) 15g, *chuān xiōng* (Rhizoma Chuanxiong) 15g, *guī jiǎ* (Carapax et Plastrum Testudinis) 15g, *sān léng* (Rhizoma Sparganii) 10g, *é zhú* (Rhizoma Curcumae) 10g, *sāng zhī* (Ramulus Mori) 10g, *guì zhī* (Ramulus Cinnamomi) 10g, and *shēng gān cǎo* (raw Radix et Rhizoma Glycyrrhizae) 5g. For cases complicated by wind-damp, *sān léng* (Rhizoma Sparganii), *é zhú* (Rhizoma Curcumae), and *guī jiǎ* (Carapax et Plastrum Testudinis) were removed, and *qiāng huó* (Rhizoma et Radix Notopterygii), *dú huó* (Radix Angelicae Pubescentis), *cāng zhú* (Rhizoma Atractylodis), and *fáng fēng* (Radix Saposhnikoviae) were added; for damp-heat *huáng bǎi* (Cortex Phellodendri Chinensis) and *yì yǐ rén* (Semen Coicis) were added, for phlegm-turbidity, *tǔ fú líng* (Rhizoma Smilacis Glabrae), *jiāng cán* (Bombyx Batryticatus), and *zhú rú* (Caulis Bambusae in Taenia) were added. Total efficacy = 90.63%.

2. Pattern Differentiation and Corresponding Treatment

Currently, the pattern differentiation of lame *bi* basically follows that of general *bi* syndromes. Usually, lame *bi* involves the contraction of external evils and right qi deficiency (right qi deficiency and evil excess). In 1983, the 11 patterns of *bi* syndromes established during the national meeting for the discussion of *bi* syndromes were: damp-heat obstructing the collaterals, cold-damp obstructing the collaterals, cold-heat complex, static blood obstructing the collaterals, dual deficiency of the liver and kidney, prevalence of wind evil, prevalence of dampness evil, prevalence of heat evil, phlegm-damp obstructing the collaterals, disharmony of nutritive and defensive qi, and dual deficiency of qi and yin.

Wang Ji-xue[9] classified RA into 3 types according to his own experience:

(1) Damp-heat obstruction: Swollen, hot, and painful joints with inhibited bending and stretching, heavy limbs, fever, vexation, a red tongue with greasy coating, and a rapid pulse. Formula: *hàn fáng jǐ* (Radix Stephaniae Tetrandrae) 12g, *cāng zhú* (Rhizoma Atractylodis) 12g, *huáng bǎi* (Cortex Phellodendri Chinensis) 12g, *tǔ fú líng* (Rhizoma Smilacis Glabrae) 12g, *dú huó* (Radix Angelicae Pubescentis) 12g, *bì xiè* (Rhizoma Dioscoreae Hypoglaucae) 12g, *hǎi tóng pí* (Cortex Erythrinae) 12g, *yì yǐ rén* (Semen Coicis) 20g, *Xuān mù guā* (Fructus Chaenomelis) 15g, and *sōng jié* (Lignum Pini Nodi) 10g.

(2) Cold-damp obstruction: Cold pain and swelling of the joints (aggravated by rest and cold), inflexible joints with cold limbs and fear of the cold, no thirst, a pale tongue with white coating, and a wiry, tight pulse. Formula: *zhì chuān wū* (Radix Aconiti Praeparata) 6g, *guì zhī* (Ramulus Cinnamomi) 6g, *shēng má huáng* (Herba Ephedrae) 6g, *fù zǐ* (Radix Aconiti Lateralis) 3g, *xì xīn* (Radix et Rhizoma Asari) 3g, *bái sháo* (Radix Paeoniae Alba) 12g, *wēi líng xiān* (Radix et Rhizoma Clematidis) 12g, *zhū líng* (Polyporus) 12g, *chuān niú xī* (Radix Cyathulae) 12g, *fú líng* (Poria) 15g, and *sāng jì shēng* (Herba Taxilli) 15g.

(3) Phlegm-stasis obstruction with internal *zang* depletion: Stabbing pain and swelling of the joints that feels hard to the touch, darkening of the skin around the joints, subcutaneous nodules, stiff and deformed joints, and a dusky or purple tongue. Signs of qi and blood deficiency can be seen in this pattern, e.g., a lusterless facial complexion, pale lips and tongue, shortness of breath, spontaneous sweating, and a deep, thready,

and weak pulse. Formula: *jī xuè téng* (Caulis Spatholobi) 20g, *hé shǒu wū* (Radix Polygoni Multiflori) 20g, *huáng qí* (Radix Astragali) 9g, *dāng guī* (Radix Angelicae Sinensis) 9g, *táo rén* (Semen Persicae) 9g, *hóng huā* (Flos Carthami) 9g, *dǎn nán xīng* (Arisaema cum Bile) 9g, *chì sháo* (Radix Paeoniae Rubra) 12g, *chuān xiōng* (Rhizoma Chuanxiong) 12g, *bái jiè zǐ* (Semen Sinapis) 12g, *dì lóng* (Pheretima) 12g, *bàn xià* (Rhizoma Pinelliae) 6g, *quán xiē* (Scorpio) 6g, and *wú gōng* (Scolopendra) 6g.

Jiang Shao-yi[10] classified RA into the following 3 patterns:

(1) Kidney qi deficiency with blood stasis and retention of dampness in the joints: Tonify the kidney, invigorate blood, dispel wind, drain dampness, strengthen the sinews, and dissipate nodules. Formula: *huáng qí* (Radix Astragali) 40g, *xiān máo* (Rhizoma Curculiginis) 9g, *yín yáng huò* (Herba Epimedii) 15g, *hóng huā* (Flos Carthami) 5g, *chuān xiōng* (Rhizoma Chuanxiong) 12g, *guì zhī* (Ramulus Cinnamomi) 15g, *sāng zhī* (Ramulus Mori) 20g, *xì xīn* (Radix et Rhizoma Asari) 5g, *léi gōng téng* (Tripterygium Wilfordii) 15g, *huái niú xī* (Radix Achyranthis Bidentatae) 20g, *sōng jié* (Lignum Pini Nodi)10g, *wū shāo shé* (Zaocys) 15g, and *shā rén* (Fructus Amomi) 10g.

(2) Kidney yang deficiency with cold congealing and dampness obstruction in the lumbus and legs: Warm the kidney, invigorate the blood, dispel wind, unblock the collaterals, disperse phlegm, and expel dampness. Formula: *lù jiǎo piàn* (Cornu Cervi) 10g, *xiān máo* (Rhizoma Curculiginis) 10g, *yín yáng huò* (Herba Epimedii)15g, *dù zhòng* (Cortex Eucommiae) 15g, *gǒu jǐ* (Rhizoma Cibotii) 15g, *léi gōng téng* (Tripterygium Wilfordii) 15g, *chì sháo* (Radix Paeoniae Rubra) 10g, *hóng huā* (Flos Carthami) 5g, *dān shēn* (Radix et Rhizoma Salviae Miltiorrhizae) 15g, *wū shāo shé* (Zaocys) 20g, *shā rén* (Fructus Amomi) 10g, and *gān cǎo shāo* (Radix et Rhizoma Glycyrrhizae) 10g.

(3) Yin and yang deficiency with phlegm-stasis: Enrich the kidney, invigorate blood, clear heat, expel phlegm, disperse swelling, relieve

pain, soften hardness, and dissipate nodules. Formula: *zhī mǔ* (Rhizoma Anemarrhenae) 15g, *dì gǔ pí* (Cortex Lycii) 15g, *shān yú ròu* (Fructus Corni) 20g, *bái jiè zǐ* (Semen Sinapis) 10g, *dǎn nán xīng* (Arisaema cum Bile) 10g, *lù jiǎo piàn* (Cornu Cervi) 15g, *yín yáng huò* (Herba Epimedii) 15g, *léi gōng téng* (Tripterygium Wilfordii) 15g, *chuān shān jiǎ* (Squama Manis) 15g, *wū shāo shé* (Zaocys) 20g, black ants 7g, (baked on the tile and ground into fine powder and mixed with decoction) *sān qī* (Radix et Rhizoma Notoginseng, ground into powder and taken with decoction) 20g, *hóng huā* (Flos Carthami) 5g, *shén qū* (Massa Medicata Fermentata) 15g, and *shā rén* (Fructus Amomi) 10g.

Li Shao[11] believes that in the early stage (acute attack) of RA, the invasion of external evils (e.g., wind, cold, damp, heat) is the main factor, while disharmony of nutritive and defensive qi is the internal factor. In this stage, focus should be placed on determining whether the pattern is of cold or heat, and of the exterior or interior. In the middle and late stages, the phlegm and stasis bind together, forming a cold-heat deficiency-excess complex. Over time, the chronic illness will give rise to the depletion of qi, blood, yin and yang. During these stages, pattern differentiation should revolve around cold and heat, and the state of the *zang-fu*, qi, and fluids.

3. Specific Formulas

Encouraged by the promising future of the internationalization and industrialization of Chinese medicine, the personal experiences of many (ancient and modern) doctors in the treatment of RA have been propagated. Some research have been conducted to study the pharmacological, anti-inflammatory, analgesic, and immunoregulatory effects of empirical formulas. Examples of these empirical formulas include: *Jiǔ Zhì Shǐ Xī Yì Wán* (九制豕稀益丸) by Wang Yi-min, *Shū Guān Wēn Jīng Chōng Jì* (舒关温经冲剂) and *Shū Guān Qīng Luò Chōng Jì* (舒关

清络冲剂）by Zhou Xue-ping, *Kè Bì Jiāo Náng*（克痹胶囊）by Li Ping, *Sān Hŭ Wán*（三虎丸）by Kuang Hui-tao, *Léi Luò Zhĭ Piàn*（雷络酯片）by Du Xiu-lan, *Zàng Yào 25 Wèi Lǘ Xuè Wán*（藏药 25 味驴血丸）by Ma De-bao, *Fēng Shī Yù Jiāo Náng*（风湿愈胶囊）by Lin Zhe, *Yào Wáng Tōng Bì Săn*（药王通痹散）by Zhao Hai-xia, *Lèi Fēng Shī Líng*（类风湿灵）by Gao Mei, *Lèi Fēng Shī II Kŏu Fú Yè*（类风湿 II 号口服液）by Zhang De-jing, *Jīn Mă Tōng Luò Jiāo Náng*（金马通络胶囊）by Rao Guang-li, *Fēng Shī I*（风湿 I 号）by Zang Dong-lian, *Xīn Guì Tōng Bì Jiāo Náng*（辛桂通痹胶囊）by He Jiang-cheng, *Dú Bù Wán*（独步丸）by Zhang Rui-ming, *Lì Jié Piàn*（历节片）by Shi Hai-bo, *Fù Fāng Qīng Bì Piàn*（复方清痹片）by Li Yong Min, *Fù Fāng Mă Qián Zĭ Piàn*（复方马钱子片）by Shi Yu-shan, *Bì Tòng Líng Jiāo Náng*（痹痛灵胶囊）by Shi Jing-jing, *Fēng Shī Yè*（风湿液）by Chen Li-min, *Wāng Bì Jiàn Bù Tāng*（尫痹健步汤）by Liu Yu-xuan, *Lèi Fēng Shī Hé Jì*（类风湿合剂）by Zhang Wei-xing, *Liù Chóng Juān Bì Chōng Jì*（六虫蠲痹冲剂）by Huang Qi, *Shè Mă Lèi Fēng Shī Wán*（麝马类风湿丸）by Li Bao-chao, *Ruăn Jiān Sàn Jié Wán*（软坚散结丸）by Jin Yong-jun, *Yăng Xuè Qū Fēng Qīng Rè Shèng Shī Tāng*（养血祛风清热胜湿汤）by Zhou Xing-zhi, *Kāng Bì Jiāo Náng*（康痹胶囊）by Guo Shu-yun, *Fēng Shī Kāng Jiāo Náng*（风湿康胶囊）by Wu Yun-qing, *Sān Lóng Fēng Shī Băo Kŏu Fú Yè*（三龙风湿宝口服液）by Tang Ao-li, *Sān Lóng Sān Chóng Tāng*（三龙三虫汤）by SunYan-chun, *Yáng Zhí Zhū Gēn Piàn*（羊踯躅根片）by LuoYong-yan, *Wāng Bì Kāng Fù* I and II（尫痹康复 I 号、II 号）by Li Yang-zhen, *Xiāo Bì Líng Dài Pào Jì*（消痹灵袋泡剂）by Fan Bing and Zhou Cui-ying, *Fēng Shī Sān Kāng*（风湿三康）by Li Kun-san, *Bì Xiāo Tāng*（痹消汤）by Zhang Liang, *Chú Shī Tōng Bì Tāng*（除湿通痹汤）by Wang Lie-sheng, *Tōng Bì Líng*（通痹灵）by Xiong Mao-lin, *Xiāo Fēng Tōng Bì Líng*（消风通痹灵）by Liu Xu-mei, *Juān Bì Hé Jì*（蠲痹合剂）by Zhou Rui-qiu, *Fù Fāng Zhú Jié Shēn Piàn*（复方竹节参片）by Chen Yun-long, *Qín Jiāo Wŭ Téng Yĭn*（秦艽五藤饮）by Wu Feng-hai, *Shè Xiāng Wū Lóng Wán*（麝香乌龙丸）by Wang Zhi-wen, *Bŭ Shèn Juān Bì Wán*（补肾蠲痹丸）by Li Jin-song, *Qū Shī Chú Bì Jiāo Náng*（祛

湿除痹胶囊) by Pang Xue-feng, *Zhuī Fēng Tòu Gŭ Wán* (追风透骨丸) by Zhang Jing-lun, *Zì Nĭ Sān Lóng Léi Gōng Wán* (自拟三龙雷公丸) by Wei Shu-xiang, *Jīng Zhū Fēng Shī Jiāo Náng* (晶珠风湿胶囊) by Fu Hong-wei, *Kè Bì* II (克痹 II 号) by Hu Xiao-hui, *Bì Zhŏng Xiāo Tāng* (痹肿消汤) by Liang Qing-hua, *Léi Bì Tài* (雷痹泰) by Wang Li-jun, *Qīng Bì Săn* (清痹散) by Zhou Fu-bo, *Sān Wū Qū Bì Tāng* (三乌祛痹汤) by He Li-zhong, *Guī Qí Biē Chóng Tāng* (归芪鳖虫汤) by Huang Ai-yun, *Qīng Bì Kē Lì Chōng Jì* (清痹颗粒冲剂) by Li Ming, *Lián Téng Yĭn* (连藤饮) by Zhang Mao-lei, *Qí Dăn Tōng Bì Tāng* (芪胆通痹汤) by Gu Xiao-hong, *Bì Kāng Piàn* (痹康片) by Hong Jin-qi, *Lóu Hŭ Èr Jīn Èr Téng Tāng* (蒌虎二金二藤汤) by Mo Ke-yuan, *Tiān Lóng Tāng* (天龙汤) by Qin Yin-zhong, and *Bān Lóng Tāng* (斑龙汤) by Zheng Hong-ling.[12-70]

Studies on the mechanism of these formulas in the treatment of RA have been conducted clinically, and attempts have been made to improve their therapeutic effects and reduce their side effects.[71-76]

Other treatment modalities introduced for the treatment of RA include Huang Di-jun's method of wheat-grain moxibustion plus tapping and cupping, Zhu Wei's apitoxin therapy, of Xiao Xue-lü's intravascular laser irradiation therapy, and Li Chang-you's foot plate therapy.[77-80]

4. Acupuncture and Moxibustion

Acupuncture and moxibustion are praised by the world medical field as miraculous external treatment modalities, and are effective therapies for eliminating disease and promoting health recovery. Modern medical studies show that acupuncture and moxibustion can increase leu-enkephalin and regulate the metabolism of free radicals in RA patients. Acupuncture can lower the ESR and the RF titer, and benefits immunoregulation to achieve the goal of dispelling wind, unblocking the collaterals, moving qi, invigorating blood, eliminating inflammation, and relieving pain.

(1) *Shùn Shì Fú Zhēn* Method (顺势伏针法)

Han Jian-zhong[81] used this method to treat 30 patients with rheumatoid arthritis. DU 14, DU 12, DU 11, DU 9, DU 8, BL 20, BL 23, RN 4, BL 40, GB 34, ST 36, KI 3, and GB 40 were selected. Treatment was given in the summer and administered once every other day. 10 sessions equaled a course, and 2 courses were given each year. The needling technique used was even supplementation and drainage. If there was no noticeable improvement, the treatment was repeated again in the following summer. Results: 8 (26.7%) showed excellent improvement, 19 (63.3%) showed some improvement, and 3 showed no change. Total efficacy = 90.0%.

(2) "Snake" Moxibustion and Acupuncture

Wei Fu-liang[82] used this treatment modality to treat 60 RA patients.

Snake moxibustion: With the patient lying prone, the area of the back from DU 14 to DU 2 were properly disinfected. Purple-skinned garlic was selected and ground into a paste. The garlic paste was spread on the back from DU 14 to DU 2, resembling a snake. The width of the paste was approximately 2.5cm, and the thickness was 1.5cm. The skin surrounding the garlic paste was covered with paper. 4-5 soybean-sized moxa cones were burned on DU 14, DU 2, and DU 4. Treatment was administered once every other day, with 10 sessions totalling a course. There was a 7-day gap between courses. Other points, e.g., DU 13, DU 12, DU 11, DU 10, DU 9, DU 8, DU 7, DU 5, and DU 3, were selected to replace the previous ones in rotation. If there were blisters on the skin after moxibustion, a three-edge needle was used to drain the blisters, followed by the application of *Lǜ Yào Gāo* (绿药膏).

Acupuncture: LI 11, LI 5, SI 6, and *bā xié* (EX-UE9) were selected in the upper limbs, and LV 7, GB 34, ST 36, BL 58, ST 41 were selected in the lower limbs, according to the parts of the body affected by the disease.

Drainage was applied by rotating the needle. Treatment was given once every other day, in alternation with "snake" moxibustion.

(3) Fire Needling

Wu Hong-dong[83] uses this method to treat RA. If the upper limbs are affected, *ashi* points and *shī shì jǐng jiā jǐ* (师氏颈夹脊) are selected; for shoulder pain, SJ 14, LI 15, and LI 14 are used; for elbow pain, LI 12, LI 11, and LI 10 are selected; for wrist pain, SJ 4, LI 5, and SI 5 are selected; if the lower limbs are involved, *ashi* points and *shī shì yāo jiā jǐ* (师氏腰夹脊 ; located 0.5 *cun* lateral from the lumbar spine) are selected; for knee pain, *xī yǎn* (EX-LE5), ST 34, ST 36, and GB 34 are selected; for ankle pain, ST 41, KI 3, and GB 40 are selected; for pain in the hands and feet, *ashi* points are chosen, and shallow and swift needling are applied. Deep and quick needling are used on large joints. Treatment is given once every other day, with 15 sessions totalling a course. After 1-3 courses, the total efficacy = 91.11%.

(4) Warming Needle Method

Gu Gao-ming[84] used this treatment method to treat 32 RA patients (efficacy rate = 93.75%).

Point combination: LI 15, SI 9, SJ 14, SJ 4, SJ 5, LI 11, LI 4, *xī yǎn* (EX-LE5), ST 36, GB 34, SP 6, ST 41, BL 60, *bā fēng* (EX-LE10), and *bā xié* (EX-UE9).

Method: For each treatment session, select 6-8 points according to the location of affected joints. Choose 30-gauge, 1.5 inch filiform needles. Insert the needle quickly, and twirl the needle until there is a sensation of qi arrival. Then, place a moxa cone (1.5-2 cm long) on the needle handle. Use 2 cones, which should last approximately 20 minutes. *Bā fēng* (EX-LE10), and *bā xié* (EX-UE9) are needled obliquely (15 degrees). Do not apply warming needle on these two sets of points; instead, apply even supplementation and drainage. Administer one treatment session per day. 30 sessions equal a course of treatment. The patient should also take *Guì Zhī Sháo Yào Zhī Mǔ Tāng* (桂枝芍药知母汤) while undergoing acupuncture treatment. Observe the patient for 3 treatment courses.

Conclusion: Warming needle is an effective therapy for treating RA. The author presumes that this method is a type of stress stimulation, which affects the immune system through the neuroendocrine system, or that it can activate T cells to produce IL-2 and regulate the T cells and B cells to bring "yin and yang to a state of relative equilibrium." Studies show that warming needle method can increase IL-2 and decrease elevated levels of immunoglobulin without affecting the normal levels of immunoglobulin, which means that the warming needle regulates the immune function in two ways.

(5) Electro-acupuncture Combined with Western Drugs to Treat Active RA

Ai Zhou used this method to treat RA. 146 RA patients were randomly divided into treatment and control groups. Point combination for the treatment group: LI 11, LI 4, GB 34, BL 11, BL 18, BL 23, ST 36, LV 3, LI 15, SJ 14, SI 9, TE 4, LI 5, SI 5, ST 41, GB 40, LV 4, *bā xié* (EX−UE9). 1.5-inch stainless steel filiform needles were used. Electro-acupuncture was applied, at a continuous wave of 60 Hz frequency. The intensity was adjusted according to the patients' tolerance levels. Treatment was administered once a day for 5 consecutive days, 25 minutes per session. The patients would have 2 days of rest and then given another 5 days of treatment. 1 month equaled a course. The patients in the treatment group also took meloxicam, sulfasalazine, and methopterin in addition to the electro-acupuncture. The patients in the control only took the drugs. Results: The efficacy of the treatment group was 79.73%, while that of the control group was 51.39% ($P<0.05$).

Electro-acupuncture has the effect of promoting the flow of qi and blood in the channels and collaterals. The combination of the drugs with electro-acupuncture for the treatment of active RA provides analgesia and relieves inflammation. It is an effective therapeutic regimen of the integration of Chinese medicine and biomedicine.

(6) Cold Moxibustion

Yu Rui-ping[90] used this method to treat interphalangeal joint inflammation in RA. 576 patients were randomly divided into a treatment group (290 patients to be treated with cold moxibustion) and a control group (286 patients to be treated with drugs). The course was 2 months. Patients in the treatment group were given external applications of Yu's self-composed *Bān Xīn Săn* (斑辛散).

Preparation method: The formula consisted of 1 portion of *bān máo* (Mylabris), 2 portions of *xì xīn* (Radix et Rhizoma Asari), 2.5 portions of *bái jiè zĭ* (Semen Sinapis), 2 portions of *dăn nán xīng* (Arisaema cum Bile), and 2.5 portions of *yán hú suŏ* (Rhizoma Corydalis). After baking the medicinals and grinding them into powder, they were filtered through an 80-mesh sifter. The powder was stored in a wide-mouthed bottle. The powder was mixed with an adhesive plaster for external application. Approximately 4-8 hours after application, there was local burning pain or itching of the skin with exudation. Another 0.5-1 hour later, the plaster was removed to reveal more than 10 small blisters or 4-6 large blisters. When the fluid in the blister turned light yellow, the plaster was removed. 5-7 days later, the epidermis healed, and the treatment was repeated again. 5 sessions equaled a course, with a 7-day interval between courses. During the interval, no other anti-rheumatic treatments were administered.

Results: Total remission rate by the end of the 2nd course was 77.2% in the treatment group, and 23.4% in the control group. Conclusion: Cold moxibustion is more effective than anti-inflammatory drugs for the treatment of RA.

(7) Acupuncture and Chinese Medicinal Wash

Luo Xiang-jun adopted this method to treat 98 RA patients.

Acupuncture: The patients in the treatment group were given acupuncture therapy with deep insertion and many needles to treat chronic cold-damp lingering in the sinews and bones. The acupoints selected were SI 4, LI 5, LI 11, SJ 5, LI 4, SJ 3, ST 36, GB 34, SP 6, LV 3, GB 41, *bā xié* (EX-UE9), ST 41, and *Hua Tuo jia ji* points. 28-30 gauge stainless steel filiform needles were used, and even supplementation and drainage was applied. The needles were retained for 30 minutes per session, and 10 sessions were considered a course. There was an interval of 4 days between courses.

Chinese medicinal wash: The formula for the medicinal wash consisted of *shēng chuān wū* (raw Radix Aconiti), *shēng cǎo wū* (raw Radix Aconiti Kusnezoffii), *shēng nán xīng* (raw Rhizoma Arisaematis), *shēng bàn xià* (raw Rhizoma Pinelliae), *xì xīn* (Radix et Rhizoma Asari), *rǔ xiāng* (Olibanum), *mò yào* (Myrrha), *qīng fēng téng* (Caulis Sinomenii), *kū fán* (Alumen Dehydratum), and *bīng piàn* (Borneolum Syntheticum). All the medicinals, except for *bīng piàn*, were soaked in water for 1 hour and then decocted. After boiling for 15 minutes, the *bīng piàn* was added, and the decoction was boiled for another minute. The patients in the treatment group were instructed to steam the affected areas of the body with the hot decoction, and then to wash the affected areas with the decoction once it has cooled down to a tolerable temperature. Each treatment session lasted 30-40 minutes. Treatment was given once a day.

The patients in the control group were only given acupuncture. The total efficacy of the treatment group was 88.73%, while that of the control group was 54% ($P<0.01$).

(8) Chinese Medicinal Atomization Combined with Acupuncture

He Yang adopted this method to treat 54 patients of RA.

Atomization: Medicinals that dispel wind, disperse cold, invigorate blood, and transform stasis were selected, i.e., *fáng feng* (Radix Saposhnikoviae), *chuān wū* (Radix Aconiti Praeparata), *cǎo wū* (Radix Aconiti Kusnezoffii Praeparata), *chuān xiōng* (Rhizoma Chuanxiong), and *hóng huā* (Flos Carthami). The medicinals were soaked in a mixture of vinegar and yellow rice wine. Absorbent cotton was used to soak up the medicinal liquid and then wrapped around the affected joints. Use an ultrasonic atomization machine to warm the area. Adjust the temperature according to the patient's tolerance level.

Acupuncture: After the atomization, patients were treated with acupuncture. The needles were retained for 20 minutes. Main points for wind-cold pattern: BL 12 and BL 17; main points for cold-damp pattern: BL 23, RN 4, and SP 9. For upper limb involvement, LI 15, LI 11, SJ 5, *bā xié* (EX-UE9), and LI 4 were added; for lower limb involvement, *bā fēng* (EX-LE10), KI 6, GB 40, and *xī yǎn* (EX-LE5) were added. Treatment was administered once a day, except on Sundays. Half a month equaled a course, and 3 courses were given. The patients in the control group were treated with hydrotherapy, magnet therapy, and audiofrequency electrotherapy. The difference of the efficacy of the two groups was significant ($P<0.05$).

Experimental Studies

In recent years, there have been many studies and research papers on RA etiology and pathogenesis. Some achievements have been made in providing new diagnostic methods for this complex disease.

1. Research on the Efficacy of Herbal Prescriptions

Xu Jia-liu[93] explored the mechanism of action of *Guì Zhī Sháo Yào Zhī Mǔ Tāng* (桂枝芍药知母汤). He found that this formula can inhibit the writhing response in mice caused by acetic acid, inhibit granuloma hyperblastosis in rat, reduce the capillary permeability in the abdominal cavity of mice, and significantly suppress primary and secondary arthritis in rats. Studies indicated that *Guì Zhī Sháo Yào Zhī Mŭ Tāng* can greatly reduce the content of PGE2 in the inflammatory tissue of rats and inhibit leukocytopenia in inflammatory reactions.

Su Xian-hong believes that RA is a chronic, recurrent systemic autoimmune disease that mainly involves the joints. In the advanced stage, the patient's daily life is severely affected by the joint deformity. Su Xian-hong proposed that *Jiāo Téng* No. 1 (艽藤 I 号) has a satisfactory effect on RA and conducted a study to show the formula's effect on the immune system. Results: The weight of the rats in the control group was decreased by 14%, while that of the *Wāng Bì Chōng Jì* (尪痹冲剂) group was decreased by 9%, and that of the *Jiāo Téng* No. 1 was decreased by only 3%. The immune index (CH50) was decreased by 2.5% in the *Jiāo Téng* No. 1 group, decreased by 21.5% in the *Wāng Bì Chōng Jì* (尪痹冲剂) group, and by 25.6% in the control group. Thus it is shown that *Jiāo Téng* I (艽藤 I 号) can strengthen the constitution, increase the ability to resist disease, and relieve inflammation.

2. Research on the Efficacy of Single Chinese Medicinals

(1) *Jīn Tiĕ Suŏ* (Psammosilene Tunicoides)

Jīn tiĕ suŏ was first recorded in the book *Materia Medica of Yunnan Province* (滇南本草 , *Diān Nán Bĕn Căo*). It is one of the essential ingredients of *Yún Nán Bái Yào* (云南白药).

Xu Jian-yang experimented with the use of large, medium, and small dosages of *jīn tiĕ suŏ* in the treatment RA, and found that the medicinal has notable analgesic effects. It greatly elevated the pain threshold and decreased the serum NO/NOS.

Du Xiu-lan found that *Xiāo Bì Gāo* (消痹膏) can inhibit the auricle swelling of mice caused by dimethyl benzene and suppress the formation of granuloma in mice. In addition, the formula can elevate the pain threshold in mice. Hence, the formula is considered to have anti-inflammatory and analgesic effects.

(2) *Chuān Wū* (Radix Aconiti)

Modern pharmacological studies have shown that the therapeutic effects of *chuān wū* (Radix Aconiti) are connected to aconite alkaloids. However, the toxic side effects of the medicinal are also linked to the same substance. The aconite alkaloids include double ester aconitine (aconitine), benzoyl single aconitine (secondary aconitine), and aconine. In addition, there are tala stibamine, chuan-wu base A and chuan-wu base B. The most toxic of them all is double ester aconitine, and the second most toxic is benzoyl single aconitine. The toxicity of aconine is very weak (or non-existent). There are many methods of processing *wū tóu* (Radix Aconiti Kusnezoffii), of which steaming and boiling are the main ones. Processing reduces the toxicity level of the herb.

The main pharmacological actions of *chuān wū* (Radix Aconiti) are the following:

➢ Analgesia and tranquilization: Aconitine and its breakdown products have an analgesic effect. *Chuān wū* (Radix Aconiti) has been used to treat pain for thousands of years. For instance, *Dà Wū Tóu Jiān* (大乌头煎) of *Essentials from the Golden Cabinet* (金匮要略, *Jīn Guì Yào Lüè*) was used to treat periumbilical pain of cold hernia.

➢ Local anesthesia: Aconitine can stimulate sensory nerve endings in the skin and mucosa. It stimulates the nerves to produce the initial sensations of itchiness and burning, and then it exerts anesthesia and loss of consciousness. Hence, in ancient times, *chuān wū* (Radix Aconiti) was adopted as the main external anesthetic and analgesic. *Chuān wū* was also mentioned in *Golden Mirror of the Medical Tradition* (医宗金鉴, *Yī Zōng Jīn Jiàn*) as one of the ingredients of an external formula for local anesthesia in surgery.

➢ Strengthens the heart and expands coronary arteries: Aconitine can selectively stimulate vagus nerves to slow the heart rate and directly stimulate cardiac muscle to strengthen the heart beat. It also strengthens the effect of adrenaline on cardiac muscle and resists the inverted T wave caused by barium chloride.

➢ Anti-inflammatory effect: Whether it is taken orally or administered via subcutaneous injection or intramuscular injection, aconitine can greatly reduce the content of antiscorbic acid in the adrenal glands of rats. The effect cannot be blocked by pentobarbital promazine, thus exhibiting an ACH-like inflammatory effect. In Chinese medicine, it is frequently used to treat rheumatic arthritis and rheumatoid arthritis, both of which fall under the category of *bi* syndromes. Zhang Zhong-jing used *Wū Tóu Tāng* (乌头汤) to treat joint-running disease with pain and inability to bend and stretch.

(3) *Léi Gōng Téng* (Tripterygium Wilfordii)

Studies have shown that *léi gōng téng* (Tripterygium Wilfordii) has notable anti-inflammatory and analgesic effects. Since the 1960s, it has been used extensively for the treatment of RA. Because of high toxicity in its crude form, it has been replaced by Tripterygium glycosides. Many doctors and scholars have continued to investigate the method of external use to reduce the side effects of *léi gōng téng*. Dr. Deng created the patents composed of the following medicinals to treat active RA patients: *léi gōng téng* (Tripterygium Wilfordii), *rŭ xiāng* (Olibanum), *mò yào* (Myrrha), *shēng nán xīng* (raw Rhizoma Arisaematis), and *chuān xiōng* (Rhizoma Chuanxiong). Results showed that there was more improvement in joint swelling, pain, tenderness, and morning stiffness in the treatment group than in the biomedicine control group. Total efficacy = 56.7%.

Dr. Zhang used Tripterygium glycosides in the treatment of 144 cases of RA. Results: After treatment, the duration of morning stiffness was shortened significantly, grip strength improved, walking speed returned to normal, and RF titer became negative. Total efficacy = 97.3%. Dr. Lao treated 50 cases of RA with the combination of small doses of Tripterygium glycosides granules with Sinomenium acutum. It is proved that the combination of the two preparations can reduce the dose and side effects of *léi gōng téng* (Tripterygium Wilfordii).

3. Research on New Formulas

(1) Granules

Since Chinese medicinal granules have the advantages of rapid effect, small volume, convenient administration and easy storage, their annual use increased by 40.9% through the 1980s. They are also the most rapidly developing form of solid Chinese medicinals in recent years. Among the 443 new types of Chinese medicinal products, granules occupy 17.2%, ranking 3rd place. As medicinal preparations continue to develop in the direction of "high performance, readily available, and prolonged effect" with "mild toxicity, few side effects, and small doses," along with new appliances such as high-speed stirring granulation, spray-drying granulation, and rolling condensation granulation, new types of Chinese medicinals granules have hit the market, e.g., sugarless granules, effervescent granules, coated granules, and swallowable granules. Current granule formulas produced by domestic factories include *Wāng Bì Chōng Jì* (尫痹冲剂), *Hán Shī Bì Chōng Jì* (寒湿痹冲剂), and *Yū Xuè Bì Chōng Jì* (瘀血痹冲剂).

Yang Feng[100] researched the effects of *Xiān Lóng Kē Lì* (仙龙颗粒) on immunoreactive inflammation, T cell subgroups, phagocytosis of macrophage, and specific antibodies. Results: *Xiān Lóng Kē Lì* (仙龙颗粒), in large, medium, or small doses, can treat primary adjuvant-induced arthritis and prevent secondary pathological changes, indicating that

Xiān Lóng Kē Lì (仙龙颗粒) has an inhibitory effect on immunoreactive inflammation. *Xiān Lóng Kē Lì* (仙龙颗粒) in large doses inhibits CD4 cells, improves CD8 expression, and reduces the ratio of CD4/CD8 cells, while prednisone inhibits both CD4 and CD8 cells and causes an abnormal CD4/CD8 ratio. This indicates that the anti-rheumatism effect of the granules is better than that of prednisone. Medium doses of *Xiān Lóng Kē Lì* (仙龙颗粒) inhibits only the CD4 cells and have no apparent effect on CD8 cells. Small doses of the granules had little effect on both the CD4 and CD8 cells. The different doses of the granules had no apparent effect on the phagocytosis of macrophage and serum hemolysin.

(2) Pills

Pills are made by grinding medicinals into fine powder, and then mixing the powder with honey, water, flour and water paste, wine, or vinegar. The commonly used pills in the clinic are honey pills, watered pills, and concentrated pills. There are differences between large pills and small pills. The main characteristics of pills are slow absorption, long-term effects, small volume, and convenience (easy to store and take). Pills are the common form of oral medicinals for patients with weak constitutions and for long-term treatment. Examples of modern pill formulas for RA: *Huá Tuó Zài Zào Wán* (华佗再造丸), *Yì Shèn Juān Bì Wán* (益肾蠲痹丸), and *Tiān Má Wán* (天麻丸).

(3) Medicinal Wine

Liquor can promote gastric and intestinal secretion and absorption, invigorate blood, promote tissue metabolism, and increase cellular energy. From a Chinese medical perspective, liquor has the effects of regulating qi and blood, connecting the channels and collaterals, tonifying yang, dispersing cold, dissipating wind, and dispelling dampness. In *Han History*, Annals of Food and Commodities (汉书 · 食货志 , *Hàn Shū, Shí*

Huò Zhì), wine is praised as being "the chief of the hundred medicinals." The main ingredient of liquor is ethanol, which has good penetrativity and thus easily enters the cells of the medicinals to dissolve most of the water soluble substances and the non-water soluble organic substances that can only be dissolved in nonpolar solvents. This special function of liquor enhances the original therapeutic effects of medicinals.

Since wine has antiseptic and disinfectant properties, it can delay the hydrolysis of medicinals and thereby strengthen their stability (if the volume of the alcohol is 40% or above). Therefore, medicinal wine is convenient because of its extremely long shelf-life. In addition, wine can dispel the bad odors of some medicinals. For instance, when *wū shāo shé* (Zaocys) and *qí shé* (Agkistrodon) are used to make medicinal wine, their fishy smell is reduced.

It should also be noted that wine, when consumed in moderate amounts, is beneficial for the health.

(4) Injection

Injection therapy has the advantages of accurate dosage, rapid action, noticeable effects, and good compliance. This treatment modality is suitable for the treatment of many diseases. The injections used for the treatment of RA include *dāng guī* (Radix Angelica Sinensis) injection and *fù shé* (蝮蛇 ; Agkistrodon Halys) injection. Cai Qing, et al.[104] used AFT intravenous drip infusion therapy along with common NSAIDs and DMARDs to treat RA patients. The control group consisted of those who tested positive with an allergic reaction during the AFT skin test, and were treated with *Dāng Guī* Injection instead of AFT. After 3 weeks of treatment, patients in both groups showed significant improvement on the swelling index, tenderness index, VAS, HAQ, and ESR ($P<0.05$ or $P<0.01$); the total efficacy rate of the treatment group was better than that of the control group ($P<0.05$).

REFERENCES

[1] Yu Jiang-di. Understanding Pattern Differentiation and Treatment of RA (辨证分型治疗类风湿性关节炎的体会). *Zhejiang Journal of Chinese Medicine* (浙江中医杂志). 2002: 485-486.

[2] Ji Hai-wang, Yao Shu-lian, Luo Qiang. The Clinical Observation of the Treatment of 43 Cases of RA by Tonifying the Kidney and Invigorating Blood (补肾活血法为主治疗类风湿性关节炎43例临床观察). *Journal of Chinese Medicine* (中医杂志). 2001,42 (10): 609-610.

[3] Zhou Xue-ping, Zhou Zhong-ying. An Exploration into the Pattern Differentiation and Treatment of RA due to Yin Deficiency (类风湿性关节炎阴虚证辨治初探). *Jiangsu Journal of Chinese Medicine* (江苏中医). 2001, 22 (1): 14-15.

[4] Ying Sen-lin. The Clinical Observation of the Treatment of 26 Cases of Active RA by Clearing Heat and Resolving Toxins (清热解毒法治疗活动性类风湿关节炎26例临床观察). *Sichuan Journal of Chinese Medicine* (四川中医). 2003, 21 (3): 42.

[5] Wang Zhen-qing. A Clinical Study of the Treatment of 202 Cases RA by Invigorating Blood and Clearing Heat (活血清热法治疗类风湿性关节炎202例临床研究). *Journal of Chinese Medicine* (中医杂志). 2002, 43 (7): 511-513.

[6] Huang Lie-sheng. The Treatment of 58 Cases of RA by Eliminating Dampness and Unblocking the Collaterals (除湿通痹汤治疗类风湿性关节炎58例). *Sichuan Journal of Chinese Medicine* (四川中医). 2001, 19 (11): 40.

[7] Chen Xiao-zhen. Treatment of 168 Cases of RA by Invigorating Blood and Transforming Stasis (活血化瘀法治疗类风湿性关节炎168例). *Shanxi Journal of Chinese Medicine* (陕西中医). 2001, 22 (3): 140-141.

[8] Wang Yong-jun, Hu Shun-jin. The Treatment of 32 Cases of RA by Transforming Stasis, Unblocking the Collaterals, and Dissipating Nodules (化瘀通络散结法治疗类风湿性关节炎32例).

[9] Wang Ji-xue. The Clinical Observation of the Treatment of 48 Cases of RA on the Basis of Pattern Differentiation (辨证分型论治类风湿性关节炎48例疗效观察). *Anhui Journal of Clinical Chinese Medicine* (安徽中医临床杂志). 1997, 9 (2): 82-83.

[10] Jiang Shao-yi. Understanding the Treatment of RA by Tonifying the Kidney and Invigorating Blood (益肾活血法治疗类风湿性关节炎的体会). *Journal of Chinese Medicine* (中医杂志). 1997, 38 (12): 721-722.

[11] Li Shao, Lü Ai-ping, Hu Yin-qi. An Overview of the Study of the Pattern Differentiation and Treatment of RA Using Chinese Medicinals (中医药对类风湿性关节炎的临床分证论治研究概况). *Journal of Chinese Medicine Fundamentals* (中国中医基础医学杂志). 2001, 7 (2): 71-73.

[12] Wang Yi-min. Introduction to an Effective Formula for Fixed *Bi* -- *Jiu Zhi Shi Xi Yi Wan* (介绍着痹效方--九制豕稀益丸). *Jiangsu Journal of Chinese Medicine* (江苏中医). 1961 (3).

[13] Zhou Xue-ping, Zhou Zhong-ying, Jin Miao-wen. Clinical Research on the Treatment of the Middle and Late Stages of RA by Boosting the Kidney, Alleviating *Bi*, Dispersing Phlegm, and

Transforming Stasis (益肾蠲痹、消痰化瘀法治疗中、晚期RA的临床研究). *Journal of Chinese Medicine* (中医杂志). 1998 (10): 606-609.

[14] Li Ping, Zhu Yong-xian, Qian Chao-yu. Observation of the Therapeutic Effects of *Ke Bi Capsule* on 80 Cases of *Bi* Syndromes (克痹胶囊治疗痹证80例疗效观察). *Journal of Anhui University of Chinese Medicine* (安徽中医学院学报). 1998, 17(2): 31-32.

[15] Kuang Hui-tao. Experimental Research on the Effect of *San Hu Wan* on RA (三虎丸对RA治疗作用的实验研究). *China Journal of Chinese Medicine News* (中国中医药信息杂志). 1998, 5 (11): 16-18.

[16] Du Xiu-lan, Zhang Hong, Fu Xin-li. Clinical Observation of the Treatment of RA with *Lei Luo Zhi Pian* (雷络酯片治疗RA的临床观察). *China Journal of Integrative Medicine* (中国中西医结合杂志). 1998, (2): 88-91.

[17] Ma De-bao. Clinical Observation of the Treatment of 120 Cases of RA with *Lü Xue Wan* [A Formula Consisting of 25 Tibetan Medicinals] (藏药25味驴血丸治疗RA120例临床观察). *China National Journal of Medicine* (中国民族医药杂志). 1998, (3): 14.

[18] Lin Zhe, Sun Dong-mei, Li Jian-ping. Research on the Principle Pharmacodynamics of *Feng Shi Yu Capsule* (风湿愈胶囊的主要药效学研究). *Journal of Changchun University of Chinese Medicine* (长春中医学院学报). 1998, 14 (2): 53-54.

[19] Zhao Hai-xia, Sun Rong. The Pharmacodynamic Study of *Yao Wang Tong Bi San* (药王通痹散的药效学研究). *Primary Journal of Chinese Medicinals* (基层中药杂志). 1998, 12 (2): 47-48.

[20] Gao Mei, Nan Jin-yi, Xu Li. The Effects of *Lei Feng Shi Ling* on the Immune Function of Mice (类风湿灵对小鼠免疫功能的影响). *Journal of Changchun University of Chinese Medicine* (长春中医学院学报). 1998, 14 (1): 56.

[21] Zhang De-jing, Lin Qi-xiu, Cheng Chun-lin. Research on the Treatment of Wind Cold Damp *Bi* with *Lei Feng Shi* Oral Liquid No. 2 (类风湿二号口服液治疗风寒湿痹的研究). *Beijing Journal of Chinese Medicine* (北京中医). 1998, 17 (1): 41-42.

[22] Rao Guang-li, Guo Yun-qing, Chen Jian-ping. Observation of the Effects of *Jin Ma Tong Luo Capsule* on AS (金马通络胶囊治疗AS效果观察). *The People's Military Surgeon* (人民军医). 1997, 40 (12): 705-707.

[23] Zang Dong-lian. A Study of the Antiinflammatory and Analgesic Effects of *Feng Shi* No. 1 (风湿一号的抗炎镇痛作用研究). *Journal of Changchun University of Chinese Medicine* (长春中医学院学报). 1998, 14 (1): 54-55.

[24] He Jian-cheng. A Study of the Antiinflammatory and Analgesic Effects of *Xin Gui Tong Bi Capsule* (辛桂通痹胶囊镇痛抗炎作用研究). *Practical Journal of Integrative Medicine* (实用中西医结合杂志). 1997, 10 (21): 2057-2059.

[25] Zhang Rui-ming. A Clinical Study of *Du Bu Wan* in the Treatment of Lumbar Pain and *Bi* Syndromes: Clinical Analysis of 120 Cases (独步丸治疗腰痛、痹证的临床研究：附120例临床分析). *Huaxi Journal of Chinese Medicine* (华西医学). 1997, 12 (4): 433-435.

[26] Shi Hai-bo. The Antiinflammatory and Analgesic Effects of *Li Jie Pian* (历节片的抗炎镇痛作用). *Chinese Herbal Medicine* (中草药). 1998, 29 (4): 249-251.

[27] Li Yong-min. An Elementary Pharmacological Study of *Fu Fang Qing Bi Pian* (复方清痹片药理学的初步研究). *Hunan Journal of Chinese Medicine* (湖南中医杂志). 1999, 15 (2): 53-54.

[28] Shi Yu-shan, Zhang Hong, Du Xiu-lan. A Double Blind Study of the Treatment of RA with *Fu Fang Ma Qian Zi Pian* (复方马钱子片治疗RA的双盲观察). *Journal of Chinese Medicine* (中医杂志). 1997, 38 (7): 411-413.

[29] Shi Jing-jing. The Clinical Observation and Pharmacological Study of the Treatment of *Bi* Syndromes with *Bi Tong Ling Capsule* (痹通灵胶囊治疗痹证的临床观察及药理实验研究). *Guizhou Journal of Chinese Medicine* (贵州医药). 1997, 21 (4): 250-252.

[30] Chen Li-min. A Pharmacological Study of *Feng Shi Ye* (风湿液药理研究). *Primary Journal of Chinese Medicine* (基层中医杂志). 1997, 11 (3): 29-30.

[31] Liu Yu-xuan. The Clinical Observation of the Treatment of the Second and Third Stages of RA with Bi Jian Bu Tang (痹健步汤治疗二、三期RA的临床观察). *Journal of Hunan University of Chinese Medicine* (湖南中医学院学报). 1997, 17 (3):8-10.

[32] Zhang Wei-xing. The Clinical Observation of *Lei Feng Shi He Ji* (类风湿合剂的临床观察). *Chinese Patent Medicine* (中成药). 1997, 19 (12): 24-25.

[33] Huang Qi. The Clinical Observation of The Treatment of 62 Cases of RA with *Liu Chong Juan Bi Chong Ji* (六虫蠲痹冲剂治疗RA62例临床观察). *Zhejiang Journal of Chinese Medicine* (浙江中医杂志). 1997, (7): 320-321.

[34] Li Bao-chao. The Treatment of 300 Cases of RA with *She Ma Lei Feng Shi Wan* (麝马类风湿丸治疗RA300例). *New Chinese Medicine* (新中医). 1997, 29 (9): 31-32.

[35] Jin Yong-jun. A Random Control Study on the Treatment of RA with *Ruan Jian San Jie Wan* (软坚散结丸治疗RA随机对照研究). *Practical Journal of Integrative Medicine* (实用中西医结合杂志). 1997, 10 (17): 1637-1638.

[36] Zhou Xing-zhi. The Treatment of 105 Cases of RA with *Yang Xue Qu Feng Qing Re Sheng Shi Tang* (养血祛风清热胜湿汤治疗RA105例). *Chinese Medical Science and Technology* (中国中医药科技). 1998, 5 (3): 185.

[37] Guo Shu-yun. The Clinical Observation of the Treatment of 82 Cases of RA with *Kang Bi Capsule* (康痹胶囊治疗RA82例临床观察). *China Journal of Chinese Medicine News* (中国中医药信息杂志). 1998, 5 (4):37-38.

[38] Wu Yun-qing. The Effects of *Feng Shi Kang Capsule* on the Bone Density of RA Patients (风湿康胶囊对RA骨密度的影响). *The People's Military Surgeon* (人民军医). 1997, 40 (2): 82-84.

[39] Tang Ao-li. The Clinical Observation of the Treatment of RA with *San Long Feng Shi Bao Kou Fu Ye* (三龙风湿宝口服液治疗RA的临床观察). *Chinese Patent Medicine* (中成药). 1998, (5): 22-24.

[40] Sun Yan-chun. The Treatment of 75 Cases of RA with *San Long San Chong Tang* (三龙三虫汤治疗RA75例). *China Journal of Integrative Medicine* (中国中西医结合杂志). 1998, (5): 312-313.

[41] Wu Jun-yu, Bai Yong-bo. Chinese Medical Diagnosis and Treatment of Modern Obstinate Diseases (现代难治病中医诊疗学). *Beijing: Chinese Medical Classics Publishing House* (中医古籍出版社). 1993.

[42] Li Yang-zhen. The Treatment of 600 Cases of Lame *Bi* with *Wang Bi Fu Kang* No. 1 and 2 (尪痹复康(Ⅰ号、Ⅱ号)治疗尪痹600例). *Journal of Anhui University of Chinese Medicine* (安徽中医学院学报). 1998, 17 (5): 11-13.

[43] Fan Bing, Zhou Cui-ying. The Clinical and Experimental Study of the Treatment of RA with *Xiao Bi Ling Dai Pao Ji* (消痹灵袋泡剂治疗RA的临床及实验研究). *Journal of Shandong University of Chinese Medicine* (山东中医药大学学报). 1998, (6): 428-431.

[44] Li Kun-san. The Treatment of 50 Cases of RA with *Feng Shi San Kang* (风湿三康治疗RA50例). *Hunan Guide to Chinese Medicine* (湖南中医药导报). 1997, 3 (1): 14-16.

[45] Zhang Liang. The Treatment of 42 Cases of RA with the Integration of Chinese Medicine and Biomedicine (中西医结合治疗类风湿性关节炎42例). *Shandong Journal of Chinese Medicine* (山东中医杂志). 2003, 22 (4): 222-223.

[46] Wang Lie-sheng. The Treatment of 58 Cases of RA with *Chu Shi Tong Bi Tang* (除湿通痹汤治疗类风湿性关节炎58例). *Sichuan Journal of Chinese Medicine* (四川中医). 2001, 19(11): 40-41.

[47] Xiong Mao-lin. The Effects of *Tong Bi Ling* on the Expression of MCP-1 and m-RNA in the Synovial Cells of Rats with RA (通痹灵对佐剂性关节炎大鼠滑膜细胞MCP-1. m-RNA表达的影响). *Chinese Medicinals* (中药材). 2002, 25 (10): 722-724.

[48] Liu Xue-mei. The Treatment of RA with *Xiao Feng Tong Bi Tang* (自拟消风通痹汤治疗类风湿性关节炎). *Sichuan Journal of Chinese Medicine* (四川中医). 2002, 20 (7): 52.

[49] Zhou Rui-qiu, Liu Di-xing. The Treatment of 106 Cases of RA with *Juan Bi He Ji* (蠲痹合剂治疗类风湿性关节炎106例). *China Journal of Integrative Medicine* (中国中西医结合杂志). 2002, 22 (5): 386-387.

[50] Chen Yun-long. The Clinical Study of the Treatment of 30 Cases of RA with *Fu Fang Zhu Jie Shen Pian* (复方竹节参片治疗类风湿性关节炎30例临床研究). *Journal of Chinese Medicine*. 2003, 44 (5): 362-363.

[51] Wu Feng-hai. The Clinical Observation of the Treatment of RA with *Qin Jiao Wu Teng Yin* (秦艽五藤饮治疗类风湿性关节炎的临床观察). *China Journal of Integrative Medicine* (中国中西医结合杂志). 2003, 23 (8): 622-623.

[52] Wang Zhi-wen, Han Bing-sheng, Jia Xiu-rong. Observation of the Therapeutic Effects of Using *She Xiang Wu Long Wan* to Treat RA (麝香乌龙丸治疗类风湿性关节炎150例疗效观察). *Sichuan Journal of Chinese Medicine* (四川中医). 2000, 18 (4): 18-19.

[53] Li Jin-song. The Treatment of 200 Cases of RA with *Bu Shen Juan Bi Wan* (补肾蠲痹丸治疗类风湿性关节炎200例). *China Journal of Integrative Medicine* (中国中西医结合杂志). 2001, 21 (10): 783.

[54] Pang Xue-feng, Meng Yu-hua. The Treatment of 86 Cases of RA with *Qu Feng Chu Bi Jiao Nang* (祛风除痹胶囊治疗类风湿性关节炎86例). *Shaanxi Journal of Chinese Medicine* (陕西中医). 2002, 23 (12): 1073-1075.

[55] Zhang Jing-lun, Zheng Guang-yong, Chen ji-quan. The Clinical Observation of the Treatment of 69 Cases of RA with *Zhui Feng Tou Gu Wan* (追风透骨丸治疗类风湿性关节炎69例临床观察). *Chinese Patent Medicine*(中成药). 2001, 23 (12): 922-924.

[56] Wei Shu-xiang and Wei Hong-bin. The Treatment of 54 Cases of RA with *San Long Lei Gong Wan* (自拟三龙雷公丸为主治疗类风湿性关节炎54例). *Journal of Chinese Medicine* (中医杂志). 2001, 42 (9): 569.

[57] Fu Hong-wei , Yang Hu-tian. The Clinical Observation of the Treatment of 45 Cases RA with *Jing Zhu Feng Shi Capsule* (晶珠风湿胶囊治疗类风湿性关节炎45例临床观察). *Shanghai Journal of Chinese Medicine*(上海中医药杂志). 2001, 933-934.

[58] Hu Xiao-hui, Wang Tao, Wang Jie. An Experimental Study on the Regulation of Natural Immunity in RA Patients Using *Ke Bi* No. 2 (克痹Ⅱ号调节初发类风湿性关节炎患者天然免疫试验研究). *Chinese Herbal Medicine* (中草药). 2000, 31 (2): 120-121.

[59] Liang Qing-hua, Tang Tao, Zhang Hua-xian. The Clinical Observation of the Treatment of Active RA with *Bi Zhong Xiao Tang* (痹肿消汤治疗活动期类风湿性关节炎的临床研究). *Journal of Hunan Medical College* (湖南医科大学学报). 2000, 25 (5): 449-502.

[60] Wang Li-jun. Observation of the Therapeutic Effect of *Lei Bi Tai* in the Treatment of 45 Cases of RA (“雷痹泰”治疗类风湿性关节炎45例疗效观察). *Jiangsu Journal of Chinese Medicine* (江苏中医). 2001, 22 (2): 20-21.

[61] Zhou Fu-bo. Observation of the Therapeutic Effect of *Qing Bi San* in the Treatment of 81 Cases of RA (清痹散治疗类风湿性关节炎81例疗效观察). *New Chinese Medicine* (新中医). 2002, 34 (3): 24-25.

[62] He Li-zhong, Yan Chao-zhong. 43 Cases of RA Treated by San Wu Qu Bi Tang (三乌祛痹汤治疗类风湿性关节炎43例). *Shaanxi Chinese Medicine* (陕西中医). 2002, 23 (3) 239-240.

[63] Huang Ai-yun. The Therapeutic Observation on 38 Cases of RA Treated by Gui Qi Bie Chong Tang (“归芪鳖虫汤”治疗类风湿性关节炎38例疗效观察). *Jiangsu Chinese Medicine* (江苏中医). 2001, 22 (11) 35.

[64] Li Ming. The Clinical Observation of the Treatment of 60 Cases of RA with *Qing Bi Ke Li Chong Ji* (清痹颗粒冲剂治疗类风湿性关节炎活动期60例临床观察). *New Chinese Medicine* (新中医). 2001, 33 (8): 14-15.

[65] Zhang Mao-lei. The Treatment of 46 Cases of Active RA with *Lian Teng Tang* (连藤汤治疗活动期类风湿性关节炎46例). *Shandong Journal of Chinese Medicine* (山东中医杂志). 2001, 20 (1): 22-23.

[66] Gu Xiao-hong. An Experimental Study on the Therapeutic Mechanism of *Qi Dan Tong Bi Tang* in the Treatment of RA (芪胆通痹汤治疗类风湿性关节炎作用机理的试验研究). *Journal of Beijing University of Chinese Medicine* (北京中医药大学学报). 2003, 26 (5): 39-41.

[67] Hong Jin-qi. The Preparation and Clinical Effects of *Bi Kang Pian* (痹康片的制备及临床疗效). *Chinese Hospital Journal of Pharmacology* (中国医院药学杂志). 2001, 21 (2): 118-120.

[68] Mo Ke-yuan. The Treatment of 45 Cases of RA with *Lou Hu Er Jin Er Teng Tang* (蒌虎二金二藤汤治疗类风湿性关节炎45例). *Sichuan Journal Chinese Medicine* (四川中医). 2002, 20 (2): 28-29.

[69] Qin Yin-zhong. The Treatment of 45 Cases of RA with *Tian Long Tang* (天龙汤治疗类风湿性关节炎45例). *Shaanxi Journal of Chinese Medicine* (陕西中医). 2001, 22 (12): 732-739.

[70] Zheng Hong-ling. The Treatment of 75 Cases of RA with Modified *Ban Long Tang* (斑龙汤加

减方治疗类风湿性关节炎75例). *Sichuan Journal of Chinese Medicine* (四川中医). 2002, 20 (8): 31-32.

[71] Deng Zhao-zhi. An Experimental Study of the Antiinflammatory and Analgesic Effects of *Fu Fang Lei Gong Teng Tu Mo Ji* on RA (复方雷公藤涂膜剂对RA的抗炎和镇痛实验研究). *China Journal of Medicine* (中国医药学报). 1998, (3): 14-16.

[72] Dai Min. A Discussion on Immunology, Toxicology, and Clinical Effects of *Lei Gong Teng Tie Gao* (雷公藤贴膏免疫学、毒理学及临床疗效探讨). *Chinese Patent Medicine* (中成药). 1998, 20 (8): 36-38.

[73] Zhang Gen-zhu. An Experimental Study on the Antiinflammatory and Analgesic Effects of *Tong Bi Tie* (痛痹贴抗炎镇痛作用的实验研究). *Beijing Journal of Chinese Medicine* (北京中医). 1998, 17 (5): 55-57.

[74] Du Xiu-lan. A Clinical Study of the Treatment of RA with *Xiao Bi Gao Tie* (消痹膏贴敷治疗类风湿性关节炎的临床研究). *Shandong Journal of Chinese Medicine* (山东中医杂志). 1999, 18 (4): 150-155.

[75] Ji Hai-wang, Cao Xiao-ju, Luo Qiang. The Clinical Observation of the Treatment of 125 Cases of Wind Cold Damp *Bi* with *Qu Feng Shi Ling Capsule* (祛风湿灵胶囊治疗风湿寒痹125例临床观察). *China Journal of Chinese Medical Science and Technology* (中国中医药科技). 1998, 5 (6): 380-381.

[76] Sun Gang. The Study on the Inflammatory Effect of *Feng Shi Yao Jiu* (风湿药酒抗炎作用研究). *Henan Chinese Medicine* (河南中医). 1997, 17 (4): 212-214.

[77] Huang Di-jun. Wheat Grain Moxibustion Plus Tap-Needling and Cupping Therapy in the Treatment of RA (麦粒灸加叩刺拔罐法治疗类风湿性关节炎). *Sichuan Journal of Chinese Medicine* (四川中医). 2000, 18 (3): 53-54.

[78] Zhu Wei. Developments in the Study of Apitoxin (蜂毒素的研究进展). *Journal of Bai Qiu-en Medical College* (白求恩医科大学学报). 2001, 27 (2): 212-214.

[79] Xiao Xue-lü, Liang Xiao-ping, Xiao xue-chang. The Therapeutic Effects of Intervessel Laser Treatment on Elderly Patients of RA (激光血管内照射对老年类风湿性关节炎的治疗作用). *China Journal of Rehabilitation and Recovery* (中华无力医学与康复杂志). 2003, 25 (3): 174-176.

[80] Li Chang-you, Fan Guang-yu, Zhi-bo Zhi-ren. The Effects of Foot Plate on the Plantar Pressure of RA Patients (足底板对类风湿性关节炎患者足底压的影响). *Journal of China Medical College* (中国医科大学学报). 2000, 29 (1): 33-34.

[81] Han Jian-zhong. The Treatment of 30 Cases of RA with "*Shun Shi Fu Zhen*" Method ("顺势伏针法"治疗类风湿性关节炎30例). *Jiangsu Journal of Chinese Medicine* (江苏中医). 1999, 20 (7): 40.

[82] Wei Fu-liang, Zhang You-gui. The Treatment of 60 Cases of RA with Acupuncture and Snake Moxibustion (长蛇灸配合针刺治疗类风湿性关节炎60例). *Journal of Anhui University of Chinese Medicine* (安徽中医学院学报). 2002, 21 (2): 30-31.

[83] Wu Hong-dong, Tian wen-hai, Fu huo-bin. The Treatment of 45 Cases of RA with Fire Needle (火针治疗类风湿性关节炎45例). *Shanxi Journal of Chinese Medicine* (山西中医). 2002, 18 (5): 40-41.

[84] Gu Ming-gao. The Treatment of 32 Cases of RA with Warming Needle (温针为主治疗类风湿性关节炎32例). *New Chinese Medicine* (新中医). 1999: 24.

[85] Liu Yuan-yuan, Jiang Gang-hui. Therapeutic Observation on 30 Cases of RA Treated by

Warm Needle (温针灸为主治疗类风湿性关节炎30例疗效观察). *Heilongjiang Chinese Medicine* (黑龙江中医药). 2005, 1: 34-35.

[86] Xiao Qun. The Effects of Acupuncture on IL-2 in the Treatment of 41 Cases of RA (针灸治疗41例类风湿性关节炎疗效分析及对白细胞介素2的影响). *Chinese Acupuncture and Moxibustion* (中国针灸). 1992, 12 (6): 26.

[87] Ai Zhou, Liu Yuan-yuan, Yang Lian. Observation of the Treatment of Active RA with Electroacupuncture and Medicinals (电针配合药物治疗类风湿关节炎活动期疗效观察). *Chinese Acupuncture and Moxibustion* (中国针灸). 2005, 25 (8): 531-533.

[88] Pert A, Dionne R, Bragin E, et a1. Alteration in Rat Central Nervous System Endorphins Following Transauricular Electroacupuncture. *Brain Res*, 1981, 224: 83.

[89] Liu Jin-hong, Fang Jian-qiao. An Exploration into the Treatment of RA with Acupuncture (针灸治疗类风湿性关节炎研究思路探讨). *Chinese Acupuncture and Moxibustion* (中国针灸). 2002, 22 (1): 59.

[90] Yu Rui-ping. Observation of the Treatment of Interphalangeal Joint Inflammation with Cold Moxibustion (冷灸治疗类风湿性指间关节炎疗效观察). *Chinese Acupuncture* (中国针灸). 2003, 23 (2): 85-86.

[91] Luo Xiang-yun, Chen Mei-ren. 98 Cases of RA Treated with Acupuncture and Chinese Medicinal External Wash (针灸配合中药外洗治疗类风湿性关节炎98例). *Hunan Journal of Chinese Medicine* (湖南中医杂志). 2004, 20 (3): 42.

[92] He Yang, Xu Hong-xia. Observation of the Therapeutic Effects of RA Medicinal Atomization with Acupuncture in the Treatment of RA (中药雾化加针灸治类风湿性关节炎疗效观察). *Clinical Journal of Acupuncture and Moxibustion* (针灸临床杂志). 2004, 20 (l0): 11-12.

[93] Xu Jia-liu, Luo Xiao-shan, Zhang Cheng-guang. A Pharmacodynamic Study of *Gui Zhi Shao Yao Zhi Mu Tang* (桂枝芍药知母汤抗风湿的药效学研究). *Chinese Medicinals* (中药材). 2003, 26 (9): 662-664.

[94] Su Xian-hong, Wang Lian-zhi. An Experimental Study of the Effects of *Jiao Teng* No. 1 on the Immune Function of RA Patients (艽藤Ⅰ号对RA免疫功能作用的实验研究). *Chinese Medicine Periodical* (中医药学刊). 2003, 21 (3): 391-392.

[95] Xu Jian-yang, Wang Fa-qiang, Zheng Wei-fa. The Effects of *Jin Tie Suo* on Serum NO/NOS Content and Pain Threshold in Laboratory Mice with RA (金铁锁对实验性RA小鼠痛阈及血清NO/NOS含量的影响). *Chinese Medicine Periodical* (中医药学刊). 2004, 22 (1): 82-84.

[96] Du Xiu-lan, Li Da-ke, Ma Cheng-tai. An Experimental Study of the Antiinflammatory and Analgesic Effects of *Xiao Bi Gao* (消痹膏抗炎镇痛作用的实验研究). *Journal of Shandong University of Chinese Medicine* (山东中医药大学学报). 2004, 28 (1): 63-65.

[97] Deng Zhao-zhi, Lin Yuan-chang, He Yi-ting. Repeated Observation of the Treatment of Active RA with *Fu Fang Lei Gong Teng Tu Mo Ji* (复方雷公藤涂膜剂对活动期类风湿关节炎的临床再观察). *Guangzhou Chinese Medical College Journal* (广州中医药大学学报). 1998, 15 (3): 180.

[98] Zhang Man-hua. The Clinical Observation of the Long-term Use of *Lei Gong Teng Zong*

Dai in 144 Cases of RA (雷公藤总甙长期治疗类风湿关节炎144例临床观察). *Journal of Suzhou Medical College* (苏州医学院学报). 1994, 14 (4): 321.

[99] Lao Zhi-ying. 50 Cases of RA Treated with a Combined Small Dose of *Lei Gong Teng Chong Ji* and *Mao Qing Teng Jian* (小剂量雷公藤冲剂和毛青藤碱联合治疗类风湿关节炎50例). *China Journal of Integrative Medicine* (中国中西医结合杂志). 1993, (9): 554.

[100] Yang Feng, Li Yan-min, Li Yin-gang. An Experimental Study of the Treatment of RA with *Xian Long Ke Li* (仙龙颗粒治疗类风湿性关节炎的实验研究). *New Chinese Medicine* (现代中医药). 2005, 25(5): 67-69.

[101] Suo De-quan, Pan Wen-jun, Yu Da-hai. A Pharmacodynamic Study of *Yu Xue Bi Chong Ji* in the Treatment of RA (瘀血痹冲剂治疗类风湿性关节炎的药理研究). *Journal of Shenyang Medical College* (沈阳药科大学学报). 2001, 18 (6): 431-435.

[102] Bao Cai-jun, Han Jin-yan, Huang Yong-kai. A Study of the Mechanism of *Ruan Jian San Jie Wan* in the Treatment of RA (软坚散结丸对类风湿性关节炎作用的机理研究). *Inner Mongolia Journal of Chinese Medicine* (内蒙古中医药). 2001, 1: 38-39.

[103] Sun Ying-chun, Ji Zhong-yu, Fu Hong-he. An Experimental Study of *Zhi Bi Tong* Wine in the Treatment of RA (止痹痛酒治疗类风湿性关节炎的实验研究). *Chinese Medicine News* (中医药信息). 2005,22 (1): 56-58.

[104] Cai Qing, Meng Ji-ming, Han Xing-hai. The Clinical Observation of the Therapeutic Effects of AFT in the Treatment of RA (蝮蛇抗栓酶辅助治疗类风湿性关节炎临床疗效观察). *China Journal of Integrative Medicine* (中国中西医结合杂志). 2002, 22 (3): 166.

Index by Disease Names and Symptoms

Index by Chinese Medicinals and Formulas

D

W

X

Y

Z

General Index

D

G

H

M

N

S

Notes

图书在版编目（CIP）数据

中医临床实用系列：痛风与类风湿性关节炎（英文）/邓兆智主编．—北京：人民卫生出版社，2008.3

ISBN 978-7-117-09485-6

Ⅰ．中…　Ⅱ．邓…　Ⅲ．①痛风—中医治疗法—英文②类风湿性关节炎—中医治疗法—英文　Ⅳ．R259.897 R259.932.2

中国版本图书馆 CIP 数据核字（2007）第 177431 号

中医临床实用系列：痛风与类风湿性关节炎（英文）

主　　编：邓兆智
出版发行：人民卫生出版社（中继线 +8610-6761-6688）
地　　址：中国北京市丰台区方庄芳群园三区 3 号楼
邮　　编：100078
网　　址：http://www.pmph.com
E - mail：pmph @ pmph.com
发　　行：zzg@pmph.com.cn
购书热线：+8610-6769-1034（电话及传真）
开　　本：787×1092　1/16
版　　次：2008 年 3 月第 1 版　2008 年 3 月第 1 版第 1 次印刷
标准书号：ISBN 978-7-117-09485-6/R・9486